Spinal Cord Stimulation II

Svante Horsch · Luc Claeys
Editors

Spinal Cord Stimulation II

An Innovative Method in the Treatment of PVD and Angina

STEINKOPFF
DARMSTADT

Springer

The Editors:
Prof. Dr. Svante Horsch
Dr. Luc Claeys
Krankenhaus Porz am Rhein
Akademisches Lehrkrankenhaus der
Universität zu Köln
Abteilung für Allgemeinchirurgie –
Gefäßchirurgie und Traumatologie
Urbacher Weg 19
51149 Köln

Die Deutsche Bibliothek – CIP-Einheitsaufnahme

Spinal cord stimulation II : an innovative method in the treatment of PVD and angina / Svante Horsch ; Luc Claeys (ed.). – Darmstadt : Steinkopff, 1995

ISBN-13: 978-3-642-72529-6 **e-ISBN-13: 978-3-642-72527-2**

DOI: 10.1007/ 978-3-642-72527-2

NE: Horsch, Svante [Hrsg.]

Softcover reprint of the hardcover 1st edition 1995

Medical Editor: Sabine Ibkendanz – English Editor: James C. Willis – Production: Heinz J. Schäfer
Cover Design: Erich Kirchner, Heidelberg

Typesetting: Typoservice, Griesheim

Printed on acid-free paper

Foreword

This volume contains proceedings of the second International Symposium on Spinal Cord Stimulation in the treatment of vascular diseases.

Almost 10 years ago, I became acquainted with the method of epidural stimulation. I was told that neuro-surgeons in Scandinavia noticed, as a side-effect of pain treatment with this method, a positive influence on peripheral circulation demonstrated by a warming of the legs.

After I started vascular surgery in my own department in the Academic Teaching Hospital in Cologne-Porz in January 1986, I tried to learn more about epidural stimulation, which I considered a possible alternative in limb salvage. Already in 1986, we implanted 10 spinal cord stimulators.

In the following years, we had an increasing number of patients with good results and we succeeded in more precisely determining the indication for this treatment.

To clarify the physiological background and the clinical possibilities was the major aim of the first symposium on Spinal Cord Stimulation in the treatment of PVD. The response to that symposium was so encouraging that we decided to hold another one. This time the participants focused not only on the clinical results in the treatment of PVD, but also on angina pectoris, Buerger's and Raynaud's dieases.

We have not yet succeeded in elucidating the way in which stimulation works, although there are many investigations that point to a reduction of peripheral vascular resistance improving the microcirculation. Yet, it is my opinion that surgery is an empirical science with a unique opportunity to make interesting and relevant observations.

Last but not least, I want to express my thanks to the Medtronic Company which sponsored both the first and the present symposium.

Cologne, October 1995 S. Horsch

Welcoming Address

It is an honor and pleasure for me to welcome you to Cologne on behalf of the German Society for Surgery and the German Society for Vascular Surgery – at this 2nd Symposium on Spinal Cord Stimulation. First, I'd like to thank the organizers Svante Horsch and Luc Claeys, that they did not spare any effort to prepare this meeting. They, in fact, succeeded in gathering more than 35 experts from all over the world – from 15 countries – who will either give one of the 29 presentations or preside over a session, or do both. All these papers are concerned with SCS or are about this innovative therapy.

The reports and discussions wil address: How does SCS work? When is SCS indicated? Results according to pain, claudication, critical tissue ischemia, Buerger's disease, and angina pectoris; comparison to other treatments, cost-benefit relationship, and more.

Progress in our profession is necessary for the good of our patients' sake. We are living in a fascinating time of progress in all sectors of surgery: for instance, endoscopic surgery in the abdomen or chest, arthroscopic operations in joints, endoluminal grafting in vascular surgery, new methods to replace blood transfusion, our speciality, spinal cord stimulation to treat patients with chronic pain and peripheral ischemia.

There is another aspect to this meeting in Cologne: This city is one of the important cultural centers of Germany. If you are new here, I hope you will find the time to look around, to pay a visit to the famous gothic cathedral, or to some of the 12 rebuilt Romanesque churches in the middle of the old city, or to some of the museums. I hope we will experience a rewarding conference of high quality, renewal personal friendships, and make new friends with persons who have the same interest: SCS.

Let me also express sincere thanks in the name of all participants to the sponsor of this meeting: Mr. Bornschein and his staff from Metronic Corp. It is not possible to organize symposia like this one without the support of industry. We thank them for their generosity.

Prof. Dr. med. H.-M. Becker
President of the German Society for Surgery
Chief of Vascular Surgery
Academic Teaching Hospital Munich-Neuperlach
of the University Munich
Oskar-Maria-Graf-Ring 51
D-81737 Munich

Contents

Spinal Cord Stimulation for Angina Pectoris

Buerger's Disease – Miscellaneous

Spinal Cord Stimulation for Chronic Pain

Physiological mechanisms activated by stimulation of the spinal dorsal columns

M. H. T. Roberts

School of Molecular and Medical Bioscience University of Wales, College of Cardiff, Cardiff, Wales, United Kingdom

Introduction

The gate theory (9) proposes that activity in large diameter primary afferents inhibits inputs from small diameter primary afferents. As noxious sensation is transmitted by fine fibres, any method of activating large fibre inputs to the appropriate segment of the spinal cord should reduce the perception of pain. This theory has generated immense interest during the last three decades and support for the proposal has come from many lines of study. Perhaps the most striking is the observation that stimulation of the dorsal columns is useful in the clinical treatment of several painful conditions (24). Collaterals from the large diameter primary afferent fibres ascend in the dorsal columns to terminate in the gracile and caudate nuclei. It is thought that the stimulation of these fibres sets up action potentials that pass antidromically down the columns to enter the spinal cord and operate the gating mechanism described above.

Recent work on animals in the laboratory has indicated that alternative explanations for the effectiveness of dorsal column stimulation should be given serious consideration. This paper outlines some of these experiments and the conclusions that may be drawn from them.

Analgesia from deep brain stimulation

Stimulation of several deep brain sites has been shown to cause analgesia in man and animals. Reynolds (18) is usually credited with the first clear demonstration that in the rat, stimulation of the periaqueductal gray (PAG) gave sufficient analgesia to perform laparotomy. Clinical relief from pain was subsequently demonstrated to result from PAG stimulation (7). Laboratory studies have shown many sites in the hindbrain, midbrain and thalamus from which various degrees of inhibition of responses to noxious stimuli may be evoked. The stimulation of many of these sites has been shown to inhibit the responses of spinal neurones to noxious stimuli and a detailed concept of a "pain inhibitory system" (5) has been developed. In essence, this consists of midline midbrain structures projecting to midline and lateral hindbrain structures that, in turn, project to the spinal cord in the dorsolateral funiculus. Activating this system inhibits the responses to noxious stimuli of multireceptive, lamina V spinal neurones.

It is quite apparent that dorsal column stimulation may well activate this brain system to cause descending inhibition of spinal neurones. This possibility was well recognised by the gate theory that included a supraspinal loop even in the earliest descriptions of the theory. However, none of the structures in the brain that modulate the perception of pain were known to have significant inputs from the dorsal column nuclei and gating of spinal inputs from high threshold nociceptors was known to occur in spinalised animals. Both of these facts argue against a supraspinal loop being important to the pain-relieving effects of dorsal column stimulation. Recent research in my laboratory and others has identified a novel part of the brain from which analgesia may be evoked by brain stimulation and an important characteristic of this area is that it receives a strong innervation from the dorsal column nuclei (16). This observation reopens the possibility that dorsal column stimulation may have an important analgesic effect due to action potentials ascending to the brain. The rest of this paper reviews these studies and describes the physiological mechanisms that may be activated by dorsal column stimulation.

The anterior pretectal nucleus

Prado and Roberts (11) conducted a survey of the brain of unanaesthetised rats in which the analgesic effects of stimulating 114 sites were assessed. Many sites lay in areas known to modulate pain sensations and stimulation of these sites caused effective analgesia. To our surprise however, electrode locations in the pretectal area were found to have the lowest thresholds for inhibition of the tail flick response to noxious heat. These thresholds were very low, and analgesia was seen with 15 μA of 50 Hz sine wave stimulation applied for only 15 s. The stimulation appeared not to be aversive to the animal and often the only sign of stimulation was a nystagmus.

Subsequent studies (13, 19) showed that the animals suffered no motor deficits that could explain the failure to remove the tail from the noxious heat. Responses to innocuous stimuli (light, touch, sound) were apparently unaffected. The duration of the analgesia was up to 1 h following 15 s of stimulation at 35 μA. The analgesia could be demonstrated with the paw pressure test, the hotplate test and the formalin test (27).

Detailed studies of the precise locations of the electrodes that gave the strongest analgesia showed that they lay in the anterior pretectal nucleus (APtN). In the rat, the APtN is close to the dorsal surface of the rostral midbrain on the diencephalic/mesencephalic border. It is the largest nucleus of the pretectal complex. This complex is known for its participation in visually guided behaviours, pupillary reflexes and optical tracking (4) but retinal and other visual nuclei connections go principally to the dorsal group of pretectal nuclei and not to the APtN itself. The APtN is therefore not considered to be part of the visual group (6). Although rather little was known of the functions of the APtN, neuronal tract tracing of the afferents and efferents suggested to some that it may have a sensorimotor function (2). The major inputs to the APtN are from the somatosensory cortex, dorsal column nuclei, periaqueductal gray, spinal lamina I cells, spinothalamic tract cells, hypothalamus, deep mesencephalon, pontine parabrachial region, inferior olive and trigeminal sensory nuclei (20). The outputs from the APtN are to zona incerta, centrolateral nucleus of the thalamus, ventrobasal thalamus, deep mesencephalon, ventrolateral medulla and sensorimotor cortex. Taken together with the observed analgesia from stimulation of the APtN, these connections are indicative of a somatosensory function for the APtN and a role in the processing of noxious stimuli.

Electrophysiological experiments were conducted in anaesthetised rats in which the lumbar spinal cord had been exposed by laminectomy. Microelectrodes recorded dorsal horn cell responses to noxious stimuli applied to the cutaneous receptive field. Brief stimulation of the APtN caused the inhibition of the nociceptive responses of deep multireceptive neurones. These neurones projected towards the brain in the ventrolateral funiculus. The responses of these neurones to brush/touch stimulation of the receptive field were not affected by stimulating the APtN. Transection of the ipsilateral dorsolateral funiculus (DLF) abolished the inhibition from the APtN. These data suggest that activation of the APtN selectively inhibits spinothalamic tract cells via fibres descending in the DLF.

Many pharmacological, physiological and behavioural experiments investigated the nature of this inhibition. The microinjection into the APtN of morphine, some cholinergic agonists, 5-hydroxytryptamine or excitatory amino acids, all activated the descending inhibition (10, 17) and studies are being conducted at present of the effects of these neurotransmitters on the intracellularly recorded membrane properties of APtN cells [Li and Roberts, unpublished]. The inhibition produced by electrical stimulation of the APtN can be antagonised by systemic injection of antagonists at opiate, cholinergic and noradrenergic receptors (12). These studies will reveal the neurotransmitters that act on the cells in the APtN, and elsewhere in the descending pathway, to cause analgesia.

The anatomical route of the descending inhibition has been investigated with lesion studies. The APtN itself does not project directly to the spinal cord, but does project densely to ventrolateral parts of the mesencephalon and medulla (22, 23). Lesions positioned in either of these areas significantly reduced the analgesic effects of stimulating the APtN. As both areas project to the dorsal horn of the spinal cord and cause analgesia when stimulated, we presume that these brainstem areas relay the effects of APtN stimulation to the cord.

Dorsal column input to the APtN

The APtN differs from other nuclei in the brain from which analgesia can be obtained in that it has a dense input from the dorsal column nuclei. This suggests a functional relationship between the APtN and the dorsal columns. We have investigated this in the rat using electrophysiological techniques. Stimulation of the gracile fasciculus of the dorsal columns at twice the threshold intensity for activation of A fibres strongly excited cells in the APtN (14). Cells in the rostral pole of the APtN were excited with a long latency and for a long period. We had previously shown that stimulation in the rostral pole gave the longest lasting analgesia, whereas stimulation more posteriorly in the main body of the nucleus gave a strong but shorter lasting effect (13). APtN cells in this main body of the nucleus were driven by dorsal column nucleus stimulation with a short latency of about 8 ms. The response was brief however, usually being little more than a burst of 4 – 20 spikes. We believe that the pathway between the gracile nucleus and the APtN was direct because it was possible to stimulate the APtN and record action potentials from the gracile nucleus that had the characteristics of antidromic action potentials. That is to say, we were stimulating the nerve terminals in the APtN and recording from cell bodies in the gracile nucleus, with no synapse between the two. The characteristics of an antidromic action potential are that it follows high frequencies of stimulation, has a very constant latency and antidromic and orthodromic action potentials collide (the "collision test", see (15)).

These experiments can only be done in anaesthetised animals with exposure of the brain and spinal cord. It is difficult, therefore, to demonstrate behavioural analgesia but if recordings are made of the responses of dorsal horn neurones to cutaneous noxious stimuli, it is possible to show if these responses are inhibited. We have done this and observed that dorsal column stimulation applied 30 – 60 s before a noxious stimulus, inhibited the nociceptive response of dorsal horn neurones. This inhibition could be mediated either via the supraspinal loop that includes the APtN or via action potentials that descend in the dorsal columns to enter the cord and operate the segmental "gate". We were able to test which of these routes caused the antinociception by surgically transecting the dorsal columns and stimulating above or below the transection (15). We observed that stimulating above the transection evoked an antinociception that was very similar to that obtained from the intact spinal cord. Stimulating below the transection, however, had no effect. We concluded that the antinociceptive effects of dorsal column stimulation were principally mediated via an ascending supraspinal loop.

At first glance these data seem to throw doubt upon the "gate theory", but by modifying our technique we were able to confirm that dorsal column stimulation does operate a segmental spinal gating mechanism. We recorded the nociceptive responses of dorsal horn cells using multibarrelled glass microelectrodes. One of the barrels contained an excitatory amino acid that was ejected into the environment of the recorded cell by microiontophoresis. This caused the cell to produce action potentials at a steady rate. When we stimulated the dorsal columns, it was clear that the cell was inhibited because the rate at which it fired action potentials was reduced. As soon as we stopped stimulating the cord, the inhibition stopped and the firing rate of the cell returned to the original level. The series of experiments (described above) that showed no effect from stimulating the dorsal columns below the transection, tested for antinociceptive effects of the stimulation 30 – 60 s after the stimulation was stopped. Clearly, at this time the descending effects of cord stimulation on the gate were no longer effective. If we test for antinociception during the stimulation period we observe a weaker, but distinct inhibition.

Our conclusions from this series of experiments are that both spinal gating mechanisms and supraspinal loops are activated by dorsal column stimulation but that the antinociceptive effects of activating the supraspinal loop are longer lasting and, we feel, more likely to be the major source of clinical benefit from cord stimulation.

The involvement of the APtN in the antinociceptive supraspinal loop was investigated by us by temporarily blocking function in the APtN. We did this by microinjecting the inhibitory amino acid, gamma amino butyric acid (GABA) into the APtN (15). This evokes a powerful hyperpolarisation and, therefore, inhibition of APtN cells. We found that this abolished the antinociceptive effects of dorsal column stimulation. We conclude that indeed, the APtN is a necessary relay in the antinociceptive effects of dorsal cord stimulation.

APtN function in chronic pain states

The studies described above relate particularly to the effects of dorsal column stimulation. Many other studies have been made and described elsewhere (16). In particular, the role of spinal lamina I cells in controlling the excitability of the APtN is important. Many lamina I cells project in the contralateral dorsolateral funiculus (DLF) to terminate in the pontine parabrachial region and the APtN (3, 8, 25, 26, 28). Stimulating the axons of these cells in the contralateral DLF strongly excites APtN cells. This suggests that noxious inputs will activate the APtN to limit the response of deep multireceptive spinal cells to the noxious input. We therefore conducted experiments on the interaction between APtN, superficial lamina I cells and deep multireceptive cells. We confirmed that stimulation of the APtN inhibited the responses of deep multireceptive cells as reported above. We were surprised to find, however, that APtN stimulation failed to inhibit lamina I cells and caused a marked potentiation of the response of these cells to noxious stimuli (Rees and Roberts, in press).

We conclude from this that the analgesic actions of APtN stimulation are associated with an inhibition of spinothalamic tract cells and a potentiation of the responses of lamina I cells that project to the APtN and parabrachialis. We therefore proposed that the normal response to a noxious stimulus consisted of the following sequence: 1) The noxious stimulus drives lamina I and multireceptive cells in the dorsal horn of the spinal cord. 2) The multireceptive cells activate thalamic and other neurones to trigger the perception of pain. 3) The lamina I cells activate parabrachial and APtN neurones. 4) The APtN cells inhibit multireceptive spinal neurones and facilitate the responses of lamina I neurones. This recurrent supraspinal loop will act, therefore, to limit the duration of perceived pain following injury. Importantly, in chronic pain states, where lamina I cells are tonically active, the descending inhibition will become tonically active also.

We have tested one aspect of this postulate. Rats received unilateral transection of two dorsal roots and were observed carefully for the subsequent 45 days. After 20 days or so it was observed that they started to nibble at the toe nails on the foot of the denervated limb. This response to denervation has been extensively studied and is well known to signal the onset of a more extensive mutilation of the insensate foot referred to as autotomy (21). It has been closely argued by others (1) that autotomy in rats is an indication of the onset of a chronic pain condition resulting from the deafferentation. The clinical equivalents of this condition are well recognised. It must be stressed that severe mutilation of the foot was never allowed to occur and the animals were immediately killed as soon as all five toes were affected or as soon as more extensive damage was done.

We studied two groups of six animals all with cut dorsal roots. One group had extensive bilateral lesion of the APtN and the other group were sham-operated controls. In the control group the first signs of autotomy were seen at day 20 and at the end of the period only six toes had been attacked. In the group of animals with APtN lesions, the first sign of autotomy occurred at day 13 and 23 toes had been attacked. These data show that lesions of the APtN dramatically increase the observed onset and severity of a chronic pain condition. We propose that the APtN is part of a feedback pathway that delays and attenuates the severity of chronic pain conditions. Disruption of this pathway exacerbates the condition.

Conclusions

It seems clear from these experiments in the laboratory that ascending pathways in the dorsal columns may have important antinociceptive effects. We have not studied the role of these pathways in peripheral vascular disease or angina pectoris. It is important to study the effects of dorsal column stimulation on those areas of the brain that control sympathetic neurones in the spinal cord. Inhibition and excitation of spinal neurones seems to be part of the complex response to analgesic stimulation of the dorsal columns. It is impossible to predict what effect this stimulation would have on cells controlling sympathetic outflows. Appropriate experiments to identify this are not difficult to design or conduct.

Physiological studies of the type described here are of great potential value to the clinical application of spinal cord stimulation. Once the circuits are understood and the neurotransmitters identified at each synapse, it should be possible to administer drugs that enhance transmission at the appropriate synapses. This would be expected to increase the frequency and degree of success obtained with therapeutic cord stimulation.

References

1. Basbaum AI, Wall PD (1976) Chronic changes in the response of cells in adult cat dorsal horn following partial deafferentation: the appearance of responding cells in a previously non-responsive region. Brain Res 116: 181–204
2. Berkley KJ, Mash DC (1978) Somatic sensory projections to the pretectum in the cat. Brain Res 158: 445–449
3. Cliffer KD, Burnstein R, Geisler GJ (1991) Distribution of spinothalamic, spinohypothalamic and spinotelencephalic fibers revealed by anterograde transport of PHA-L in rats. J Neurosci 11: 852–868
4. Collewjin H (1978) Direction selective units in the rabbits nucleus of the optic tract. Brain Res 100: 489–508
5. Fields HL, Basbaum AJ (1984) Endogenous pain control mechanisms. In: Wall PD, Melzack R (eds) Textbook of Pain. Churchill Livingstone. pp 142–152
6. Gregory KM (1985) The dendritic architecture of the visual pretectal nuclei of the rat: a study with the Golgi-Cox method. J Comp Neurol 234: 122–135
7. Hosobuchi Y (1980) The current status of analgesic brain stimulation. Acta Neurochirurgica (suppl) 30: 219–227
8. Ma W, Blomqvist A, Berkley KJ (1989) Spino-diencephalic relays through the parabrachial nucleus in the cat. Brain Res 480: 37–50
9. Melzack R, Wall PD (1965) Pain mechanisms: A new theory. Science 150: 971–979
10. Prado WA (1989) Antinociceptive effects of agonists microinjected into the anterior pretectal nucleus of the rat. Brain Res 493: 147–154
11. Prado WA, Roberts MHT (1985) An assessment of the antinociceptive and aversive effects of stimulating identified sites in the rat brain. Brain Res 340: 219–228
12. Rees H, Prado WA, Rawlings S and Roberts MHT (1987) The effects of intraperitoneal administration of antagonists and development of morphine tolerance on the antinociception induced by stimulating the APtN of the rat. Br J Pharmacol 92: 769–779
13. Rees H, Roberts MHT (1987) Anterior pretectal stimulation alters the responses of spinal dorsal horn neurones to cutaneous stimulation in the rat. J Physiol 385: 415–436
14. Rees H, Roberts MHT (1989) Activation of cells in the anterior pretectal nucleus by dorsal column stimulation in the rat. J Physiol 417: 361–373

15. Rees H, Roberts MHT (1989) Antinociceptive effects of dorsal column stimulation in the rat: involvement of the anterior pretectal nucleus. J Physiol 417: 375–388
16. Rees H, Roberts MHT (1993) The anterior pretectal nucleus: a proposed role in sensory processing. Pain 53: 121–135
17. Rees H, Roberts MHT, Sherwood CA (1987) Antinociceptive effects of D,L homocysteic acid into the anterior pretectal nucleus of the rat. J Physiol 394: 415–436
18. Reynolds DV (1969) Surgery in the rat during electrical analgesia induced by focal stimulation. Science 164: 444–445
19. Roberts MHT, Rees H (1986) The antinociceptive effects of stimulating the pretectal nucleus of the rat. Pain 25: 83–93
20. Roberts MHT, Rees H (1994) Physiological basis of spinal cord stimulation. Pain Reviews 1: 184–198
21. Saade NE, Atweh SF, Jabbur SJ, Wall PD (1990) Effects of lesions of the anterolateral columns and dorsolateral funiculi on self mutilation behaviour in rats. Pain 42: 313–321
22. Terenzi MG, Rees H, Morgan SJS, Foster GA, Roberts MHT (1991) The antinociception evoked by anterior pretectal nucleus stimulation is partly dependent upon ventrolateral medullary neurones. Pain 47: 231–239
23. Terenzi MG, Rees H, Roberts MHT (1992) The pontine parabrachial region mediates some of the descending inhibitory effects of stimulating the anterior pretectal nucleus. Brain Res 594: 205–214
24. Wall PD, Sweet WH (1967) Temporary abolition of pain in man. Science 155: 108–109
25. Wiberg M, Blomqvist A (1984) The spinomesencephalic tract in the cat: its cells of origin and termination pattern as demonstrated by intraaxonal transport method. Brain Res 291: 1–18
26. Willis WD (1989) Projections of the superficial dorsal horn to the midbrain and thalamus. In Cervero F, Bennett GJ, Headley PM (eds) Processing of sensory information in the dorsal horn of the spinal cord. Plenum Press, New York pp 217–237
27. Wilson DG Rees H, Roberts MHT (1991) The antinociceptive effects of anterior pretectal stimulation in tests using thermal, mechanical and chemical noxious stimuli. Pain 44: 195–200
28. Yesierski RP (1988) Spinomesencephalic tract: projections from the lumbrosacral spinal cord of the rat, cat and monkey. J Comp Neurol 267: 131–146

Author's address:
Dr. M. H. T. Roberts
School of Molecular and Medical Bioscience
University of Wales, Cardiff
PO Box 911
Cardiff CF1 3US
United Kingdom

Central nervous mechanisms involved in neuropathic and nociceptive pain

B. Olausson

Dept. of Clinical Neurophysiology, Sahlgren University Hospital, Göteborg, Sweden

Introduction

In the nociceptive pathway, from the peripheral receptor up to the cortex a variety of physiological control mechanisms have been described. The most well-known is the gate-control hypothesis proposed by Melzack and Wall (1965) (7). The importance of this hypothesis has primarily been its impact in the development of pain relieving treatments such as transcutaneous electrical nervous stimulation (TENS) and spinal cord stimulation (SCS). The gate control hypothesis postulates a segmental pain control influenced by segmental and supraspinal input.

Mechanisms that mimic the segmental control has been described both at a thalamic and a cortical level (8, 9). These control mechanisms have been suggested to be involved in the pain-relieving effects following TENS, SCS, and intracranial electrical stimulation.

In the thalamus a variety of nuclear structures which receive nociceptive afferents have been described, including the ventrobasal (VB) complex and the intralaminar (IL) nuclei. Cells in the VB complex usually have limited cutaneous receptive fields while cells in IL often have large cutaneous receptive fields. The nociceptive cells in the VB complex have been denoted as a sensory-discriminative function, while cells in the intralaminar nuclei have been ascribed to a function in the cognitive-affective mechanism related to pain.

Under pathological conditions such as chronic inflammation or peripheral nerve injury the reaction-pattern of the thalamic cells may change. The normally silent cells in IL may become spontaneously active (5). Nociceptive cells in the VB complex may change their receptive field properties and become excited from larger skin areas and by non-noxious stimuli (6). Under such conditions normally non-noxious stimuli can induce painful sensations.

The current contribution emphasizes the interacion between nociceptive and non-nociceptive afferents in the thalamus of the cat and the involvement of GABA-ergic mechanisms.

Methods

Paralyzed chloralose anaesthetized cats were used. Craniotomy was made to reveal the area overlying the right thalamus and laminectomies were performed to expose the spinal C1 and Th10–L1 segments. After surgery each cat was placed in a stereotaxic frame. Stimulating electrodes were placed in the dorsal column nuclei (DCN) at the C1 segment, and in the spinothalamic tract (STT), at Th10–L1 level.

Electrical stimulation was given to the DCN and the STT, at a low current. A lesion of the dorsal column was performed at the right side of the Th10 spinal segment using either a small sharp knife or fine forceps.

The recording electrode was stereotaxically placed in the posterior thalamus and cells characterized as nociceptive if activated by electrical tooth pulp (TP) and/or (STT) stimulation and activated mainly by pinch or pricking in the cutaneous receptive fields.

Single unit recordings in the thalamus were made with a multi-barreled glass electrode (six barrels), with a central tungsten core. The barrels were filled with: 5 mM bicuculine (pH 3.0); 5 mM picrotoxin (pH 3.0); 5 mM saclofen (pH 3.0), 0.2 M DLH (pH 7.0); GABA 1 M (pH 7.0) all in 150 mM NaCl. Two barrels were filled with NaCl (150 mM pH 7.0), one of these acted as an electrical balance channel, and the other was used for iontophoretic application of NaCl as a control substance. Current for ejection was usually 20–100 nA. During advancement of the electrode, retaining currents of at least 5 nA of appropriate polarity were applied to prevent diffusion of the drugs.

A conditioning-test paradigm was used. The cellular response evoked by stimulation of TP or STT was used as a test and was preceded by electrical activation of DCN as a conditioning stimulus. Each series was started by collecting data to construct post-stimulus histograms with test stimuli alone and used as controls. The conditioning stimulation was then delivered at delays in fixed steps from 25 to 400 ms preceding the test stimulus. The same paradigm was used during iontophoresis of drugs to test their effect on the interaction.

The experimental protocol was accepted by the ethical committee at the University of Göteborg.

Results

Nociceptive cells (n = 13) localized to the VB complex or to the intralaminar nuclei in the posterior thalamus of the cat were studied. All of the studied cells showed spontaneous activity and iontophoretic administration of DLH increased the firing rate of the cells. Administration of GABA decreased the firing rate of the cells (Fig. 1) and administration of picrotoxin or saclofen did not affect their firing rate. In five out of eight tested cells where GABA was given simultaneous to picrotoxin, the GABA-induced inhibition was partly antagonized. This effect was not observed during GABA and saclofen administration (Fig. 1).

Evoked activity

Evoked cellular responses to TP stimulation consisted of early spikes with stable latencies and later occurring spikes with variable latencies. Administration of GABA reduced both the early and the late responses. No significant changes of the responses to TP stimulation could be detected during simultaneous administration of picrotoxin or saclofen.

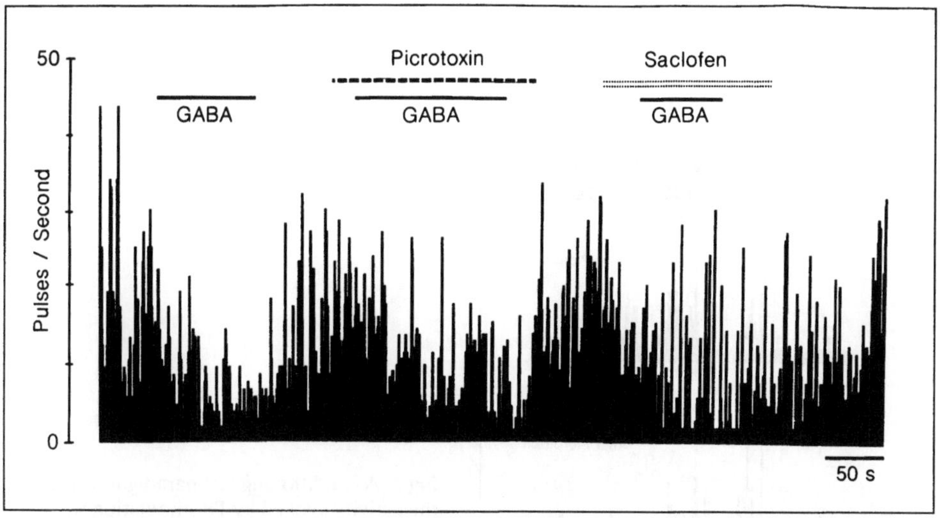

Fig. 1. Example of a WDR cell in the posterior thalamus. Iontoforesis of GABA augmented the spontaneous activity. The effect of GABA was partially reversed by simultaneous administration of picrotoxin while sactofen induced a burst-like activity in the cell.

Evoked cellular responses following stimulation in the STT consisted of early spikes with stable latencies and later occurring spikes with variable latencies.

Administration of GABA during STT stimulation did not significantly influence the early response, but reduced the late response. Administration of picrotoxin or saclofen simultaneous to STT stimulation did not significantly influence either the early or the late responses.

Action potentials evoked by DCN stimulation showed short latencies and a late response commonly seen after STT and TP stimulation was not present following DCN stimulation.

Administration of GABA reduced the cellular response to DCN stimulation. The evoked responses increased when picrotoxin was administered, while saclofen administration had no significant effect.

Conditioning test paradigm

All cells excited by TP stimulation showed a reduced evoked cellular activity by preceding stimulation given to the DCN. The depressing effect following DCN stimulation lasted up to 100 ms and 150 ms of the early and late TP evoked responses respectively (Fig. 4).

Administration of GABA did not affect the depression of the early TP evoked response by DCN stimulation, but increased the depression of the late response (Fig. 4). Picrotoxin significantly disinhibited the effect of DCN stimulation on both the early and the late TP evoked responses (Fig. 2). Saclofen did not influence the depression either of the early or the late TP evoked response to DCN stimulation (Fig. 4).

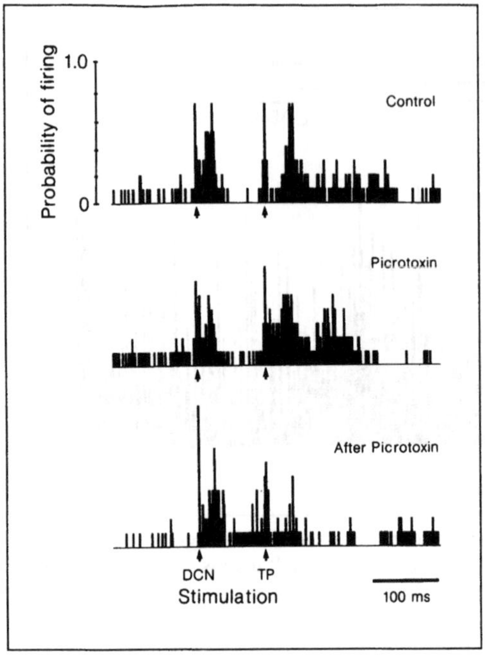

Fig 2. A conditioning test paradigm where the activity evoked by TP stimulation was inhibited by preceeding DCN stimulation (control). Iontophoresis of picrotoxin partially blocked the DCN induced inhibition (picrotoxin). After recovery the inhibition returns (after picrotoxin).

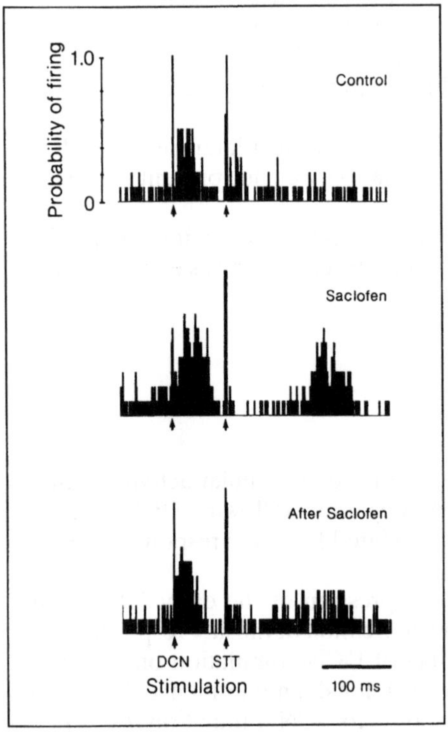

Fig. 3. The same paradigm as in Fig. 2 was used. The activity evoked by STT stimulation was inhibited by preceeding DCN stimulation (control). Iontophoresis of saclofen partially blocked the DCN induced inhibition, particularly the late response (saclofen). After recovery the inhibition returns (after saclofen).

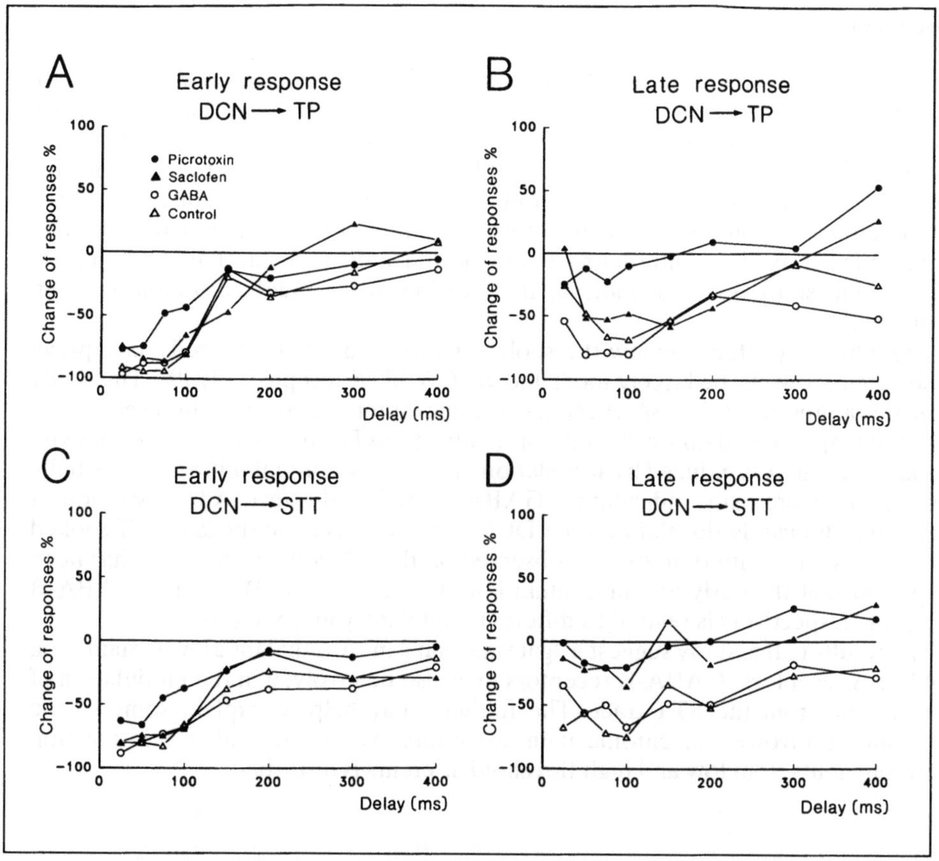

Fig. 4. Mean effects on early and late TP and STT induced responses by preceding DCN stimulation at delays from 25 to 400 ms, during iontophoretic drug application. A and B) A significant disinhibition at 75 – 100 ms ($p < 0.05$) and at 50 – 100 ms ($p < 0.01$) delays on the early (A) and late (B) responses to TP stimulation, respectively, during picrotoxin administration. C and D) A significant disinhibition at 75 – 100 ($p < 0.05$) and at 25 – 50 ms ($p < 0.01$) delays on the early (C) and late (D) responses to STT stimulation, respectively, during picrotoxin administration. The late response following STT stimulation was disinhibited by saclofen at 25 ($p < 0.05$) and at 100 ($p < 0.01$) ms delays.

All cells excited by STT stimulation showed a reduced cellular activity by preceding stimulation given to the DCN. The depression lasted up to 100 ms and 150 ms of the early and the late responses to STT stimulation respectively (Fig. 4).

The depression by DCN stimulation of the early and the late response to STT stimulation were not significantly affected by GABA administration (Fig. 4). On the other hand, picrotoxin significantly disinhibited both the early and the late response to STT stimulation by preceding DCN activation (Fig. 4). Saclofen disinhibited the late response to STT stimulation at 25 ms and at 100 ms delays, but did not influence the early (Fig. 3).

Discussion

Results from previous studies with intracellular recording from units in the VB complex following stimulation of cutaneous low threshold afferents, revealed excitatory postsynaptic potentials (EPSPs) of short latency followed by a pronounced, long lasting inhibitory postsynaptic potentials (IPSPs) (2). A feedback and a feed forward inhibition are indicated by previous studies (1) in related thalamic nuclei, and the interneurones responsible for the feed forward inhibition are located in the VB-complex, while the feedback interneurones are located in the reticular thalamic complex. The present study does not indicate the location of the involved inhibitory interneurones.

The inhibitory effects on low threshold somatosensory thalamic cells have previously been shown to be largely mediated via GABA-A receptors (4, 10). This study indicates a presence a GABA-A mediated tonic inhibition normally induced by low threshold input to thalamic cells. Inhibitory effects on TP and on STT evoked activity in thalamic cells was induced by stimulation of the DCN. This inhibition was partially reversed by picrotoxin, indicating a GABA-A mediated effect. Administration of saclofen significantly disinhibited the DCN induced effects on the late STT evoked activity. Such disinhibition was not observed on the TP evoked activity. It has been suggested that the early and late inhibition mediated via GABA-A and GABA-B receptors respectively is related to different modulatory mechanisms (3).

The results in this study suggest a "gate-mechanism" at a thalamic level, mainly via GABA-A receptors. GABA-B receptors may also be involved in the modulation of information from the STT tract. The findings may help to explain some of the mechanisms involved in chronic pain conditions where the thalamic interaction between inputs from low and high threshold afferents is disturbed.

Acknowledgements

This work was supported by the Swedish Medical Research Council (Project No. 55), The Bank of Sweden Tercentenary Foundation, CIBA-GEIGY Sweden, and The Medical Faculty, University of Göteborg. Excellent technical assistance was given by Mrs. Stina Morelius.

References

1. Ahlsén G, Lindström S, Lo FS (1985) Interaction between inhibitory pathways to principal cells in the lateral geniculate nucleus of the cat. Exp Brain Res 58: 134–143
2. Andersen P, Eccles JC, Sears TA (1964) The ventro-basal complex of the thalamus: types of cells, their responses and their functional organization. J Physiol (Lond) 174: 370–399
3. Crunelli V, Leresche N (1991) A role for GABA-B receptors in excitation and inhibition of thalamocortical cells. TINS 14: 16–21
4. Eaton S, Salt T (1991) Sensory stimuli evoke inhibitory post-synaptic potentials mediated by GABA in the ventrobasal thalamus in vivo. Eur J Neurosci 3: 296–300
5. Jeanmonod D, Magnin M, Morel A (1994) A thalamic concept of neurogenic pain. In: Proceedings of the 7th World Congress on Pain: Progress in Pain Research and Management, Vol. 2, Eds: Gebhart GF, Hammond DL, Jensen TS, IASP Press, Seattle, pp 767–787

6. Lenz FA, Kwan HC, Dostrovsky JO, Tasker RR (1989) Characteristics of the bursting pattern of action potentials that occurs in the thalamus of patients with central pain, Brain Res 496: 357–360
7. Melzack R, Wall PD (1965) Pain mechanisms: A new theory. Science 150: 971–979
8. Olausson B (1989) Thalamo-cortical mechanisms in nociception. Thesis, University of Gothenburg
9. Rydenhag B (1985) Thalamic nociceptive mechanism. Thesis, University of Gothenburg
10. Salt TE (1989) Gamma-aminobutyric acid and afferent inhibition in the cat and rat ventrobasal thalamus. Neuroscience 28: 17–26

Author's address:
B. Olausson MD PhD
Dept. of Clinical Neurophysiology
Sahlgrenska University Hospital
University of Göteborg
S-41345 Göteborg
Sweden

Spinal cord stimulation in ischemia and ischemic pain
Possible mechanisms of action

B. Linderoth

Department of Neurosurgery, Karolinska Hospital, Stockholm, Sweden

Introduction

Spinal cord stimulation has by now been used for pain due to tissue ischemia in the extremities (peripheral vascular disease; PVD) for almost 20 years. The pioneer report by Cook et al. appeared in 1976 (12). The spread of the method for this indication was slow in the beginning, but after the presentation of the studies by Augustinsson, Jivegård, Galley, Jacobs and their collaborators (1, 16, 23–25) and others, the method has been adopted in most major centers.

The primary indication in PVD is still rest pain with no or little tissue involvement, i.e., stage III acording to the Fontaine scale. In spite of the wide acceptance of the method by now, knowledge about the mechanisms behind its beneficial effect is still scanty. It is probable that this lack of knowledge has hampered both the spread and the further development of SCS. Thus, research on these matters is urgently called for.

In a typical example of the ischemic foot in PVD, there may be several pain components present, e.g. 1) deep aching ischemic pain, 2) pain from ischemic ulcers and from the borders of gangreneous zones, both nociceptive and responsive to opioids – and in advanced states, also 3) a neuropathic component which may be opiate-resistant (cf. 5,52).

It was earlier commonly accepted that only neurogenic pain – and not nociceptive pain states – was responsive to spinal cord stimulation (19, 50). Thus, it might seem strange that nociceptive ischemic pain responds to SCS, while other nociceptive states do not. However, there are several indications that the mechanisms involved in the stimulation-induced alleviation of ischemic pain are fundamentally different from those active when neuropathic pain is treated (35, 36). This issue will be discussed in more detail below.

It is now also well-known that SCS has wide-spread effects on autonomic functions. From the observations of Meglio et al. (48, 49), we have learned that the heart rate is often slightly decreased during stimulation and, furthermore, there are many reports on the effects on peripheral circulation (e.g., 7, 38, 47). These changes may be illustrated in different ways: by demonstrating an increase in skin temperature, a change in macro- or microcirculation, elevation of peripheral blood pressures, and oxygen tension in the tissues (4, 37). An example is shown in Fig. 1 which illustrates the increase in thermoregulatory skin circulation which may result from SCS – here pictured by the thermo-camera.

Figure 2 illustrates a case of arterial occlusive disease in the right leg and SCS giving mainly right-sided paresthesiae. Both skin microcirculation measured by the laser Doppler technique and the skin temperature increase during stimulation and further on after cessation of stimulation (from (38)).

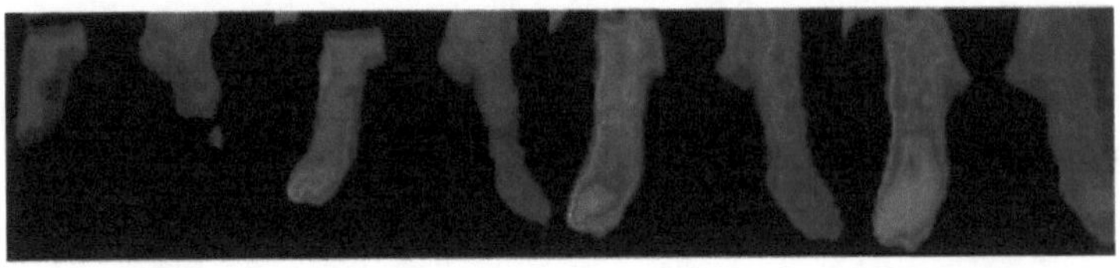

Fig. 1. This thermographic record of the skin temperature in both feet of a patient before and during SCS, as well as 20 min after treatment, illustrates how the thermoregulatory microcirculation increases during and after stimulation. The blue-green colors (lower skin temperature) present initially, successively give way to red and yellow colors (warmer), illustrating the rise in skin temperature. It is evident that the increase is detectable after only some minutes of stimulation (from (38)).

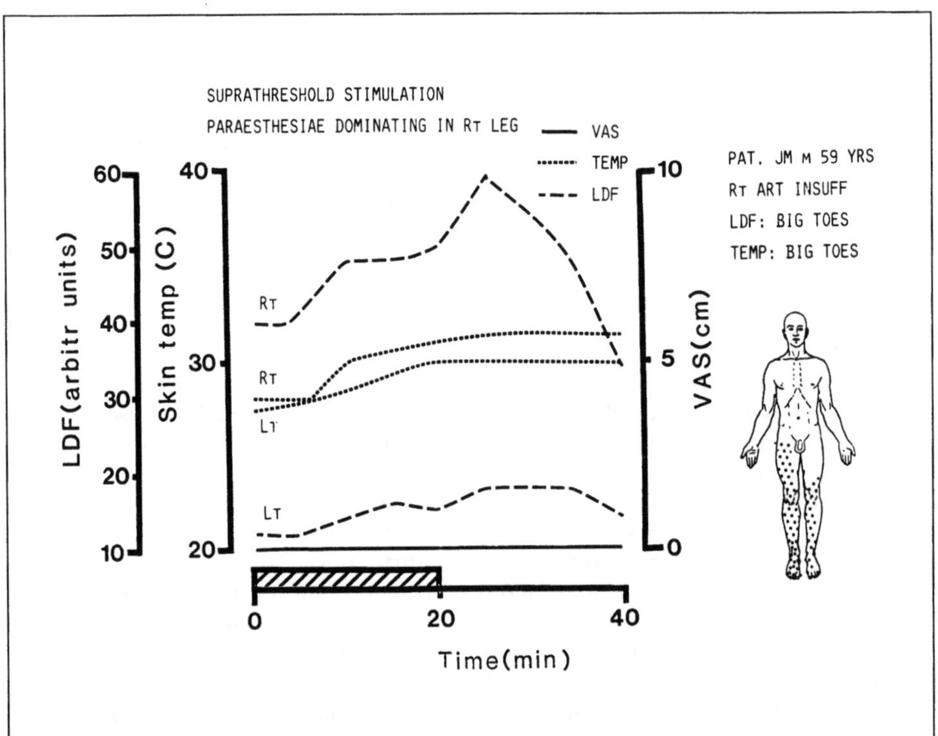

Fig. 2. This diagram illustrates changes in skin temperature as measured by thermocamera (dotted line), skin microcirculation monitored by laser-Doppler flowmetry (broken line) in a case of PVD during SCS with paresthesiae mainly in the right leg. It is readily seen that the changes are more prominent in the leg with paresthesia than in the other leg (from (38)).

There has been a continuing debate whether the processes underlying the stimulation-induced pain relief in, for example, neuropathic conditions are the same as those resulting in pain alleviation in states of tissue ischemia. However, as already mentioned, there are several fundamental differences between the pain inhibition in these two conditions, pointing to the possibility of quite different effector mechanisms (35, 36).

It is our belief that the most important pain relief following SCS in PVD and similar conditions is secondary to a relative increase in circulation in the ischemic tissue in relation to the metabolic demands, while pain inhibition in neuropathy is the result of other processes (cf. e.g., 2, 36). I will now proceed by presenting the observations on which this view is based – as well as the alternative hypotheses discussed during the 1980s and up to the present.

Hypotheses about effector mechanisms for pain relief in ischemia

The four main hypotheses about the mechanisms underlying the relief of ischemic pain by SCS are listed in Table 1 and may be summarized as follows:

1) That SCS by some mechanism directly inhibits the "pain signal".

2) That SCS induces antidromic activity in sensory nerves resulting in peripheral vasodilatation and pain relief – and this includes also the activation of small diameter high threshold fibers.

3) That SCS releases substances with effects on the peripheral vascular beds.

4) That SCS modulates the activity of the autonomic nervous system, notably the sympathetic system and that this results in vasodilatation with secondary pain alleviation.

SCS inhibits "pain signal"

The first hypothesis, that the alleviation of the ischemic pain is due to a block of the transmission of impulses transmitted from the dorsal horn to the brain via the spinothalamic tracts, has been supported by, for example, Hosobuchi (22) and by the Foreman group, Oklahoma City (9, 15).

Table 1. Hypotheses about mechanisms underlying the pain inhibitory effects of SCS in ischemia.

I	Inhibition of pain signal > decreased sympathetic activity > vasodilatation > further pain reduction, etc.
II	Antidromic activation of primary afferents > release of vasoactive substances > vasodilatation > pain reduction
III	Release of vasoactive substances (local/distant effects) > vasodilatation > pain reduction
IV	Modulation of autonomic activity > vasodilatation > decrease of pain

There are several neurophysiological studies demonstrating an inhibitory effect of electric stimuli applied to the dorsal columns on the transmission of nociceptive impulses from the dorsal horn via the spinothalamic tracts (for a review see (35)). However, most of these studies use A) acute peripheral nociception, i.e., a stimulus mode which usually does not respond to SCS, and B) electric SCS stimuli which have little similarity to those used for spinal cord stimulation clinically. In the paper by Chandler et al. (9) which describes a very elegant study, great care was taken to adapt stimulation frequency and current intensity to the clinically used parameters. However, the test situation contains still only short trains of pulses applied to the spinal cord (20 milliseconds long) preceeding the noxious stimulus by 20 – 160 ms, and thus, the experimental situation differs in relevant aspects from the clinical use of SCS, which is why the outcome from such studies also has to be interpreted with caution. Of course, they elucidate central inhibitory mechanisms, but do not explain the full effect seen in the clinical setting.

I will proceed by presenting some differences between stimulation-induced alleviation of pain in ischemia in contrast to the beneficial effect in neuropathy, thereby indicating.the possibility of fundamentally different underlying mechanisms for stimulation-induced pain relief in the two conditions. These aspects are summarized in Table 2.

First, the dominating types of pain in PVD, i.e., the deep aching ischemic pain and the pain originating from ischemic ulcers and from the ischemic penumbra surrounding the gangrene, are certainly nociceptive and responsive to opiates. The deep ischemic pain is alleviated by the stimulation, but the superficial pain components from the ulcers seem merely to be masked by the stimulation-induced paresthesiae and appear again immediately after the stimulation is switched off. Furthermore, acute pain evoked by manipulations with the ulcerated zones (e.g., changing of bandages) may be very intense and this cannot be prevented by the SCS. Thus, a block of the pain signals seems to be a less plausible explanation for the clinical effects of SCS since only certain pain components are relieved.

Second, the latency for pain relief is quite different in neuropathic pain and in PVD. In neuropathic conditions a pain decrease often is evident after only 10 min of stimulation, while in stimulation-naive ischemic cases it may take up to 2 days of protracted stimulation before a significant pain relief is present. The changes in peripheral microcirculation are more rapid (38). This indicates that a mediating mechanism, e.g., the peripheral vasodilatation and reperfusion of the ischemic tissue may need

Table 2. Differences between SCS-induced pain alleviation in neuropathic and ischemic pain states indicating different underlying mechanisms (explanation, see text)

1. Type of pain:	-nociceptive -neuropathic
2. Latency of response	
3. Concomitant sensation:	– none – warmth – cold
4. Dependence on paresthesiae	

some time to stabilize and abolish the pain-inducing mechanisms. Vasospastic pain states (e.g., Raynaud's syndrome), and angina pectoris react differently from the ischemic rest pain and are much more rapid in their response to stimulation.

Third, in neuropathic pain cases the stimulation-induced paresthesiae may be accompanied by either a sensation of warmth, cold or by no temperature sensation at all – and still the treatment is successful for the pain. On the contrary, in the ischemic cases the accompanying temperature sensation is usually warmth (or none at all) if the stimulation is effective for the pain. A feeling of cold is most often experienced as very unpleasant for the patient with ischemic leg pain (cf. e.g. (2)).

A fourth difference is that properly located paresthesiae seems to be more critical in neuropathic than in ischemic pain. There is a gross correlation between effect and paresthesiae in ischemic pain as well, but it has been demonstrated that in patients, stimulated with a low intensity unable to evoke paresthesiae, cutaneous vasodilatation may still be observed (Fig. 3). Furthermore, patients who experience unilateral paresthesiae may only have stimulation-induced vasodilatation bilaterally (Fig. 4) (from (38)).

In neuropathic pain cervical stimulation may be effective for pain in the legs given that the painful areas are covered by proper paresthesiae. In ischemic pain stimulation must be applied segmentally, i.e., for the legs, the lumbar segments have to be stimulated by an electrode at vertebral level T10-L1. Lately, some clinical observations have indicated that this might not be generally valid (51; Linderoth, unpublished observations), however, it is still the major rule.

Thus, the paresthesiae do not seem to be absolutely mandatory for the vascular effect to be demonstrated – but presently, they remain an indispensable aid in the placement of the electrode.

In summary then there are many indices that alleviation of ischemic pain is not merely "a block of the pain signal". Only certain pain components are inhibited and several traits specific to the response of pain and microcirculation in ischemia indicate that the pain reduction may be secondary to another phenomenon, e.g., the increased microcirculation.

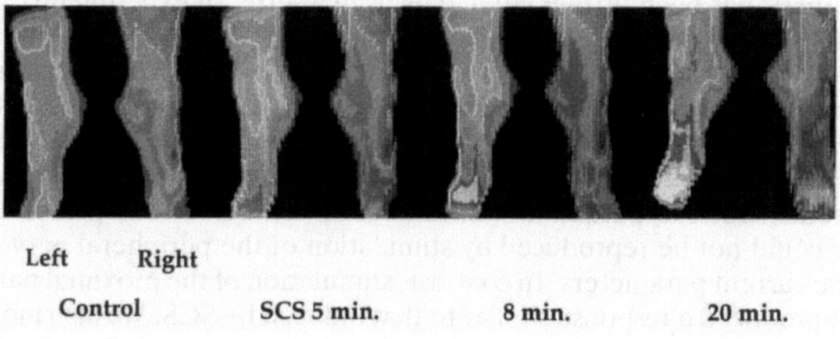

Fig. 3. In this case SCS was applied with an intensity just below the threshold for the detection of paresthesiae. Thus, the patient felt nothing of the stimulation – but nevertheless there is a detectable change in thermoregulatory flow, here illustrated by thermography (from (38)).

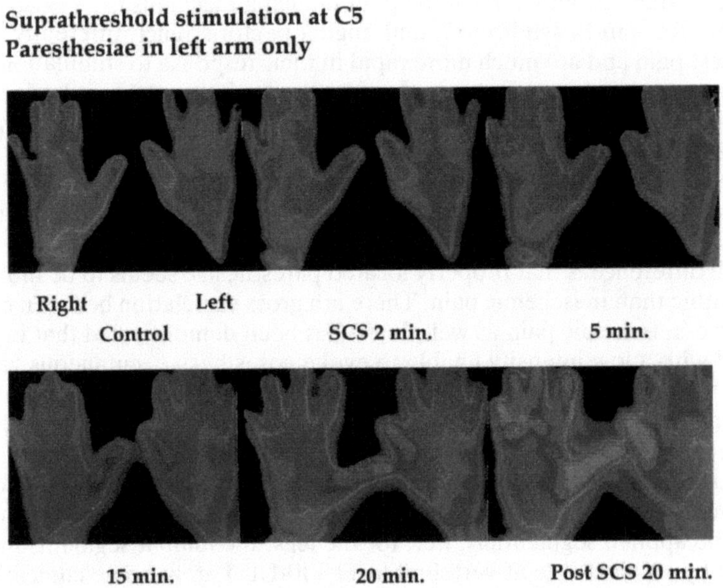

Fig. 4. In this patient paresthesiae was present in one limb only, but still the SCS resulted in a bilateral warming of the skin. Thus, the paresthesiae is not absolutely mandatory for this effect to take place (from (38)).

SCS evokes antidromic activity

The second hypothesis implies that the vasodilatation during SCS would depend on the same mechanisms that accounts for the marked vasal response recorded when dorsal roots or peripheral nerves are antidromically stimulated with very high intensity. This is actually based on old observations made by Bayliss at the turn of the century (3) and repeatedly observed by others after this (e.g., 6, 17, 21). Hilton and Marshall (20) proposed that the effect was mainly due to a release of prostacyclin from thin nerve fibers, but others have proposed other substances like substance P, CGRP, etc. (for review see 35).

This hypothesis has been further studied by us in a series of experiments.

In studies on anesthetized rats the peripheral microcirculation was investigated by laser-Doppler technique during experimental SCS applied with current parameters tailored to be similar to those used in the clinic (50 Hz; 0.2 ms; intensity 2/3 of motor threshold). In the initial experiments various pathways suggested to mediate this peripheral vasodilatation were eliminated surgically (39 – 41) (Fig. 5). We sectioned the dorsal roots, but the peripheral vasodilatation with SCS was preserved and, furthermore could not be reproduced by stimulation of the peripheral nerve stump with the same current parameters. In contrast, stimulation of the proximal part of the severed root produced a response similar to that induced by SCS. We also monitored antidromic activity in peripheral nerves observing that with stimulation of the spinal cord itself vasodilatation was obtained with stimulation parameters recruiting only large diameter, low threshold fibers. Thus, the outcome of these studies indicated that neither antidromic activation of primary afferents nor recruitment of small diameter fibers was mandatory for the SCS-induced vasodilatation.

Further on, there is a massive clinical experience from thousands of patients that SCS does not have to evoke unpleasant or painful sensations to be effective either for ischemic or for neuropathic pain. The resulting paresthesiae are instead experienced as a pleasant, sometimes warming tingling. Thus, there is neither experimentally nor clinically any support for a recruitment of high threshold, thin pain transmitting fibers in SCS.

SCS induces release of vasoactive substances

There are several vasoactive substances possibly released by electric afferent stimulation like transcutaneous electrical nerve stimulation (TENS) and by SCS. This has previously been extensively discussed by, for example, Kaada and collaborators (e.g., 31, 32) and by Kjartansson et al. (33, 34). Substances of special interest have been the vasoactive intestinal polypeptide (VIP) (e.g., 8), substance P, the calcitonin-gene-related peptide (CGRP), the prostaglandins, nitric oxide, etc. At present, there is little clear support for a role of any of these behind the effects of SCS, but some authors have formulated hypotheses about stimulation-induced CGRP release as a possible mediating mechanism (34, 44, 45). Studies are urgently needed in this area.

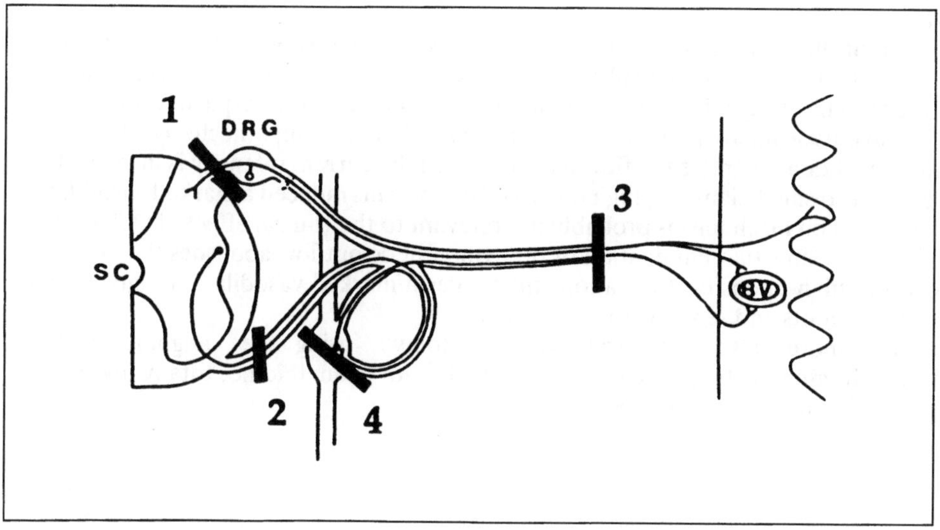

Fig. 5. Schematic diagram of the spinal cord, the ventral and dorsal roots, the paravertebral sympathetic chain and the peripheral nerve supplying the skin. Transection of dorsal roots (1) did not abolish the vasodilatory effect of SCS, but section of the ventral roots (2) or the peripheral nerve (3) depleted the effect as did previous complete bilateral lumbar sympathectomy (4); (redrawn after (33)).

SCS modulates autonomic activity

A hypothesis proposed by many researchers and clinicians in this field is that SCS might modulate the activity of the autonomic system, and especially inhibit sympathetic activity (35, 38, 40, 41, 48). Vasodilatory sympathetic fibers with acetylcholine as the postganglionic transmitter for muscle tissue, and similar fibers to the skin with hitherto unknown transmitters have been proposed, but the most plausible mechanism is that SCS acts on sympathetic vasoconstrictor fibers (for reviews see 27 – 30). Some evidence in favor of this hypothesis will be presented below.

It is well known that sympathetic blocks and sympathectomy are efficient in ischemic pain conditions, at least temporarily. However, if alteration of sympathetic activity would be a critical factor it might seem strange that SCS is effective also in cases submitted to repeated sympathetic blocks with gradually decreasing efficacy, or to surgical sympathectomy (7, 12, 22 – 24). One explanation is simply that the elimination of the autonomic activity often may be incomplete (as was also demonstrated by us in animal experiments; 41) and that SCS thus may act on the persistent autonomic activity. In properly denervated and well-controlled cases (demonstrated both in man and in the rat) the vasodilatory effect is depleted (41, 51). If following sympatectomy in a rat, regional sympathetic reflexes are still active, as e.g., demonstrated in a temperature test, this animal could also respond with vasodilatation, selectively in the same vascular bed, to the SCS to follow (41).

In order to examine the hypothesis that reduction of sympathetic activity would be responsible for the SCS-induced increase in peripheral blood flow, we surgically eliminated, in different studies, sympathetic outflow to the examined vascular beds in the following ways (cf. Fig. 5 above):

1) Cutting of ventral roots supplying the examined area; 2) Sectioning of the sciatic nerve (39, 40); 3) Bilateral lumbar sympathectomy performed 1 week before SCS (41).

Each of these maneuvers abolished the vasodilatory response otherwise induced by SCS and by themselves resulted in an increase in peripheral microcirculation.

Figure 6 illustrates the experimental set-up, and Fig. 7 shows typical recordings of skin and muscle microcirculation before and after lumbar sympathectomy. The lowermost panel demonstrates the flow increase when the current intensity is increased to recruite also small diameter, high threshold fibers. This induced a marked vasodilatation, based on mechanisms probably not relevant to the clinical effect of SCS (41).

Thus, it seems that elimination of the sympathetic outflow abolishes the effect of SCS, but high-intensity stimulation still evokes a marked vasodilatation given that the dorsal roots and sensory fibers are intact.

Furthermore, also "chemical sympathectomy", using the ganglion blocker hexamethonium or by pretreating the animals with guanethidine, totally abolished the vasodilatory effects of SCS (40, 41, 43)

Transmitters and receptor groups involved

In separate experiments (43) more selective pharmacological blocking of autonomic transmission was used both on the ganglionic and on the neuro-effector levels.

From Table 3 it is evident that inhibition of the transmission via muscarinic receptors had little effect on the stimulation-induced vasodilatation (atropine antagonizes both M_2 and M_3 subgroups), but the nicotinic receptor antagonist chlorisondamine abolished the reponse in higher doses (the initially increased SCS effect may be the result of a decreased peripheral resistance).

Non-specific block of alpha-adrenergic transmission decreased the effect in both tissues studied and this seemed to be mainly a result of inhibition of alpha-1 mediated influence on the microcirculation.

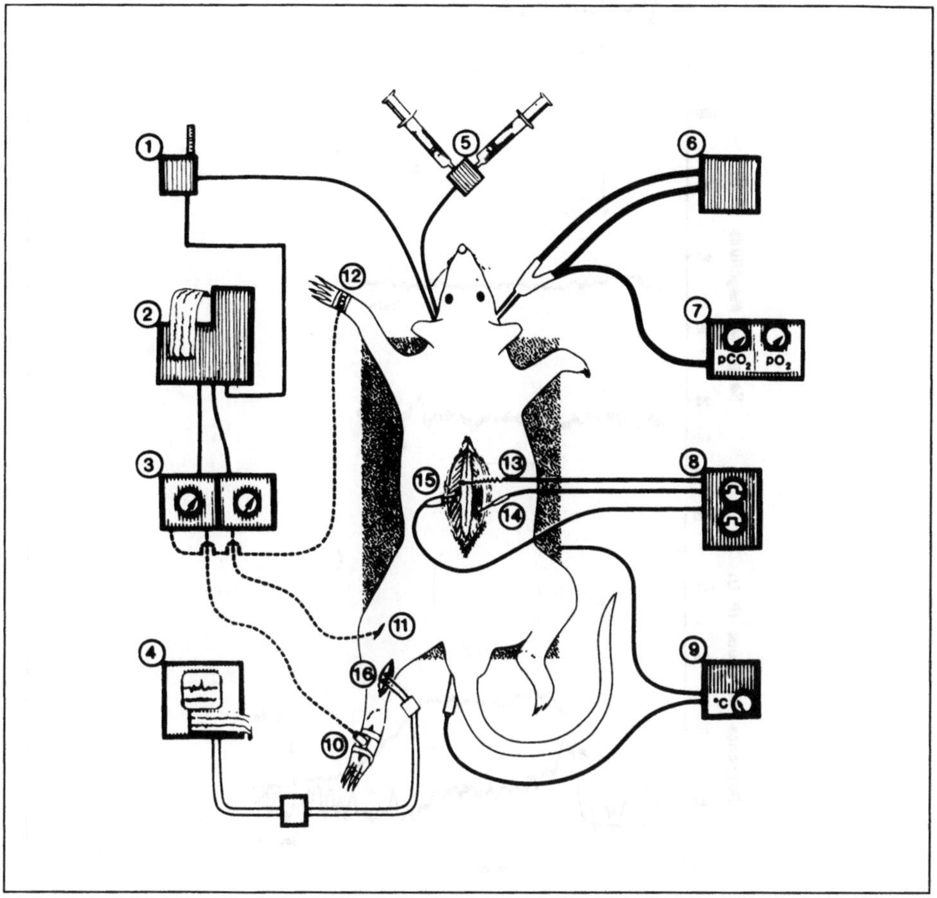

Fig. 6. Schematic illustration of the experimental set-up for studies of microcirculation during SCS. 1) Transducer for monitoring of systemic blood pressure via a carotid artery; 2) Pen recorder for LDF and systemic blood pressure; 3) Laser-Doppler flow meters; 4) Nerve activity recording unit; 5) Jugular i.v. infusion line; 6) Respirator; 7) CO_2- and O_2-analyzer; 8) Stimulator; 9) Temperature control unit; 10, 12) Laser-Doppler surface probes in plastic holders; 11) Laser-Doppler single fiber probe for monitoring of muscle microcirculation; 13) Spinal cord cathode (silver sphere; diam.: 1 mm); 14) Needle anode; 15) Bipolar stimulating electrodes for stimulation of cut and intact dorsal roots; 16) Bipolar recording electrode on sural nerve (from (35)).

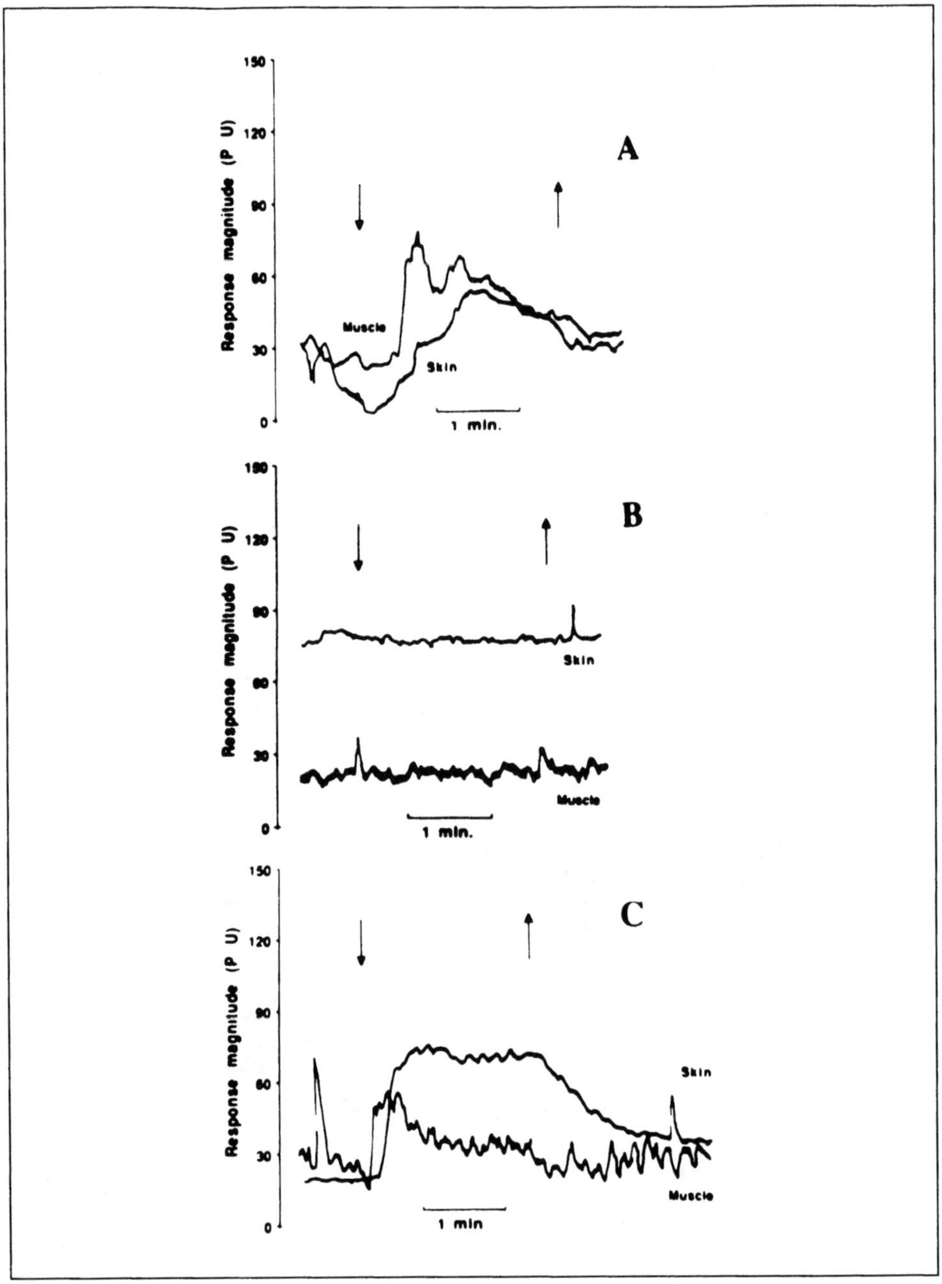

Fig. 7. Recordings of skin and muscle microcirculation with laser-Doppler flowmetry before (A: upper panel) and after (B: middle panel) lumbar sympathectomy. It is readily seen that before surgery there were marked flow increases in both vascular beds during SCS, but the vasodilatory effect was totally abolished after sympathectomy. That a reserve of vasodilatation persists is demonstrated in the lowermost panel (C) where high intensity, low frequency stimulation is applied instead. This induced a marked flow increase in both territories.
Arrow down: SCS on; Arrow up: SCS off. (from (41); with permission from Neurosurgery).

Beta-adrenergic antagonism resulted in differential effects on the micro-circulatory response to stimulation in skin and muscle respectively. As was the case with non-specific alpha-adrenergic antagonism, also unspecific blocking of beta-adrenergic receptors abolished the responses in both the vascular beds studied. However, beta-1 adrenoreceptors seemed more critical for the effect in the skin, while beta-2 receptors may mediate the effect in muscle tissue.

Table 3. Summary of the effects on muscle and skin microcirculation of different, more receptor-specific, antagonistic substances administered during SCS. The stimulation-induced vasodilatation following drug administration is coded: +: enhanced response in comparison to control; =: response amplitude comparable to control; −: reduced response compared to control; O: no vasodilatation. (extract from Linderoth et al. 1994, Table 1)

Substance	Dose (mg/kg iv)	Effect muscle	skin
Cholinergic receptor acting drugs:			
Pirenzepine	1	=	=
(muscarinic M_1-receptor antagonist)	2	=	=
	5	=	=
	10	=	=
Atropine	0.05	=	=
(muscarinic M_2/M_3-receptor antagonist)	0.2	=	=
	0.5	=	=
Chlorisondamine	0.3	+	+
(nicotinic receptor antagonist)	3	+	+
	10	−	−
	20	O	O
α-adrenergic receptor acting drugs:			
Prazosine	0.05	=	−
(α_1-receptor antagonist)	0.1	=	−
	0.5	=	O
	1	O	O
Yohimbine	0.1	=	=
(α_2-receptor antagonist)	0.5	=	=
	1	=	=
β-adrenergic receptor acting drugs:			
Atenolol	0.5	=	=
(β_1-receptor antagonist)	1	=	−
	3	=	−
	5	=	O
Butoxamine	1	=	=
(β_2-receptor antagonist)	5	−	=
	7	−	=
	10	O	=

Thus, these studies favor the view that SCS acts on sympathetic vasoconstrictor activity mainly exerted via nicotinic receptors in the ganglia and alpha-1 adrenoreceptors in the neuro-effector junction. The role of the beta receptors might be different in skin and muscle respectively.

Electrophysiological evidence

Finally, is there some neurophysiological investigations demonstrating that SCS applied with "clinical current parameters" actually decreases activity in peripheral sympathetic neurons? The evidence is hitherto scanty. However, in one pilot study, Dr. I. Fedorcsak from Budapest, in collaboration with us, earlier reported that stimulation of the dorsal spinal cord at the T2-level in cats resulted in a depression of sympathetic activity as recorded extracellularly from the paravertebral chain close to the stellate ganglion (14). Both the number of bursts and the number of spikes in a burst were diminished during stimulation (Fig. 8). The findings from this pilot study need to be repeated with refined techniques under more controlled conditions (cf. 30).

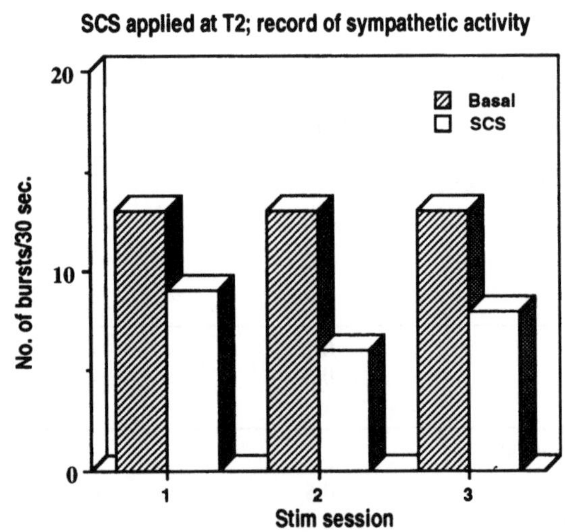

Fig. 8. Extracellular recording from the paravertebral chain close to the stellate ganglion in a cat during SCS applied at the T2 level with parameters similar to those used clinically. The diagram demonstrates the reduction in the number of bursts which resulted from the application of the SCS (from (14)).

The lack of adequate animal models

The studies described up to now have all been performed on normal animals without vascular problems. We have constantly searched for adequate models for the ischemic problems observed in our patients, but the outcome of this search has been poor. Aged rats have been investigated with little success, and also diabetic and spontaneously hypertensive animals have been considered. The only animal model of ischemia we have studied so far is a free flap model in the rat earlier used by Gherardini et al. (18).

Preliminary observations in a model of vasospasm

We used a rat model of mechanically induced vasospasm on an island flap in the groin (44). First, the rats had an electrode system for SCS (42) chronically implanted and after some days of recovery they were again anesthetized by ip chloral hydrate, a neurovascular skin flap was raised in the groin and the microcirculation monitored by laser-Doppler, both in the flap and in a control area. Vasospasm was then induced by gently, repetitively compressing the exposed feeding artery with microforceps along 5 mm of the vessel for 10 s. In pilot studies, we observed that SCS had the best effect if given before the vasospasm. In the main experiment two groups of animals were submitted to vasospasm one with and one without previous SCS for 20 min.

It was evident that both groups developed the vasospasm mirrored by a decrease in flap microcirculation, but the restoration of the basal level of microcirculation was much more rapid and complete in the SCS-treated animals. In the SCS group 100 % of the animals eventually recovered completely while the figure for the control group was only 28 %. Preliminary experiments indicate also that the outcome is similar after spasm induction by topical noradrenaline application onto the feeding artery (44).

SCS in angina pectoris

I will merely give some brief comments on the use of SCS in angina pectoris, a condition which has turned out to be a cardinal indication for SCS with 80 – 90 % success rate (13).

Also for angina there is much debate about possible effector mechanisms. Some different factors proposed to underly the pain relief are listed in Table 4.

Table 4. Beneficial effects of SCS in angina pectoris; some hypotheses about effector mechanisms

Proposed mechanisms/effects	1. Block of pain signal/masking of angina
	2. Inhibition of sympathetic activity
	3. Release of vasoactive substances a. decrease of metabolic demands b. increase / redistribution of cardiac blood flow

Foreman and collaborators (9) advocate an inhibition of the nociceptive transmission in the spinothalamic tract, while the Göteborg group propose different mechanisms in occlusive cardiac disease and in syndrome X, respectively. In arteriosclerosis, Mannheimer et al. hypothesize that a decrease of oxygen demand in the ischemic myocardial tissue may be one important component, while in syndrome X an actual increase of the regional perfusion may lie behind the beneficial effect on the angina (13, 26). Both these effects could be mediated by a depression of sympathetic activity, possibly to some part mediated via the release of endogenous opioids as demonstrated by the same group (46). There is also some evidence that such stimulation-induced changes might be neurally mediated since TENS, in a recent report, has been demonstrated to increase coronary flow in normal humans, while those with transplanted – and denervated – hearts presented no such effect (10, 11).

Conclusions

In conclusion, today there are clear indications that a major part of the relief of ischemic pain by SCS is secondary to the increased peripheral circulation.

The data presented here support the hypothesis that inhibition of sympathetically maintained peripheral vasoconstriction constitutes an important factor behind the stimulation-induced vasodilatation in skin and muscle. The vasoconstriction seems to be mediated by several receptor groups. The role played be other vasoactive substances released from autonomic and from other perivascular nerve fibers remains unknown, but hopefully data are forthcoming.

Future research should be directed onto further exploration of the importance of modulation of sympathetic activity by SCS using microelectrode technique applied to peripheral sympathetic neurons – as also proposed by Jänig (30), and to the search for suitable animal models for ischemia.

References

1. Augustinsson LE, Carlsson CA, Holm J, Jivegård L (1985) Epidural electrical stimulation in severe limb ischemia. Ann Surg 202: 104–110
2. Augustinsson LE, Linderoth B, Mannheimer C (1992) Spinal cord stimulation in various ischaemic conditions. In: Illis L (ed) Spinal Cord Dysfunction, Vol III. Functional Stimulation. Oxford Medical Publications, Oxford, pp 272–295
3. Bayliss WM (1901) On the origin from the spinal cord of the vasodilator fibers of the hind-limb and on the nature of these fibers. J Physiol 26: 173–209
4. Boccalon H (1994) Criteria of efficacy: the survey. In: Herreros J et al. (eds) Spinal Cord Stimulation for Peripheral Vascular Disease. Advances and Controversies. Editorial Libro del Ano, SL, Madrid, pp 57–67
5. Bonica J (1990) Pain due to vascular disease. In: Bonica JJ (ed) The Management of Pain, 2nd ed. Lea & Febiger, Philadelphia, pp 502–537
6. Brodin E, Linderoth B, Gazelius B, Ungerstedt U (1987) In vivo release of substance P in cat dorsal horn studied with microdialysis. Neurosc Lett 76: 357–362

7. Broseta J, Barbera J, De Vera JA, Barcia-Salorio JL, Garcia-March G, Gonzalez-Darder J, Rovaina F, Joanes V (1986) Spinal cord stimulation in peripheral arterial disease. J Neurosurg 64: 71–80
8. Broseta J, Sanchez-Ledesma MJ, Goncalvez J (1994) Humoral mechanisms mediating in the increase of peripheral blood flow following spinal cord stimulation. An experimental study in the dog. In: Herreros J et al. (eds) Spinal Cord Stimulation for Peripheral Vascular Disease. Advances and Controversies. Editorial Libro del Ano, SL, Madrid, pp 17–23
9. Chandler MJ, Brennan TJ, Garrison DW, Kim KS, Schwartz PJ, Foreman RD (1993) A mechanism of cardiac pain suppression by spinal cord stimulation: implications for patients with angina pectoris. Eur Heart J 14: 96–105
10. Chauhan A, Mullins PA, Taylor G, Petch MC, Schofield PM (1993) Coronary blood flow, transcutaneous electric nerve stimulation and possible mechanisms of action. Eur Heart J, Vol 14. Abstr Suppl XVth Congress Eur Soc Cardiol p 315
11. Chauhan A, Mullins PA, Thuraisingham SI, Taylor G, Petch MC, Schofield PM (1994) Effect of transcutaneous electrical nerve stimulation on coronary blood flow. Circulation, Vol 89 (2) pp 694–702
12. Cook AW, Oygar A, Baggenstos P, Pacheco S, Kleriga E (1976) Vascular disease of extremities. Electrical stimulation of spinal cord and posterior roots. N Y State J Med 76: 366–368
13. Eliasson T (1994) Spinal cord stimulation in angina pectoris. Thesis. Östra Hospital, Göteborg, 88 pp
14. Fedorcsak I, Linderoth B, Gunasekera L, Bognar L, Meyerson BA (1991) Peripheral vasodilation due to sympathetic inhibition induced by spinal cord stimulation. 3rd IBRO World Congress of Neuroscience, Montreal, p 126
15. Foreman RD, Chandler MJ, Brennan TJ, Kim KS, Garrisn DW, Schwartz PJ (1989) Does dorsal column stimulation reduce the activity of spino-thalamic tract cells that respond to cardiac input? Circulation 80 Suppl II: 552
16. Galley D, Elharrar C, Scheffer J, Rakotonarivo J, Medvedowski A, Barnay JC, Medvedowski L, Serena G (1988) Intéret de la neurostimulation épidurale dans les artériopathies des membres inférieurs. Arteres et Veines 7: 61–71
17. Gazelius B, Brodin E, Olgart L, Panopolous P (1981) Evidence that substance P is a mediator of antidromic vasodilatation using somatostatin as a release inhibitor. Acta Physiol Scand 113: 155–159
18. Gheradini G, Lundeberg T, Gazelius B, Brodda-Jansen G, Samuelson U (1994) Calcitonin gene-related peptide dose dependent increases microcirculation after mechanically induced vasospasm in an island flap in the rat. Plastic and Reconstruct Surg (submitted)
19. Gybels JM, Sweet WH (1989) Neurosurgical treatment of persistent pain. In: Gildenberg PL (ed) Pain and Headache. Karger, Basel, pp 442
20. Hilton SM, Marshall JM (1980) Dorsal root vasodilatation in cat skeletal muscle. J Physiol 299: 277–288
21. Hinsey JH, Gasser HS (1930) The component of the dorsal root mediating vasodilatation and the Sherrington contracture. Am J Physiol 92: 679–689
22. Hosobuchi Y (1990) Treatment of ischemic pain by neurostimulation. In: Lipton S, Tunks E, Zoppi M (eds) Advances in Pain Research and Therapy, Vol 13. Raven Press, New York, pp 223–226
23. Jacobs MJHM, Jörning PJG, Joshi SR, Kitslaar PJEHM, Slaaf DW, Reneman RS (1988) Epidural spinal cord electrical stimulation improves micro-vascular blood flow in severe limb ischemia. Ann Surg 207: 179–183
24. Jacobs MJHM, Jörning PJG, Beckers RCY, Ubbink DT, van Kleef M, Slaaf DW et al (1990) Foot salvage and improvement of microvascular blood flow as a result of epidural spinal cord electrical stimulation. J Vasc Surg 12: 354–360
25. Jivegård L, Augustinsson LE, Carlsson CA, Holm J (1987) Long-term results of epidural spinal electrical stimulation (ESES) in patients with inoperable severe lower limb ischaemia. Eur J Vasc Surg 1: 345–349
26. de Jongste MJL (1994) Neurostimulation as an adjuvant therapy for patients with intractable angina pectoris. Thesis. Groningen, pp 156
27. Jänig W (1985) Organization of the lumbar sympathetic outflow to skeletal muscle and skin of the cat hindlimb and tail. Rev Physiol Biochem Pharmacol 102: 119–213

28. Jänig W (1986) Spinal cord integration of visceral sensory systems and sympathetic nervous system reflexes. In: Cervero F, Morrison JFB (eds) Progress in Brain Res, Vol 67. Elsevier, Amsterdam, pp 255–277
29. Jänig W (1990) Functions of the sympathetic innervation of the skin. In: Loewy AD, Spyer KM (eds) Central Regulation of Autonomic Functions. Oxford University Press, New York, pp 334–348
30. Jänig W (1994) Spinal cord stimulation in patients: Basic anatomical and neurophysiological mechanisms. In: Horsch S, Clays L (eds) Spinal Cord Stimulation. An Innovative Method in the Treatment of PVD. Steinkopff Verlag, Darmstadt, pp 37–58
31. Kaada B (1987) Mediators of cutaneous vasodilatation induced by transcutaneous nerve stimulation in humans. In: Nobin A, Owman C, Arneklo-Nobin B (eds) Neuronal Messengers in Vascular Function. Elsevier, Amsterdam, pp 475–488.
32. Kaada B, Eielsen O (1984) In search of mediators of skin vasodilation induced by transcutaneous nerve stimulation: III. Increase in plasma VIP in normal subjects and in Raynaud's disease. Gen Pharmacol 15: 107–113
33. Kjartansson J (1988): Peripheral sensory neurons and viability of skin flaps. Thesis. Karolinska Institutet, Stockholm, pp 30
34. Kjartansson J, Lundeberg T (1990) Effects of electrical nerve stimulation (ENS) in ischaemic tissue. Scand J Plastic Reconstr Surg 24: 129–134
35. Linderoth B (1992) Dorsal Column Stimulation and Pain: Experimental studies of putative neurochemical and neurophysiological mechhanisms. Thesis. Karolinska Institutet, Stockholm, pp 67
36. Linderoth B (1993) Neurophysiological mechanisms involved in vaso-dilatation and ischemic pain relief induced by spinal cord stimulation. In: Galley D, Illis LS, Krainick JU, Meglio M, Sier JC, Staal MJ (eds) Proceedings of the 1st Congr of the Internat Neuromod Soc, Rome, May 1992. Monduzzi Editore, Bologna, pp 27–40.
37. Linderoth B (1994) Assessment of microvascular flow modifications in spinal cord stimulation. In: Herreros J et al. (eds) Spinal Cord Stimulation for Peripheral Vascular Disease. Advances and Controversies. Editorial Libro del Ano, SL, Madrid, pp 89– 92
38. Linderoth B, Meyerson BA, Skoglund CA (1987) Spinal cord stimulation for treatment of peripheral vascular disease. Review and short-term effects. Proceedings of the 13th Meeting of the Scandinavian Association for the Study of Pain, Kolding (abstr)
39. Linderoth B, Fedorcsak I, Meyerson BA (1989) Is vasodilatation following dorsal column stimulation mediated by antidromic activation of small diameter afferents? Acta Neurchir Suppl (Wien) 46: 99–101
40. Linderoth B, Fedorcsak I, Meyerson BA (1991) Peripheral vasodilatation after spinal cord stimulation: Animal studies of putative effector mechanisms. Neurosurgery 28: 187–195
41. Linderoth B, Gunasekera L, Meyerson BA (1991) Effects of sympathectomy on skin and muscle microcirculation during dorsal column stimulation: animal studies. Neurosurgery 29: 874–879
42. Linderoth B, Stiller C-O, O'Connor WT, Hammarström G, Ungerstedt U, Brodin E (1993) An animal model for the study of brain transmittor release in response to spinal cord stimulation in the awake, freely moving rat: preliminary results from the PAG. Acta Neurochir Suppl 58: 156–160. Advances in Stereotactic and Functional Neurosurgery, vol. 10, Springer-Verlag, New York
43. Linderoth B, Herregodts P, Meyerson BA (1994) Sympathetic mediation of peripheral vasodilatation induced by spinal cord stimulation. Animal studies of the role of cholinergic and adrenergic receptor subtypes. Neurosurgery 35: 711–719
44. Linderoth B, Gherardini G, Ren B, Lundeberg T (1995) Pre-emptive spinal cord stimulation reduces ischemia in an animal model of vasospasm (accepted for publ. in Neurosurgery)
45. Lundeberg T, Kjartansson J, Samuelsson U (1988) Effect of electrical nerve stimulation on healing of ischaemic skin flaps. Lancet 24: 712–714
46. Mannheimer C, Emanuelsson H, Larsson G et al (1991) Myocardial release of endogenous opioids in the human heart and the effects of epidural spinal electrical stimulation (ESES) in pacing-induced angina pectoris. J Am Coll Cardiol 17: 107
47. Meglio M, Cioni B, Sandric S (1981) Spinal cord stimulation and peripheral blood flow. In: Hosobushi Y, Corbin T (eds) Proceedings of a Symposium on Indications for Spinal Cord Stimulation. Excerpta Medica, Princeton, pp 60–66

48. Meglio M, Cioni B, Sandric S (1981) Evaluation of cardiac activity during spinal cord stimulation. In: Hosobushi Y, Corbin T (eds) Proceedings of a Symposium on Indications for Spinal Cord Stimulation. Excerpta Medica, Princeton, pp 67–72
49. Meglio M, Cioni B, Rossi GF, Sandric S, Santarelli P (1986) Spinal cord stimulation affects the central mechanisms of regulation of the heart rate. Appl Neurophysiol 49: 139–146
50. Meyerson BA (1990) Electric stimulation of the spinal cord and brain. In: Bonica JJ, Loeser JD, Chapman RC, Fordyce WE (eds) The Management of Pain, 2nd ed, Lea and Febiger, Philadelphia, pp 1862–1877
51. Naver H, Augustinsson L-E, Elam M (1992) The vasodilating effect of spinal dorsal column stimulation is mediated by sympathetic nerves. Clin Autonom Res 2: 41–45
52. Seijo F (1994) Ischemic pain: nociceptive pain or deafferentation pain. In: Herreros J et al. (eds) Spinal Cord Stimulation for Peripheral Vascular Disease. Advances and Controversies. Editorial Libro del Ano, SL, Madrid, pp 25–29

Author's address:
Assor. Prof. Bengt Linderoth, MD PhD
Dept. of Neurosurgery
Karolinska Hospital
S-17176 Stockholm
Sweden

Influence of cervical spinal cord stimulation on the vascular system

Ph. Gersbach[1], M. Hasdemir[2], D. Mettler[3]

Department of Thoracic and Cardiovascular Surgery[1], Department of Neurosurgery[2], Department of Experimental Surgery[3] of the University of Bern, Inselspital, Bern/Switzerland

Introduction

Various studies have shown that dorsal column stimulation (DCS) represents a useful alternative treatment in selected cases of unreconstructable peripheral (1, 13, 14, 22, 26) and coronary (5, 9, 19, 21, 23) artery disease. Despite good short- and long-term success rates (8, 11, 27), this method still faces some skepticism and criticism, particularly in surgical circles (18). This attitude is mainly due to three major drawbacks of DCS: 1) its supposed vascular effects can only be measured by microcirculatory tests which are often sophisticated and thus not easily reproducible; 2) the typical microcirculatory changes attributed to DCS (12, 13, 14, 15, 24) are characteristically confined to restricted body areas, and are therefore often considered as insufficient to achieve limb salvage in clinical practice; and 3) the DCS mode of action has as yet not been precisely established (1, 4, 15, 22, 23, 26). It is thus of crucial importance to demonstrate by the usual hemodynamic tests that the clinical successes obtained with DCS treatment cannot be attributed to any placebo effect, but to vasoactive mechanisms effectively elicited by DCS.

The limitations of DCS mentioned above are generally attributed to a segmental mode of action (1, 15, 16, 20). We postulated that applying DCS at the highest possible cervical level (C1/C2), near the major supraspinal centers responsible for vasomotor fiber adjustment (Fig. 1), may permit us to overcome these segmental limitations and to elicit a more generalized autonomic reaction leading to major hemodynamic changes, possibly important enough to be detected by routine hemodynamic investigations.

Method

Seventeen anesthetized (Ketamine 10 mg/kg im / Azaperon 2 mg/kg iv / Metomidate 5 mg/kg iv) and mechanically ventilated (30 % oxygen / 70 % nitrous oxide and 0.5 – 1.5 % Halothane) Göttingen minipigs were surgically instrumented for exhaustive hemodynamic testing (Table 1) (3):

An experimental bipolar electrode (Medtronic Inc., Minneapolis) with an inter-electrode distance of 4 mm was introduced through a C2/C3 laminectomy in the epidural space and pushed cranially until its tip reached the C1 segment (Fig. 1). After fixation in the midline, the electrode was connected to the stimulator (Screener

Table 1. Instrumentation and gathered parameters.

Device	Position	Recordings
3 ECG leads	chest wall – upper extremity – lower extremity	heart frequency and rate/ECG
Seldicath 13 mm	distal aorta	systemic blood pressure (systolic, diastolic, mean)
7F Swan-Ganz thermodilution catheter	right pulmonary artery	pulmonary pressure (systolic, diastolic, mean) cardiac output stroke volume central venous pressure
5,2F pigtail catheter	left ventricle	left ventricular enddiastolic pressure
Fooley catheter	bladder	urinary output

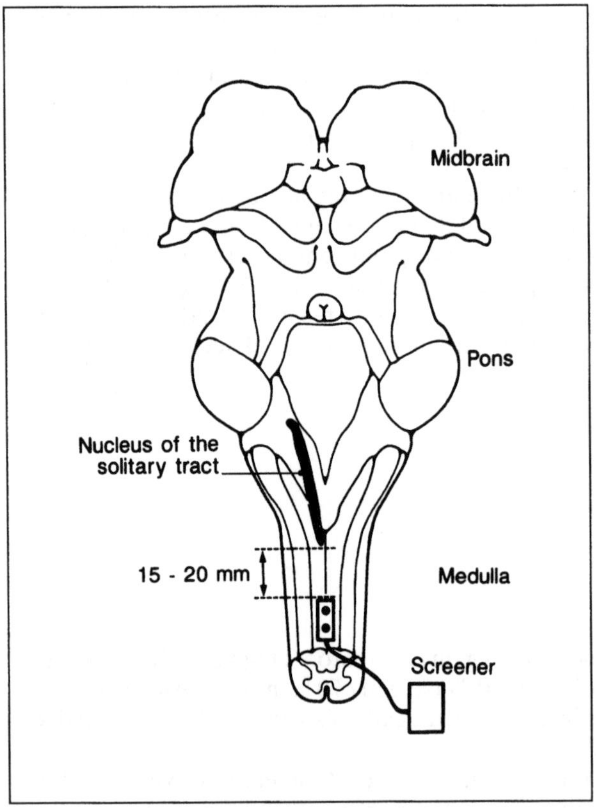

Fig. 1. Position of the stimulation electrode: Exact position of the lead tip with its relationship to the caudal part of the nucleus of the solitary tract

Kit Model 3625, Medtronic Inc., Minneapolis). After a resting period of at least 1 h, basic hemodynamic values were registered. Iterative stimulations of intensities corresponding to those used clinically in humans (2V, 5V, 10V / 50 Hz / 210 ms) were then applied for 10, 20 or 60 min. The first intensity applied changed for each animal. In order to avoid any external influence on the basic vascular tone, the body temperature, the analgesia level, the pH, and blood gas values were kept within very narrow limits during the whole experiment.

Measurements

ECG, systemic blood pressure, pulmonary artery pressure, left ventricular end-diastolic pressure, and central venous pressure were continuously displayed on an eight-channel universal monitor (SMW 611 Hellige GmbH, Freiburg, FRG). Significant tracings were printed with an eight-channel printer (SMR 821, Hellige). The cardiac output was determined (four consecutive measurements) every 15 min and by acute hemodynamic changes.

The values at rest were gathered during long resting periods after full instrumentation as well as during the resting interval between consecutive stimulations.

The pre-stimulation values were registered immediately before each stimulation and compared to the values at rest. In case of significant differences, DCS was either delayed or not taken into account for further global evaluation.

The stimulation values were systematically registered during the first minute of stimulation and after 5, 10, 15, 30, 45 and 60 min.

Statistical evaluation of the results was performed by means of the student's *t*-test for two-tailed hypothesis and the trend test was used for comparing the DCS effects at different intensities.

Results

At rest, only minor hemodynamic changes, generally not exceeding 10 % of the base value, spontaneously occurred (Fig. 2). In contrast, 87 % of the DCS induced striking hemodynamic changes which never occurred in any animal at rest (Fig. 3). These changes were not limited to a single parameter but involved the whole hemodynamic system. They were also important enough to be easily detected by basic hemodynamic tests. Significant reactions were, however, more often observed at higher intensity DCS (Fig. 4). Each animal responded to at least one of the three intensities tested, and stimulations of same intensities had very comparable effects in different animals or when repeated in the same animal after convenient resting periods (Fig. 5).

Fundamentally, DCS induces a notable rise in cardiac output (CO), stroke volume (SV), mean blood pressure (BP), heart rate (HR), urinary output, and to a lesser extent, in pulmonary pressure (PP). Comparison of the changes occurring in these different parameters at different DCS intensities, however, shows extremely important variations (Figs. 5 and 6):

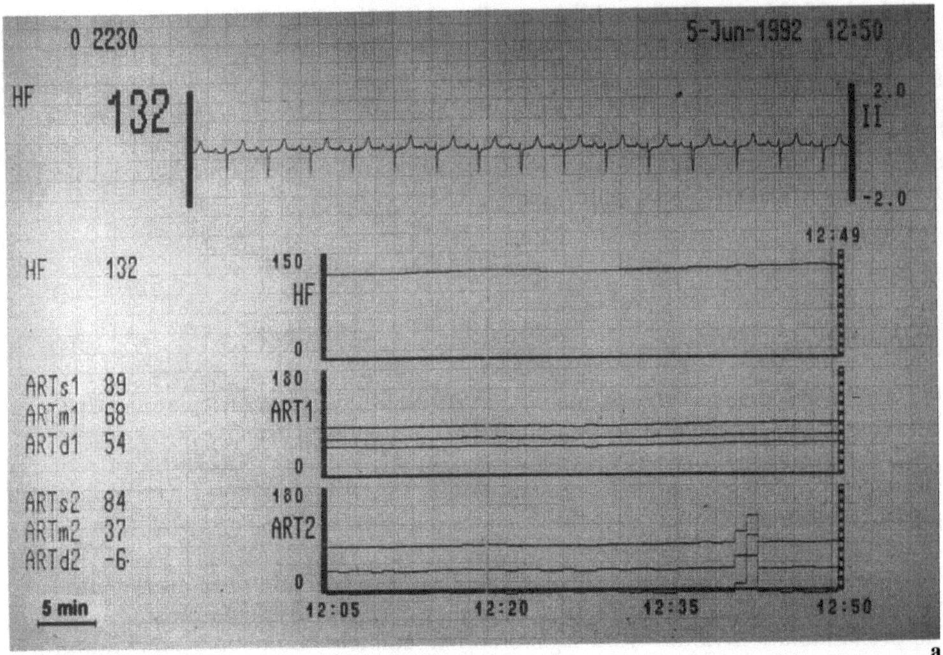

a

b

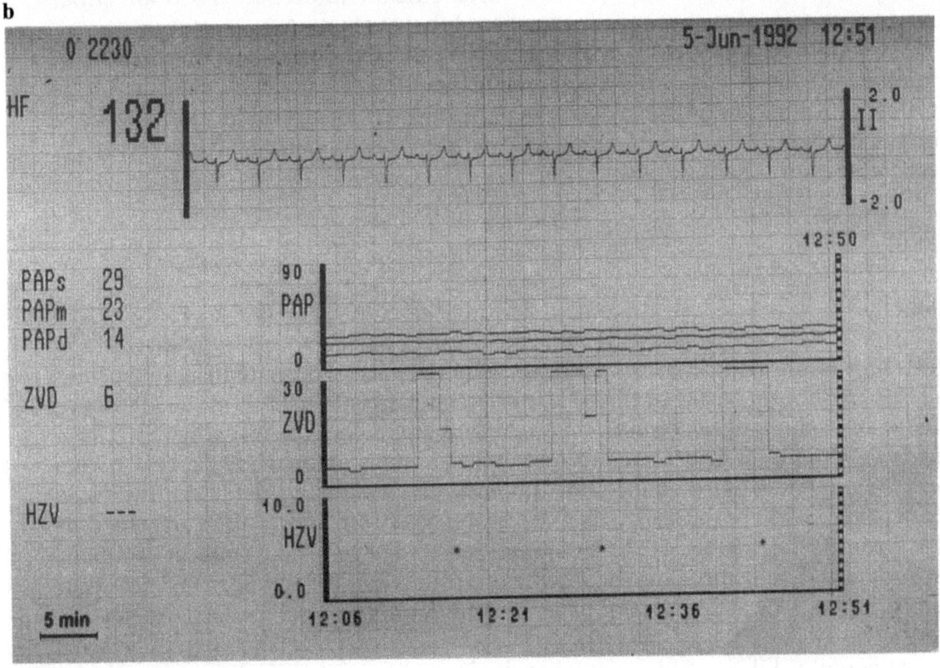

Fig. 2 a+b. Tracings at rest showing only minimal changes in HR, BP, PP, CO, LVEDP and CVP. HF = heart rate; ART1 = systemic blood pressure (systolic, mean and diastolic values); ART2 = left ventricular pressure; PAP = pulmonary artery pressure; ZVD = central venous pressure (many artifacts due to repeated CO determinations); HZV = cardiac output (scale 1 – 10 liters/min.). Time on horizontals axis.

- C1/C2 DCS at 2V mainly induces a mean increase in cardiac output which is stable and reaches more than 30 % (+ 1.3 to 1.5 l/min), while increases in blood pressure (+ 5 to + 9 %) and heart rate (+ 1 to 15 %) are less obvious (Fig. 6a).
- C1/C2 DCS at 10V is chiefly followed by an impressive rise in blood pressure (+ 20 to + 40 %) while the increase in cardiac output is less substantial (+ 8 to + 27 %) (Fig. 6b).
- C1/C2 DCS at 5V finally induces intermediate changes: an increase in cardiac output of + 16 to + 27 % and a rise in blood pressure of + 15 to + 27 % (Fig. 6c).

The important rise observed in blood pressure and, to a lesser extent, in heart rate under high-intensity DCS has as a consequence that the rate pressure product (RPP = SBP × HR) massively increases. This reflects an increase in cardiac work and in myocardial oxygen consumption (23) which is out of proportion to the increase in cardiac output observed under high intensity DCS. Conversely, the rate pressure prod-

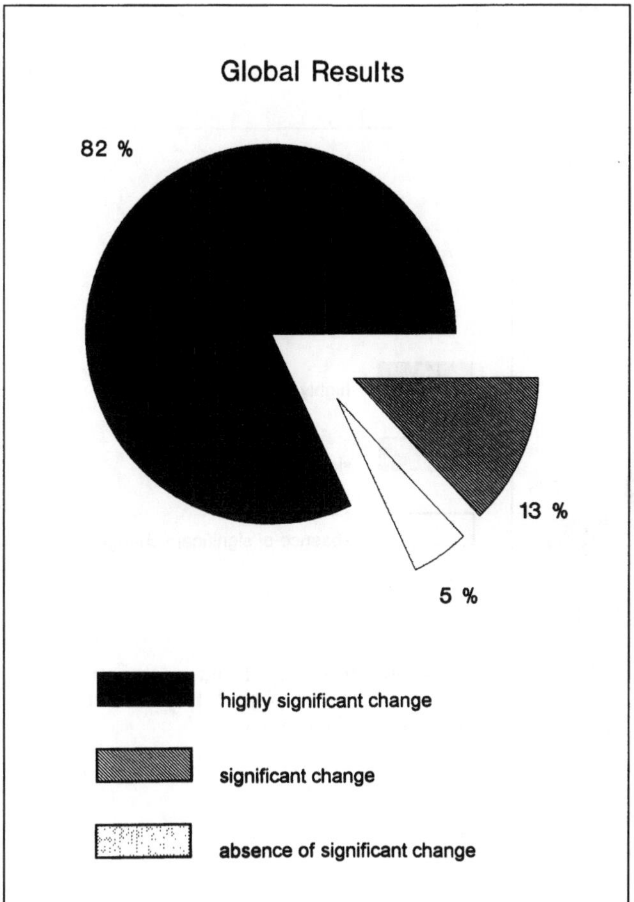

Fig. 3. Statistically significant macrocirculatory changes elicited by C1/C2 DCS (global results)

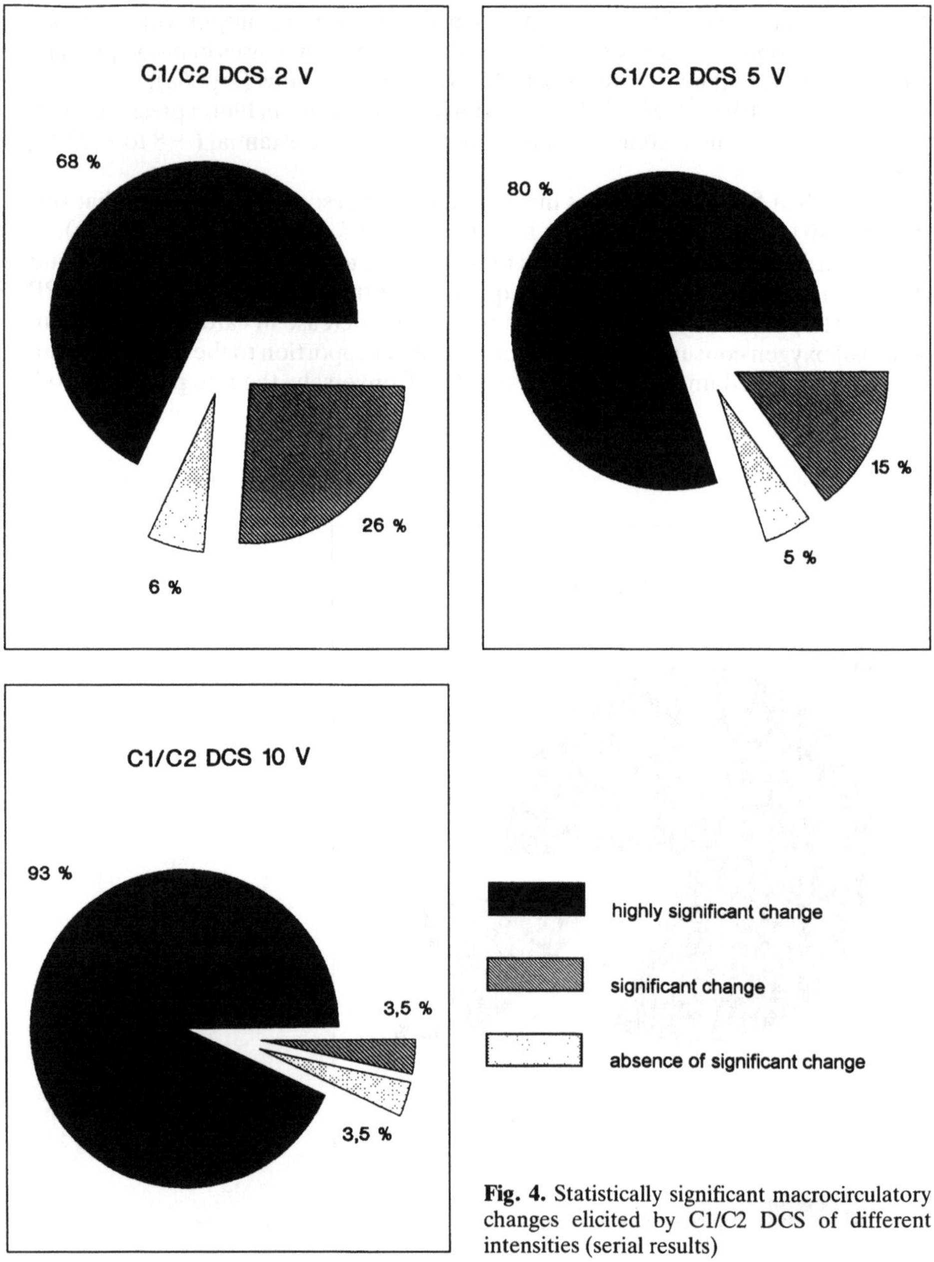

Fig. 4. Statistically significant macrocirculatory changes elicited by C1/C2 DCS of different intensities (serial results)

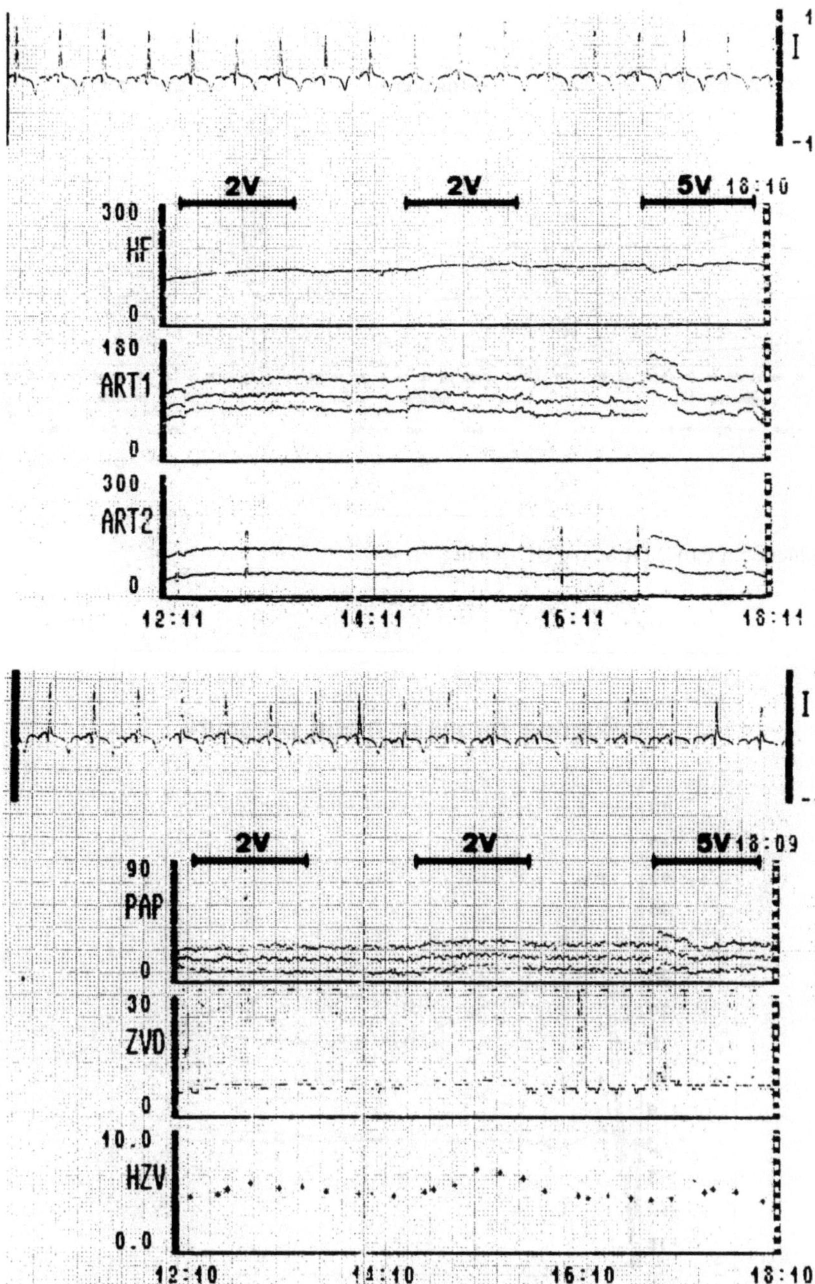

a

b

Fig. 5 a + b. Typical hemodynamic changes occurring during long-lasting (1 h) C1/C2 DCS of different intensities (2V/5V)
HF = heart rate; ART1 = systemic blood pressure (systolic, mean and diastolic values); ART2 = left ventricular pressure; PAP = pulmonary artery pressure; ZVD = central venous pressure (many artifacts due to repeated CO determinations); HZV = cardiac output (scale 1 – 10 liters/min.). Time on horizontals axis.

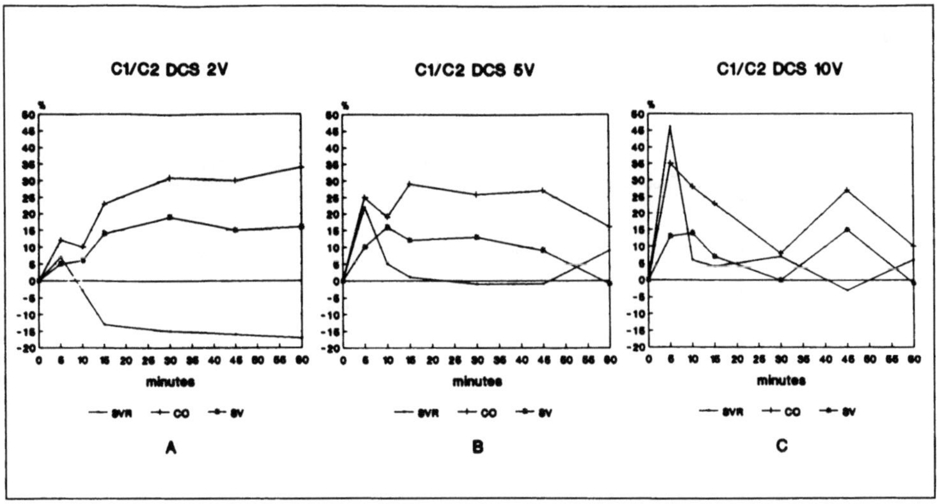

Fig. 6. Influence of C1/C2 DCS on CO, SV and SVR

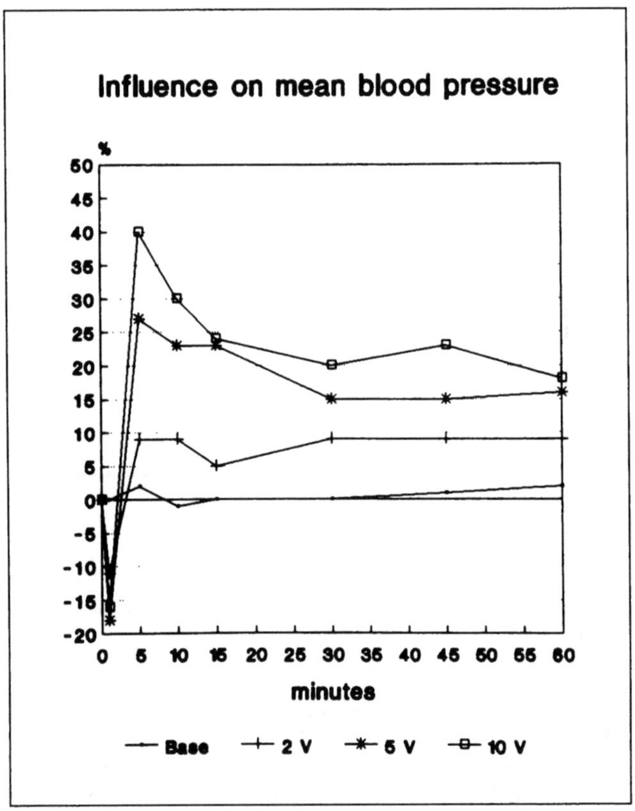

Fig. 7. Variations in mean systemic blood pressure at different C1/C2 DCS intensities

uct only moderately rises under low-intensity DCS while the cardiac output substantially increases, indicating a highly efficient and economical cardiac work. This important difference in cardiac work is related to changes in systemic vascular resistances (SVR, Figs. 6 – 8), which decreases by more than 15 % under 2V C1/C2 DCS, but increases up to + 10 % under high intensity C1/C2 DCS. A maximal rise in urinary output (+ 60 to + 80 %) also occurs under stimulation at 2V, most probably reflecting an increase in splanchnic perfusion, probably following the drop in SVR characteristic of low intensity C1/C2 DCS.

Finally, C1/C2 DCS characteristically induces an initial acute drop in heart rate and systemic and pulmonary pressures which lasts for less than 1 min. The extent of this reaction, albeit not its duration, is proportional to DCS voltage.

Discussion

This whole experiment was performed in deeply anesthetized healthy animals insensible to very strong control noxious stimuli. In this situation the major hemodynamic changes elicited by C1/C2 DCS are absolutely independent of its pain-alleviating effects (1, 16, 17, 22, 26). Vasoactive properties of DCS were often reported in restricted capillary areas (8, 13, 14, 24). Sciacca et al. (25), measuring the penile blood flow in rabbits submitted to thoraco-lumbal DCS found microcirculatory changes practically identical to those elicited in the macrocirculation by high cervical DCS, and Linderoth et al. (15), using laser-Doppler flowmetry, registered closely comparable changes in peripheral skin blood flow in rats undergoing thoraco-lumbal stimulation. These very striking similarities suggest that the changes registered in the macrocirculation under C1/C2 DCS and those occuring at capillary level during DCS at lower spinal levels are the same, and therefore that the C1/C2 level is responsible for a more diffuse effect of DCS involving much larger microcirculatory areas.

Very high cervical DCS has already been tested in clinical conditions by several authors. Barolat et al. (2) recently reported their experience in 135 patients who received an electrode at the C1/C2 level for intractable pain in the occipital area, the jaw and ear area, and in the upper limbs. Unfortunately, no hemodynamic controls are available in this group of patients. In two angina patients stimulated at the C2 level, González-Darden et al. (9) found an improvement, not only in anginal pain and in tolerance to stress, but also in concomitant lower limb claudication. This observation also strongly suggests that the positive effect of C1/C2 DCS in such different and distant territories of perfusion may well be the consequence of an improvement of the whole hemodynamic system.

The hypothesis of an influence of very high-cervical DCS on some major supraspinal autonomic centers seems to be anatomically plausible: The C1/C2 level is located only a few centimeters distal from neuronal structures supposed to be responsible for the central control of vasomotricity (3). Recent c-Fos studies have demonstrated that DCS at high-thoracic level is able to influence parts of the brain specifically involved in autonomic function control (10). It also has been reported that an important portion of the spino-thalamic tract afferents and of vagal efferents are concentrated at the C1/C2 level (7). The initial drop in heart rate and blood pressure regularly observed in this experiment during the first seconds of stimulation may therefore be indicative of an initial parasympathetic activation.

This experiment was not designed in order to determine the ultimate mode or place of action of DCS, but rather to study whether or not DCS applied at the highest possible cervical level is able to influence the microcirculation as a whole. It has allowed us to gather the basic information about the microcirculatory effects of C1/C2 DCS necessary to conceive further pharmacological tests.

Conclusions

DCS is definitely not a placebo therapy. It holds striking vasoactive properties which are absolutely independent of its pain-alleviating effects. DCS applied at a very high cervical level induces major hemodynamic changes which are easily detectable by routine hemodynamic investigations. These changes are quickly reversible and easily reproducible. They also depend qualitatively and quantitatively on the intensity applied.

Schematically, low intensity C1/C2 decreases the afterload and optimizes the cardiac work, leading thus to an important increase in cardiac output. C1/C2 DCS of higher intensities mainly induce a striking rise in blood pressure and in cardiac work which is not associated with a corresponding rise in cardiac output.

References

1. Augustinsson LE, Carlsson CA, Holm J, Jivegård M (1985) Epidural electrical stimulation in severe limb ischemia. Pain relief, increased blood flow and a possible limb-saving effect. Ann Surg 202: 104–110
2. Barolat G, Ketcik B, He J (1994) Experience with 250 epidural electrodes implanted in the cervical spine. Proceedings of the 2nd International Congress of the International Neuromodulation Society, Göteborg, June 1–4
3. Chalmers JP, Kapoor V, Llewellyn-Smith IJ, Minson JB, Pilowsky PM (1992) Central control of blood pressure. Eur Heart J; Suppl A 13: 2–9
4. Chandler MJ, Brennan TJ, Garrison DW, Kim KS, Schwartz PJ, Foreman RD (1993) A mechanism of cardiac pain suppression by spinal cord stimulation: implications for patients with angina pectoris. Eur Heart J 14: 96–105
5. DeJongste MJL, Haaksma J, Hautvast RWM, Hillege HL, Meyler PJW, Staal MJ, Sanderson JE, Lie KI (1994) Effects of spinal cord stimulation on myocardial ischemia during normal activity in patients with severe coronary artery disease. A prospective ambulatory ECG study. Br Heart J 71: 413–418
6. Foreman RD, Chandler MJ, Brennan TJ, Kim KS, Garrison DW, Schwartz PJ (1989) Does dorsal column stimulation reduce the activity of spinothalamic tract cells that respond to cardiac input? Circulation; Suppl II 80: 552
7. Foreman RD (1994) Neurophysiological mechanisms of pain relief by spinal cord stimulation in angina pectoris. Spinal cord stimulation: An innovative method in the treatment of PVD. 2nd international meeting. Köln, Oct. 28–29
8. Galley D, Rettori R, Baccalon H, Medvedowsky A, Lefebre JM, Sellier F, Chauvreau C, Serise JM, Pieronne A (1992) Spinal cord stimulation for the treatment of peripheral vascular disease of the lower limbs. A multicenter study in 244 patients. J Mal Vasc 17: 208–213

9. González-Darder JM, Canely C, González-Martinez V (1991) High cervical spinal cord stimulation for unstable angina pectoris. Stereotact Funct Neurosurg 56: 20–27
10. Hautvast RWM, DeJongste MJL, VandenBrink A, Homminga SA, Ruiters M, Lie KI, Korf J, TerHorst GJ (1994) Spinal cord stimulation and the induction of immediate early gene c-Fos and stress protein HS 72 in the central nervous system of rats. Proceedings of the 2nd International Congress of the International Neuromodulation Society Göteborg, June 1–4
11. Horsch S, Claeys L (1994) Epidural spinal cord stimulation in the treatment of severe peripheral arterial disease. Ann Vasc Surg 8: 468–474
12. Jacobs MJHM, Jörning PJG, Joshi SR, Kistlaar PJEHM, Slaaf DW, Reneman RS (1988) Epidural spinal cord electrical stimulation improves microvascular blood flow in severe limb ischemia. Ann Surg 207: 179–183
13. Jacobs MJHM, Jörning PJG, Beckers RCY, Ubbink DT, van Kleef M, Slaaf DW, Reneman RS (1990) Foot salvage and improvement of microvascular blood flow as a result of epidural spinal cord electrical stimulation. J Vasc Surg 12: 354–360
14. Jünger M, Fenchel G, Schulze M, Rahmel B, Seboldt H, Hoffmann F, Patheiger U (1990) Skin microcirculation during epidural spinal electrical stimulation (ESES) in patients with severe peripheral arterial oclcusive disease. Int J Microcirc Clin Exp 9: 223
15. Linderoth B, Fedorcsak I, Meyerson BA (1991) Peripheral vasodilation after spinal cord stimulation: Animal studies of putative effector mechanisms. Neurosurgery 28: 187–195
16. Linderoth B, Gunasekera L, Meyerson BA (1991) Effects of sympathectomy on skin and muscle microcirculation during dorsal column stimulation: Animal studies. Neurosurg 29: 874–879
17. Linderoth B, Herregodts P, Meyerson BA (1994) Sympathetic mediation of peripheral vasodilation induced by spinal cord stimulation: Animal studies of the role of cholinergic and adrenergic receptor subtypes. Neurosurgery 35: 1–9
18. LoGerfo FW (1991) Epidural spinal cord electrical stimulation: An unproven methodology for management of lower extremity ischemia. Editorial. J Vasc Surg 13: 518–519
19. Mannheimer C, Eliasson T, Andersson B, Bergh CH, Augustinsson LA, Emanuelsson H, Waagstein F (1993) Effects of spinal cord stimulation in angina pectoris induced by pacing and possible mechanisms of action. Br Med J 307: 477–480
20. Meglio M, Cioni B, Rossi GF, Sandric S, Santarelli P (1986) Spinal cord stimulation affects the central mechanism of regulation of heart rate. Appl Neurophysiol 49: 139–146
21. Murphy DF, Giles KE (1987) Dorsal cord stimulation for pain relief from intractable angina pectoris. Pain 28: 365–368
22. Nachbur B, Gersbach Ph, Hasdemir M (1994) Spinal cord stimulation for unreconstructible chronic limb ischemia. Eur J Vasc Surg 8: 383–388
23. Sanderson JE, Ibrahim B, Waterhouse D, Palmer RGB (1994) Spinal electrical stimulation for intractable angina pectoris-long-term clinical outcome and safety. Eur Heart J 15: 810–814
24. Sciacca V, Mingoli A, di Marzo L, Maggiore C, Fiume D, Cavallero A (1989) Predictive value of transcutaneous oxygen tension measurement in the indication for spinal cord stimulation in patients with peripheral vascular disease: Preliminary results. Vasc Surg 23: 128–132
25. Sciacca V, Mattioli GL, Oppido PA, Di Giugno G (1994) Epidural spinal cord electrical stimulation (ESES) effect on penile flow: An experimental study. Proceedings of the 2nd International Congress of the International Neuromodulation Society Göteborg, June 1–4
26. Tallis RC, Jacobs M, Miles J (1992) Spinal cord stimulation in peripheral vascular disease. Editorial, Brit J Neurosurg 6: 101–105
27. Zucco F, Allaria B, Vaghi M, Rizzi F, Reina W, Boselli E, Brusa S, Tacconi A (1994) Spinal cord stimulation in peripheral vascular disease treatment: Nine-year experience with 241 patients. In: Horsch S, Claeys L (eds) Spinal Cord Stimulation. An Innovative Method in the Treatment of PVD. Steinkopff, Darmstadt, Springer International, pp 183–189

Author's address:
Philippe Gersbach, MD
Department of Thoracic and Cardiovascular Surgery
University of Bern
Inselspital
3010 Bern
Switzerland

Spinal cord stimulation for chronic intractable pain

R. B. North*, P. N. Cutchis**

* Department of Neurosurgery, Johns Hopkins University School of Medicine, Baltimore, MD
** Applied Physics Laboratory, Johns Hopkins University, Laurel, MD

Introduction

The "gate theory" of pain transmission in the dorsal horn of the spinal cord, published in 1965, provided the foundation for the use of electrical stimulation for pain relief (57). The feasibility of chronic neural stimulation was greatly increased when the miniaturized highly reliable solid-state electronic technology developed for cardiac pacemakers was transferred to implantable neural stimulators.

After initially promising results, use of electrical stimulation became widespread and poor understanding of patient selection criteria yielded disappointing outcome in many cases. Recent advances in patient selection, multidisciplinary management approaches and more versatile and reliable stimulation devices have significantly improved long-term results (64, 68).

Neurophysiology of pain relief by electrical stimulation

The gate theory postulates that collaterals from large myelinated afferent axons associated with tactile sensation produce presynaptic inhibition at small diameter Aδ and C fibers which carry pain sensation. Myelinated axons have about 300 times less membrane capacitance than unmyelinated axons due to the spiral Schwann's cell membrane. Therefore, for a given stimulation current, it is much easier to reach threshold voltage in these axons ($Q = CVm$ where Q = charge, C = capacitance, Vm = membrane potential) than in smaller unmyelinated axons.

In mixed peripheral nerves the motor threshold may be very close to the sensory threshold, thus making amplitude adjustment very important. Additionally, most pain problems involve the distribution of more than one peripheral nerve. Both of these problems of peripheral nerve stimulation can be overcome by spinal cord stimulation. Fortuitously, large diameter primary afferents are segregated into the dorsal columns. Antidromic activation of these primary afferents can, through collaterals in the dorsal horn, affect activity in the distribution of multiple peripheral nerves.

While the "gate theory" is useful in explaining many clinical phenomena, it remains controversial (61) and does not explain all painful conditions. For example, hyperalgesia can be signaled by large fibers (13). Pain relief by electrical stimulation in this circumstance may be due to frequency-related conduction block. The site of action for this effect is the primary afferent branch point where dorsal column fibers and dorsal horn collaterals diverge. Clinical experience with spinal cord stimulation has shown that patients significantly prefer a minimum pulse repetition frequency of 25 pulses per second (68). Other mechanisms, including those involving interneurons in the dorsal horn or sympathetic mechanisms, may also be frequency dependent (23, 29, 49).

It is important to scale the stimulation levels in experimental models of spinal cord stimulation, both in human and animal models, to levels between the amplitude producing first perception and the level producing discomfort or motor threshold (44). Animal models have been of limited clinical use in the past due to lack of an appropriate model for chronic or neuropathic pain. However, a sciatic nerve ligation model in the rat, using stimulation levels scaled to a clinically relevant range, has been reported recently (58). This model showed relief by spinal cord stimulation of the manifestations of pain or hyperalgesia.

Computer simulations using finite element analysis have been used to model currents and voltages produced by spinal cord stimulation (15, 30). The results from these models are in general agreement with cadaver and primate measurements (76). The most critical factor in achieving stimulation at a desired segmental level is the longitudinal location of the electrodes. Additionally, bipolar stimulation has been found to be most selective for longitudinally oriented midline fibers. A contact separation of 1.4 times the combined thickness of the meninges and cerebrospinal fluid (about 7 mm) has been reported to be optimal (30). The dorsal root fibers are relatively superficial for the first few segments after entering the spinal cord (24) and decrease in diameter as they ascend (69). Both of these anatomic factors explain why more cephalad placement, which might be expected to produce more widespread pain relief, instead requires increased stimulation amplitudes and yields undesirable segmental effects (42).

Neurotransmitter and metabolite levels in cerebrospinal fluid have shown some changes in patients undergoing spinal cord stimulation (50). Naloxone, a narcotic antagonist, has no effect on pain relief by spinal cord stimulation or by peripheral nerve or transcutaneous nerve stimulation (28).

Implantable stimulation devices

Spinal cord stimulation electrodes

Figure 1 shows several electrodes, including some arrays which can be placed through a Tuohy needle and other arrays which require laminectomy. Originally, laminectomy was required for introduction of all available electrodes into the epidural, subdural, or subarachnoid space (11, 60, 79, 85). Laminectomy, especially when conducted under local anesthesia, limits longitudinal access to the spinal canal. This significantly decreases the ability to achieve the goal of eliciting paresthesias that overlap the patient's pain distribution, which is necessary for successful pain relief. The need for a less invasive procedure became evident when it was found that not all patients achieve pain relief even with satisfactory electrode placement.

In the 1970s the development of percutaneous techniques for electrode placement alleviated many of these problems (25, 31, 32). Unpleasant local segmental effects occurred in many early implants before recruitment of more caudal segments. This was caused by the high thoracic electrode placement then used (60, 79). Overlap of the patient's pain distribution with the distribution of stimulation paresthesias is critical to a successful clinical outcome. Percutaneous electrodes, by allowing free longitudinal access to the spinal cord, greatly increase the likelihood of achieving overlap by obtaining the optimal level for electrode placement. In the clinical problem of failed back syndrome low thoracic placement has proven the most efficacious for isolating painful segments (5). Percutaneous electrodes, originally utilized for temporary pain relief testing, were later adapted for chronic use (63, 93). With the early electrodes, which had only single contacts, multiple electrodes had to be inserted to apply bipolar stimulation. This was frequently complicated by migration of one electrode relative to the other, which then required surgical revision (63).

The problem of movement of electrode contacts relative to each other was largely eliminated by the development in the early 1980s of multicontact electrode arrays which could be inserted as an assembly through a Tuohy needle. These electrodes, along with the ability of present pulse generators to allow noninvasive electrode selection, polarity selection, and pulse width and amplitude adjustment has resulted in significantly improved clinical results (64, 68).

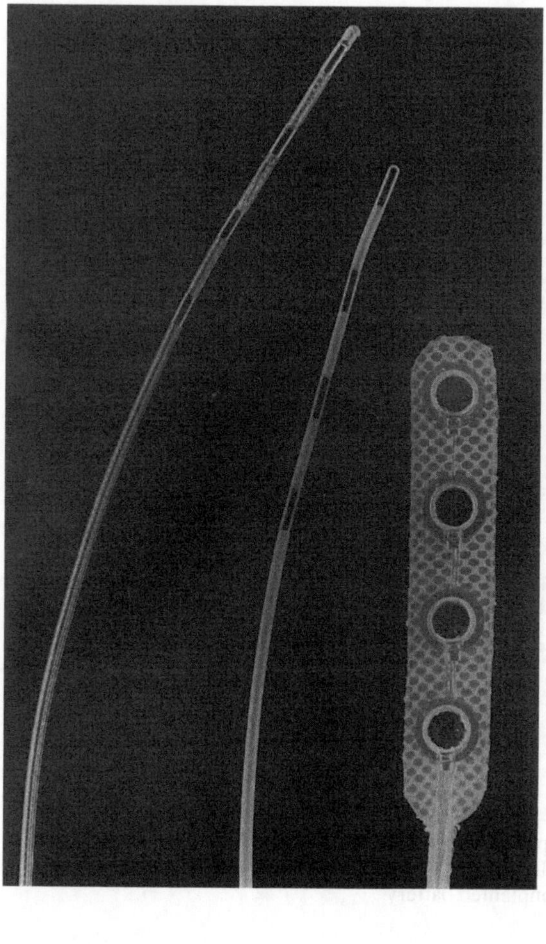

Fig. 1. Spinal cord stimulation electrodes in use today are arrays of multiple contacts and include those which are percutaneously placed through a Tuohy needle and those requiring laminectomy

Implantable pulse generators

The earliest implantable spinal cord and peripheral nerve stimulators were radiofrequency (RF) powered. These pulse generators functioned as AM radio demodulators and delivered the envelope of the RF burst to the patient. Their main advantage is that they contain no implanted battery to limit implant lifetime. There is, however, the inconvenience to the patient or an external transmitter which must be worn during stimulation. Also, variable alignment of the external transmitter antenna coil over the implant may cause variability in stimulation amplitude.

"Totally implantable" stimulators, which are powered by an internal battery, havc been available for more than a decade. While these units have obvious advantages in terms of convenience and cosmesis, they do have limited lifetimes. Additionally, compromises may have to be made in both selection of stimulation parameters as well as patient usage patterns to prolong battery life. The power requirements and patient usage pattern determined during the temporary percutaneous test phase should be used to determine the feasibility of a "totally implanted" neurostimulator. Figure 2 shows several representative pulse generators including both the "totally implanted" and RF coupled externally powered units.

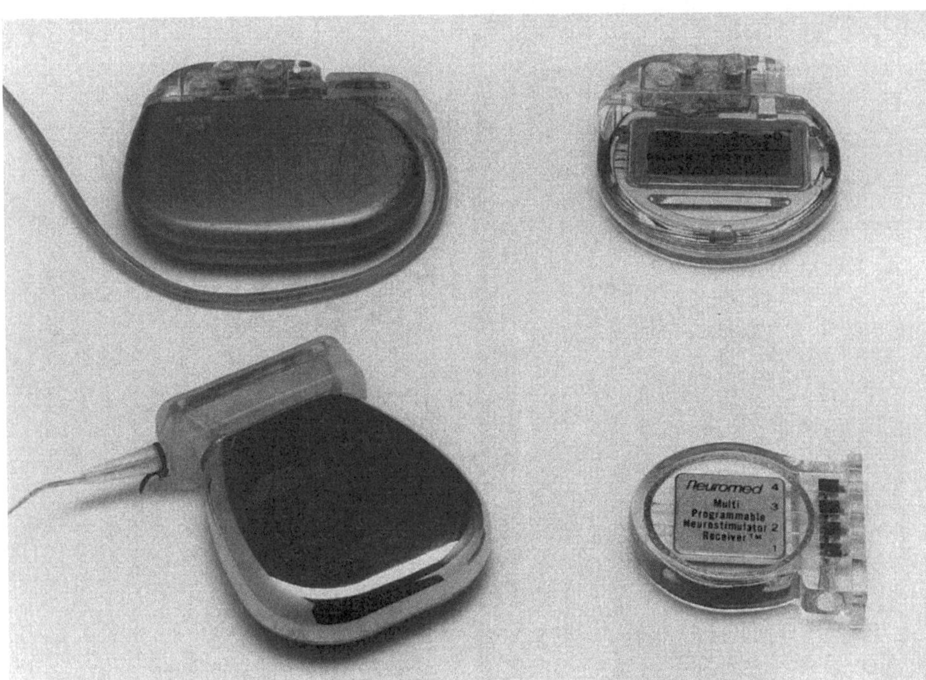

Fig. 2. Contemporary pulse generators for spinal cord stimulation permit noninvasive programming of electrode polarity from an array of multiple contacts. Some are powered externally through transcutaneous RF coupling while others use an implanted battery

Advances in circuit miniaturization have allowed stimulators to become considerably more complex over time. Encoding of commands from the external transmitter to the implant increases reliability and can virtually eliminate the chance that inappropriate pulses are delivered to the patient. In addition, the flexibility in programming is increasing; pulse generators which allow interleaving of pulses between two or more alternating locations should become available in the near future. In these devices the amplitude and pulse width of stimulation at the different locations will likely be independently programmable, thereby compensating for variability in "contact efficacy" at these positions.

Patient screening protocols

A chief advantage of spinal cord stimulation over other procedures, such as ablative procedures which attempt to disrupt pain transmission by destroying a portion of the nervous system, is that it is a reversible procedure. Furthermore, preoperative tests can be conducted that allow for the exact replication of long-term treatment. A temporary percutaneous epidural electrode may be placed fluoroscopically, allowing a therapeutic trial of spinal stimulation to be conducted. The optimal longitudinal electrode position may then be ascertained by mapping the epidural space for the location which provides the best pain relief. The results of this trial can then be used to decide whether to proceed to a permanent implant, and how best to approach it.

A criterion for reimbursement from third-party payers is "demonstration of pain relief with a temporarily implanted electrode" before permanent implantation. While this requirement might technically be met by proceeding immediately to a permanent implant from the test procedure (27), there are advantages to a longer trial with temporary electrodes. These advantages include: (a) Temporary percutaneous electrodes can be placed in a fluoroscopy suite as opposed to an operating room, thereby reducing costs and permitting evaluation of a larger number of electrode positions and stimulation parameters. (b) The pain relief can be evaluated by the patient outside of the operating room and in more real-life conditions of activity and position. (c) The experience gained by the physician and the patient with the temporary electrodes facilitates implantation of a technically superior permanent device.

Temporary electrodes may emerge from the patient in either of two ways. In the first, the electrode lead exits through the needle tract at the insertion site and is anchored by a skin suture. The alternative method is that an incision is made at the needle site, and the lead is tunneled subcutaneously and anchored as would be done for permanent implant. The latter method allows conversion of the electrode for permanent use if a percutaneous extension cable is used and later removed. While this saves the expense of an additional electrode, it has several disadvantages: (a) Two trips to the operating room are required, one for electrode placement and a second for internalization or removal. Only a single trip to the operating room is necessary with a percutaneous lead. (b) The need to return to the operating room may bias the patient or physician in their decision to implant a pulse generator. The removal of a percutaneous electrode at the bedside does not require the commitment of going to the operating room and is therefore unlikely to influence the decision to proceed to implant. (c) A subcutaneously anchored permanent electrode does not allow bedside adjustment through lead withdrawal and therefore reduces the flexibility of the therapeutic trial. (d) Pain associated with subcutaneous tunneling and the incision may affect the therapeutic trial results. (e) The risk of infection around the permanent system is increased when percutaneous lead extensions are used (37, 42).

After placement of temporary electrodes and conclusion of the therapeutic trial, the criteria for proceeding to permanent implant varied considerably. Some authors require 70 – 75 % reported pain relief (18, 47, 56) some as little as 30 % (6). The length of testing also varies greatly from only intraoperative testing (27) to 2 months of percutaneous testing (55). If long-term success is defined by a minimum reported percentage of pain relief (frequently 50 %), this success rate is increased by requiring an arbitrarily higher reported percentage of pain relief during the test phase. This may accentuate only one of a number of important outcome measures. In our practice a permanent implant is offered to patients who, after a 2.5- to 3-day trial with temporary electrodes, demonstrate improved or stable analgesic requirements and activity levels and report 50 % or greater pain relief. Extended trials are conducted on an "as needed" basis. Prolonged trials may cause additional morbidity such as infection and epidural scarring and may not produce additional information on outcome measures such as return to work, productive activity, or utilization of other health care resources.

General indications for implanted stimulation devices

The following requirements should be met before considering the surgical implantation of a spinal cord stimulator.

1. There should be an objective basis for the pain complaint. For example, in the case of "failed back syndrome" or "postlaminectomy syndrome" there should be abnormal findings on diagnostic imaging studies and/or objective findings on physical examination. Additionally, these objective findings must outweigh nonphysiologic or functional signs in the decision process (88). The findings of epidural fibrosis and diminished deep tendon reflexes, both of which may occur after successful surgery, are nonspecific and do not alone indicate the need for therapy. The indications for the original surgery are frequently not clear in cases of "failed back surgery syndrome" in which the original patient records and imaging studies are available (53).
2. Alternative therapies must have been exhausted. In the "failed back surgery syndrome" example, surgical options must still be considered, even though reoperation may carry greater risk and offer poorer yield in some cases (65).
3. Psychiatric evaluation and clearance have been obtained. Major psychiatric problems such as somatiform disorder, drug addiction, or issues of secondary gain must all be addressed (44). Standardized psychological tests may be of value in identifying poor candidates for spinal cord stimulation (16).
4. Pain relief should be demonstrated with temporary electrodes before the decision is made to proceed to a permanent pulse generator. During the testing with temporary electrodes, the ability to achieve overlap of stimulation paresthesias with the pain distribution can be evaluated, and the need for special electrode geometries can be ascertained.

Specific indications for spinal cord stimulation

1. The most frequent indication for spinal cord stimulation in the United States has been failed back surgery syndrome. Achieving overlap of paresthesias with pain distribution is technically difficult in these patients when their pain includes axial low back pain. The use of detailed psychophysical tests and complex electrode arrays may be helpful in these cases (43, 44). In cases in which axial low back pain is nociceptive or mechanical the response to spinal cord stimulation may not be as good as in those in which the pain is neuropathic or due to deafferentiation (77). In our spinal cord stimulation patients in whom low back pain was not the chief complaint, there have been only minor associations between outcome and the reported percentage of low back pain (65, 68). While it has been reported that patients with unilateral pain are more amenable to treatment than those with bilateral pain (41, 56, 72, 85), this has not been our clinical experience (68).

2. The most common indication for spinal cord stimulation in Europe has been for ischemic pain for peripheral vascular disease (10, 35). The unique feature of this application is that there are measurable changes in response to treatment as opposed to only subjective reports of pain relief. In the small series which have been reported, improvements in red blood cell flow velocity, capillary density, limb salvage rate, and perfusion pressures have been observed at levels that approached statistical significance (1, 34, 35). More recently, cardiac ischemic pain (angina pectoris) has been treated, with encouraging results (2).

3. Pain from spinal cord injury which is confined to a single segmental level is amenable to spinal cord stimulation with over 90 % of these patients proceeding to permanent implant after percutaneous trial in our practice (68).

4. Spinal cord stimulation provides effective pain relief in most cases of postamputation pain syndromes such as phantom limb pain and stump pain (38).

5. Patients with peripheral nerve injury, neuralgia, and causalgia (including reflex sympathetic dystrophy) often respond to spinal cord stimulation (4). In our clinical experience the rate of progression to permanent implant from trial electrodes is significantly less in these patients than in those with other conditions (68). However, this is of limited clinical significance since a majority of these patients have proceeded to permanent implant.

6. Intractable pain associated with spasticity of the lower extremities is often responsive to spinal cord stimulation; spasticity itself may be responsive in some cases (3).

Clinical results

A reported pain relief of 50 %, as rated by the patient, is the most frequent criterion of "success" for spinal cord stimulation. The clinical outcome of published studies may be affected by whether the source of the follow-up data is from physicians' office and hospital charts or by interviews with disinterested third parties (22, 25, 64). The latter evaluation method is being used increasingly in reported studies on spinal cord stimulation (11, 26, 37, 41, 51, 62 – 64, 68, 78, 84).

The population of patients reported is often based on the number receiving permanent implants rather than the number of patients screened with temporary electrodes. In series with a permanent implantation rate as low as 40 % (17), it is important to adjust for this factor. In our clinical experience it is less critical where the rate exceeds 75 % (68). In other surgical procedures for pain relief, usually the number of patients undergoing the definitive procedure is reported, not the number undergoing diagnostic studies such as nerve blocks or myelography, which may have comparable morbidity to percutaneous electrode placement. Spinal cord stimulation is similar to other pain relief modalities such as implantable drug delivery systems in that a low morbidity diagnostic trial accurately simulates the definitive procedure.

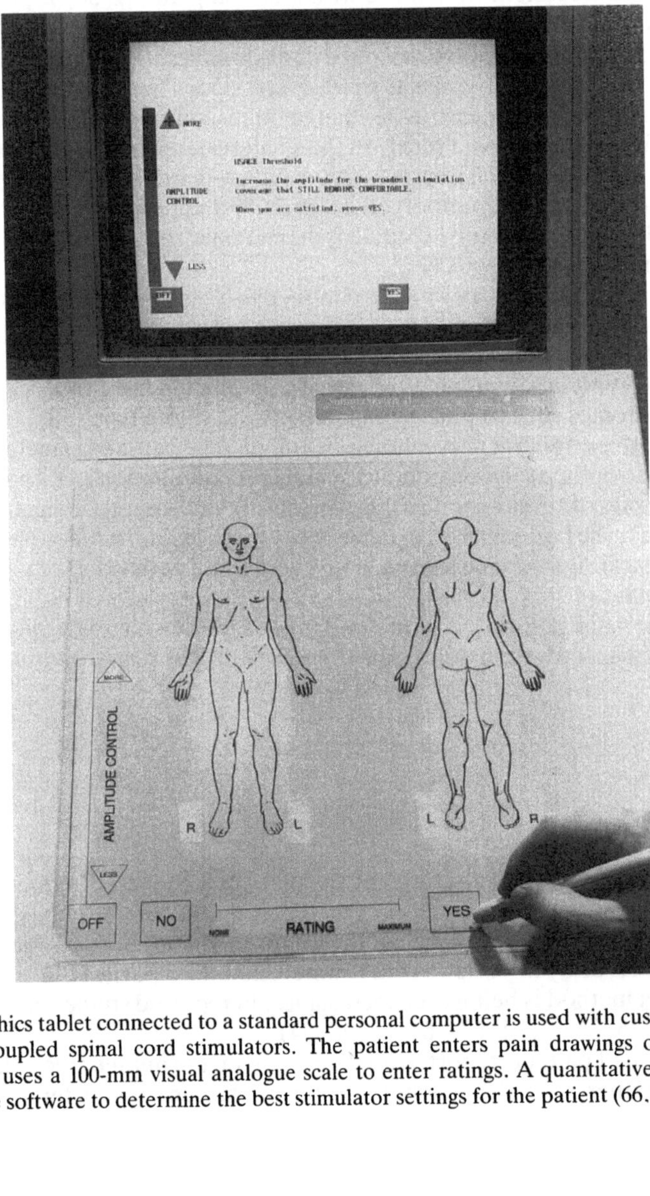

Fig. 3. A graphics tablet connected to a standard personal computer is used with custom software to control RF-coupled spinal cord stimulators. The patient enters pain drawings over a standard template and uses a 100-mm visual analogue scale to enter ratings. A quantitative analysis is performed by the software to determine the best stimulator settings for the patient (66, 67)

Other outcome measures which may be used include secondary measures such as performance of daily activities, work status, level of medication use, and neurologic symptoms (motor, sensory and bladder or bowel function).

Computer assisted methods of stimulator adjustment

Contemporary programmable pulse generators along with multiple electrode arrays have improved both the technical results and clinical outcome of spinal cord stimulation. However, the number of possible anode and cathode assignments grows rapidly as the number of available contacts increases. For example, with four electrodes there are 50 possible usable combinations (only those with at least one anode and cathode are usable), and the number rises to 6050 with eight electrodes. It is desirable to study as many of the usable combinations as possible in each patient over a range of amplitudes from first perception to discomfort, so that the amplitude at which paresthesias overlap the pain distribution may be discerned. Then a comparison may be made between different configurations of electrodes and pulse parameters to determine those which best meet the patient's needs.

The large amounts of data generated by a quantitative study of different electrode combinations and pulse parameter settings requires computerized methods (5, 43, 66, 67). The computer data can be entered by a health care professional working with the patient (5, 43) or directly by the patient (66, 67). In our practice a patient-interactive graphic interface to a personal computer has been developed and is in routine clinical use (Fig. 3). This system allows patients to control stimulation amplitude, enter ratings on an analog scale, and enter "pain drawings" over standardized templates of anterior and posterior views of the body. While it is conceivable that non-computerized methods could be used to effectively examine the available electrode combinations with four electrode contacts, the full range of parameters available with larger numbers of contacts will make computer aided evaluation essential for optimal therapy. In addition, as novel pulse sequences and modulation schemes become available, the parameter space which needs to be examined will increase even further. Presently our computer system is being programmed for clinical trials using "on the fly" reprogramming during stimulation which will allow pulse to pulse variation in amplitude, pulse width and electrode configuration under computer control.

The multichannel systems, which are technically single-channel generators gated to multiple outputs, are significantly more reliable technically and clinically than previous single channel systems. Clinical failures are less frequent, as is the need for surgical electrode revision (68). Figures 4 and 5 show analyses of hardware failures and clinical failures, respectively, over our more than 20 years of experience.

Conclusions

Several advances made over the past two decades have significantly improved the clinical outcome of spinal cord stimulation for pain relief. These include the development of programmable implantable stimulation devices, percutaneous placement of electrodes, and improved patient selection and management techniques. While

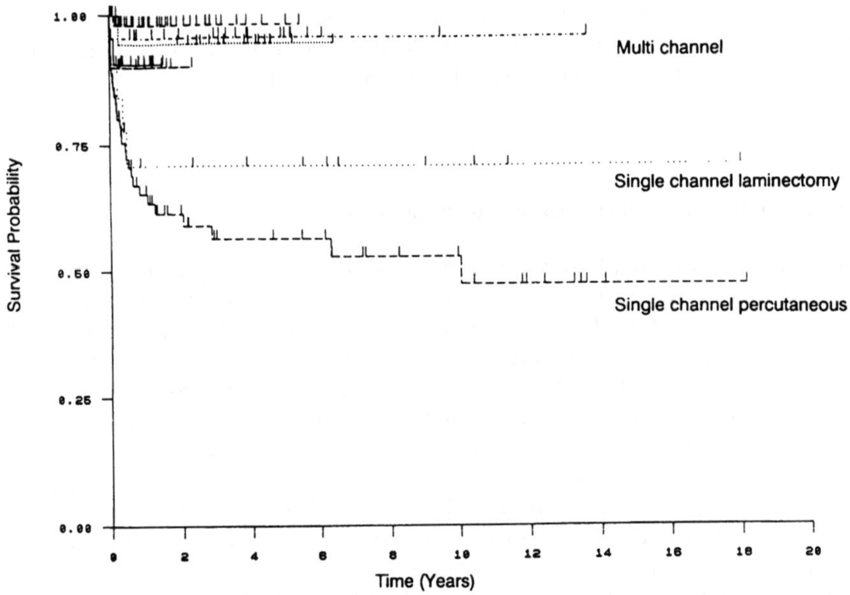

Fig. 4. Kaplan-Meier curves for different electrode combinations over the past two decades. Technical failures requiring surgical revision were the statistical endpoint. Upper curves, multicontact percutaneous electrodes; lower curves, dual independently inserted percutaneous electrodes; middle curve, bipolar electrodes placed by laminectomy

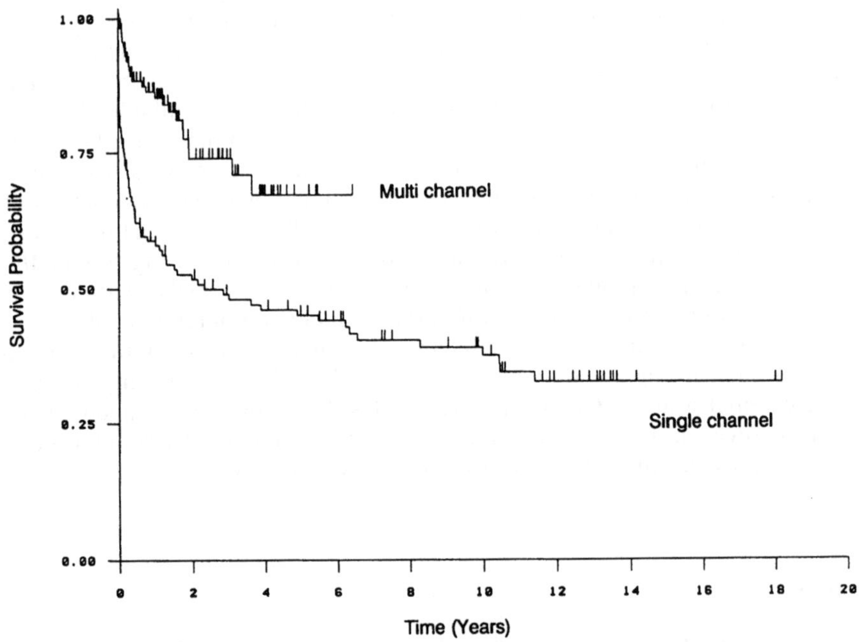

Fig. 5. Kaplan-Meier survival curves showing the lifetimes of single-channel and multichannel devices. The endpoint was clinical failure defined as cessation of patient use for any reason. The multichannel systems were significantly more reliable ($p < 0.001$). (Reproduced with permission from [68])

implantation of neurostimulators now achieves success in a majority of patients, further research is needed in optimal selection of electrode combinations and investigation of new stimulation patterns which may further increase efficacy.

Table 1. The literature on spinal cord stimulation exhibits a variety of follow-up intervals and methods, temporary electrode screening methods, and criteria for "success". Comparisons among studies or meta-analyses are difficult. An "excellent" or "good" result commonly signifies at least 50 % reported relief of pain; but this is only one of many important outcome measures.

Reference	Number implanted	Number screened	Number failed backs	Follow-up range	Follow-up mean	"Exc/good" results (≥50 % relief)	"Exc/good" FBSS results	Third-party follow-up
Bel and Bauer [6]	14		14		2 yrs.	60 %	60 %	
Blond et al. [7]	58	59	59	12–72 mos.	37 mos.	89.5 %	89.5 %	
Blume et al. [8]	20		20	≥3 yrs.		70 %	70 %	
Broseta et al. [9]	11			3–20 mos.	13 mos.	64 %		
Burton [11]	75	0	55		1 yr.	59 %		y (mfr)
Burton [12]	198		186			43 %		
Clark [14]	13		6			54 %	67 %	
De la Porte and Siegfried [17]	36	94	36	3–96 mos.	36 mos.	60 %		
De la Porte and Van de Kleft [18]	64	78	78	1–7 yrs.	4 yrs.	55 %	55 %	
de Vera [19]	110	124	18			75 %		
Demirel [20]	33	48	11	2–5 yrs.		18 %		
Devulder et al. [21]	45		23			78 %		
Devulder et al. [22]	69		43	≥8 yrs.		55 %		
Erickson and Lang [26]	70	10		≥10 yrs.		15–20 %		y (60)
Hoppenstein [31]	27		12			58 %	64 %	
Hunt et al. [33]	13		5	9 mos. – 4 yrs.		15–31 %	20–60 %	
Kälin and Winkelmüller [36]			77			88 %	88 %	
Koeze et al. [37]	26	0	5		28 mos.	46–62 %		y
Krainick et al. [31]	91	126	5	≥5 yrs.		18 %		
Kumar et al. [40]	60		54	6–60 mos.		62 %		
Kumar et al. [41]	94	121	56	6 mos. – 10 yrs.	40 mos.	66 %		y
Law [42]	81					36 – 80 %		
Leclercq and Russo [45]	20		20	1–24 mos.		50 %	50 %	
LeDoux and Langford [46]	26	32	32	≥5 years		76 %, 1 yr.	76 %, 1 yr.	
LeRoy [48]	49		49	1–63 mos.	30.7 mos.	60 %		n
Long and Erickson [51]	69		54	12–35 mos.		18 %		y
Long et al. [52]	31		24	4–7 yrs.		73 %, 3 yrs.		y
McCarron et al. [54]	22			3–24 mos.		68 %		
Meglio et al. [55]	64	109	19				23 %	n
Meilman et al. [56]	12	20	20	≥3.5 yrs.		60 %	60 %	
Mittal et al. [59]	26	31	21			46 %		
Nielson et al. [62]	130	221	79	1–35 mos.		49 %	46 %	y
North et al. [65]	50	54	50		5.0 yrs.	47 %	47 %	y
North et al. [68]	171	205	153	2–20 years	7.1 yrs.	52 %		y
Pineda [70]	76		56			43 %	43 %	
Racz et al. [71]	26	0	18	12–42.7 mos.		65 %		n
Ray et al. [72]	78		50	3–64 mos.	19.4 mos.	49 %		
Richardson et al. [73]	22	36	12	1–3 yrs.		56 %		
Shealy [80]	80	0		7 mos. – ?		25 %	15–45 %	n
Shelden et al. [81]	27		3				67 %	
Siegfried and Lazorthes [82]	89	191	75	1–8 yrs.	~4 yrs.	37 %		
Simpson [83]	56	24	7	2 wks. – 9 yrs.	29 mos.	47 %		
Spiegelmann and Friedman [84]	30	43	18	3–33 mos.	13 mos.	60 4		y
Sweet and Wepsic [85]	98	100	33			21–42 %	15–45 %	
Urban et al. [86]	7	20	9			86 %		
Vogel et al. [87]	27	50	29	>3 yrs.		18.6 %		n
Waisbrod and Gerbershagen [89]	16		16	6–30 mos.	16 mos.	75 %		n
Winkelmüller [90]	71	94	56	4 mos. – 7 yrs.			69 %	
Young and Shende [91]	27		17	16–51 mos.		66 % ≥50 %		
Young [92]	51	14	25	12–67 mos.	38 mos.	65 % ≥50 %		

FBSS, failed back surgery syndrome; third-party follow-up: mfr, device manufacturer.

References

1. Augustinsson LE, Carlsson CA, Holm J, Jivegard L (1985) Epidural electrical stimulation in severe limb ischemia: Evidence of pain relief, increased blood flow and a possible limb-saving effect. Ann Surg 202: 104–111
2. Augustinsson LE (1989) Spinal cord electrical stimulation in severe angina pectoris: surgical technique, intraoperative physiology, complications and side effects. Pace 12: 693–4
3. Barolat G, Myklebust JB, Wenninger W (1988) Effects of spinal cord stimulation on spasticity and spasms secondary to myelopathy. Appl Neurophys 51: 29–44
4. Barolat G, Schwartzman RJ, Woo R (1989) Epidural spinal cord stimulation in the management of reflex sympathetic dystrophy. Stereotact Funct Neurosurg 53: 29–39
5. Barolat G, Massaro F, He J, Zeme S, Ketcik B (1993) Mapping of sensory responses to epidural stimulation of the intraspinal neural structures in man. J Neurosurg 78: 233–239
6. Bel S, Bauer BL (1991) Dorsal column stimulation (DCS): Cost to benefit analysis. Acta Neurochir 52(suppl.): 121–123
7. Blond S, Armignies P, Parker F, Dupard T, Guieu JD, Duquesnoy B, Christiaens JL (1991) Sciatalges chroniques par désafférentation sensitive après chirurgie de la hernie discale lombaire: aspects cliniques et thérapeutiques. Neurochirurgie 37: 86–95
8. Blume H, Richardson R, Rojas C (1982) Epidural nerve stimulation of the lower spinal cord and cauda equina for the relief of intractable pain in failed back surgery. Appl Neurophysiol 45: 456–460
9. Broseta J, Roldan P, Gonzales-Darder J, Bordes V, Barcia-Salorio JL (1982) Chronic epidural dorsal column stimulation in the treatment of causalgic pain. Appl Neurophys 45: 190–194
10. Broseta J, Barbera J, DeVera J, Barcia-Salorio J, March G, Gonzalez-Darder J, Rovaina F, Joanes V (1986) Spinal cord stimulation in peripheral arterial disease. J Neurosurg 64: 71–80
11. Burton C (1975) Dorsal column stimulation: optimization of application. Surg Neurol 4: 171–176
12. Burton CV (1977) Session on spinal cord stimulation: safety and clinical efficacy. Neurosurgery 1: 164–165
13. Campbell JN, Raja SN, Meyer RA, Mackinnon SE (1988) Myelinated afferents signal the hyperalgesia associated with nerve injury. Pain 32: 89–94
14. Clark K (1975) Electrical stimulation of the nervous system for control of pain: university of Texas Southwestern Medical School experience. Surg Neurol 4: 164–166
15. Coburn B, Sin W (1985) A theoretical study of epidural electrical stimulation of the spinal cord. I. Finite element analysis of stimulus fields. IEEE Trans Biomed Eng 32: 971–977
16. Daniel M, Long C, Hutcherson M, Hunter S (1985) Psychological factors and outcome of electrode implantation for chronic pain. Neurosurgery 17 (5): 773–777
17. De la Porte C, Siegfried J (1983) Lumbosacral spinal fibrosis (spinal arachnoiditis): its diagnosis and treatment by spinal cord stimulation. Spine 8 (6): 593–603
18. De la Porte C, Van de Kelft E (1993) Spinal cord stimulation in failed back surgery syndrome. Pain 52: 55–61
19. de Vera JA, Rodriguez JL, Dominguez M, Robaina F (1990) Spinal cord stimulation for chronic pain mainly in PVD, vasospastic disorders of the upper limbs and failed back surgery. Pain (Suppl 5): S81
20. Demirel T, Braun W, Reimers CD (1984) Results of spinal cord stimulation in patients suffering from chronic pain after a two year observation period. Neurochirurgia 27: 47–50
21. Devulder J, De Colvenaer L, Rolly G, Caemaert J, Calliauw L (1990) Spinal cord stimulation and the relief of chronic non-malignant pain in 45 patients. Pain 5: S236
22. Devulder J, Vermulen H, De Colvenaer L, Rolly G, Calliauw L, Caemaert J (1991) Spinal cord stimulation in chronic pain: Evaluation of results, complications, and techincal considerations in sixty-nine patients. Clin J Pain 7: 21–28
23. Duggan AW, Foong FW (1985) Bicuculline and spinal inhibition produced by dorsal column stimulation in the cat. Pain 22: 249–259
24. Dyck PJ, Lais A, Karnes J, Sparks M, Dyck PJB (1985) Peripheral axotomy induces neurofilament decrease, atrophy, demyelination and degeneration of root and fasciculus gracilis fibers. Br Res 340: 19–36
25. Erickson DL (1975) Percutaneous trial of stimulation for patient selection for implantable stimulating devices. J Neurosurg 43: 440–444

26. Erickson DL, Long DM (1983) Ten-year follow-up of dorsal column stimulation, In: Bonica JJ (ed), Advances in pain research and therapy vol. 5, Raven, New York, pp 583–589
27. Feler C, Kaufman S (1992) Spinal cord stimulation: One stage? Acta Neurochir 117: 91
28. Freeman TB, Campbell JN, Long DM (1983) Naloxone does not affect pain relief induced by electrical stimulation in man. Pain 17: 189–195
29. Handwerker HO, Iggo A, Zimmerman M (1975) Segmental and supraspinal actions on dorsal horn neurons responding to noxious and non-noxious skin stimuli. Pain 1: 147–165
30. Holsheimer J, Strujik JJ, Rijkhoff NJM (1991) Contact combinations in epidural spinal cord stimulation: a comparison by computer modeling. Stereotact Funct Neurosurg 56: 220–233
31. Hoppenstein R (1975) Percutaneous implantation of chronic spinal cord electrodes for control of intractable pain: preliminary report. Surg Neurol 4: 195–198
32. Hosobuchi Y, Adams JE, Weinstein PR (1972) Preliminary percutaneous dorsal column stimulation prior to permanent implantation. J Neurosurg 37: 242–245
33. Hunt WE, Goodman JH, Bingham WG (1975) Stimulation of the dorsal spinal cord for treatment of intractable pain: a preliminary report. Surg Neurol 4: 153–156
34. Jacobs MJ, Jorning PJ, Joshi SR, Kitslaar P, Slaaf DW, Reneman RS (1988) Epidural spinal cord electrical stimulation improves microvascular blood flow in severe limb ischemia. Ann Surg 207: 179–183
35. Jacobs MJ, Jorning PJ, Beckers RC, Ubbink DT, Van Kleef M, Slaaf DW, Reneman R (1990) Foot salvage and improvement of microvascular blood flow as a result of epidural spinal cord electrical stimulation. J Vasc Surg 12: 354–360
36. Kälin, M-T, Winkelmüller W (1990) Chronic pain after multiple lumbar discectomies – significance of intermittent spinal cord stimulation. Pain 5: S241
37. Koeze TH, Williams AC, Reiman S (1987) Spinal cord stimulation and the relief of chronic pain. J Neurol Neurosurg Psych 50: 1424–1429
38. Krainick JU, Thoden U, Riechert T (1980) Pain reduction in amputees by long-term spinal cord stimulation: long-term follow-up study over 5 years. J Neurosurg 52: 346–350
39. Krainick JU, Thoden U 1989) Dorsal column stimulation, In: Wall PD, Melzack R (eds) Textbook of pain. Churchhill Livingstone, New York, pp 701–705
40. Kumar K, Wyant GM, Ekong CEU (1986) Epidural spinal cord stimulation for relief of chronic pain. Pain Clin 1 (2): 91–99
41. Kumar K, Nath R, Wyant GM (1991) Treatment of chronic pain by epidural spinal cord stimulation: a 10-year experience. J Neurosurg 75: 402–407
42. Law J (1983) Spinal stimulation: statistical superiority of monophasic stimulation of narrowly separated, longitudinal bipoles having rostral cathodes. Appl Neurophys 46: 129–137
43. Law JD (1987) A new method for targeting a spinal stimulator: quantitatively paired comparisons. Appl Neurophys 50: 436
44. Law JD, Kirkpatrick AF (1991) Pain management update: spinal cord stimulation. Am J Pain Management 2: 34–42
45. Leclercq T, Russo E (1981) La stimulation epidurale dans le traitement del doleurs chroniques. Neurochirurgie 27: 125–128
46. LeDoux MS, Langford KH (1993) Spinal cord stimulation for the failed back syndrome. Spine 18: 191–194
47. Leibrock L, Meilman P, Cuka D, Green C (1984) Spinal cord stimulation in the treatment of chronic low back and lower extremity pain syndromes. Nebraska Med J 69 (6): 180–183
48. LeRoy PL (1981) Stimulation of the spinal cord by biocompatible electrical current in the human. Appl Neurophysiol 44: 187–193
49. Lindblom U, Tapper N, Wiesenfeld Z (1977) The effect of dorsal column stimulation on the nociceptive response of dorsal horn cells and its relevance for pain suppression. Pain 4: 133–144
50. Linderoth B (1992) Dorsal column stimulation and pain: experimental studies of putative neurochemical and neurophysiological mechanisms. Stockholm, Kongl Carolinska Medico Chirurgiska Institutet
51. Long DM, Erickson DE (1975) Stimulation of the posterior columns of the spinal cord for relief of intractable pain. Surg Neurol 4: 134–141
52. Long DM, Erickson D, Campbell J, North R (1981) Electrical stimulation of the spinal cord and peripheral nerves for pain control. Appl Neurophysiol 44: 207–217

53. Long DM, Filtzer DL, BenDebba M, Hendler NH (1988) Clinical features of the failed-back syndrome. J Neurosurg 69: 61–71
54. McCarron RF, Racz G (1987) Percutaneous dorsal column stimulator implantation for chronic pain control. Presented at North American Spine Society meeting
55. Meglio M, Cioni B, Rossi GF (1989) Spinal cord stimulation in management of chronic pain: a 9-year experience. J Neurosurg 70: 519–524
56. Meilman PW, Leibrock LG, Leong FTL (1989) Outcome of implanted spinal cord stimulation in the treatment of chronic pain: arachnoiditis versus single nerve root injury and mononeuropathy. Clin J Pain 5: 189–193
57. Melzack P, Wall PD (1965) Pain mechanisms: a new theory. Science 150 (3699): 971–978
58. Meyerson BA, Herregodts P, Linderoth B (1992) Enhanced flexor reflex in the mononeuropathic rat is attenuated by spinal cord stimulation. Acta Neurochir 117: 88
59. Mittal B, Thomas DGT, Walton P, Calder I (1987) Dorsal column stimulation (DCS) in chronic pain: report of 31 cases. Ann Roy Coll Surg 69 (3): 104–109
60. Nashold BS Jr, Friedman H (1972) Dorsal column stimulation for control of pain, preliminary report on 30 patients. J Neurosurg 36: 590–597
61. Nathan PW (1976) The gate-control theory of pain: A critical review. Brain 99: 123–158
62. Nielson KD, Adams JE, Hosobuchi Y (1975) Experience with dorsal column stimulation for relief of chronic intractable pain. Surg Neurol 4: 148–152
63. North RB, Fischell TA, Long DM (1977) Chronic stimulation via percutaneously inserted epidural electrodes. Neurosurgery 1: 215–218
64. North RB, Ewend MG, Lawton MT, Piantadosi S (1991) Spinal cord stimulation for chronic, intractable pain: superiority of "multichannel" devices. Pain 44: 119–130
65. North RB, Ewend MG, Lawton MT, Kidd DH, Piantadosi S (1991) Failed back surgery syndrome: five-year follow-up after spinal cord stimulator implantation. Neurosurgery 28: 692–699
66. North RB, Fowler KR, Nigrin DA, Szymanski RE (1992) Patient-interactive, computer-controlled neurological stimulation system: clinical efficacy in spinal cord stimulation. J Neurosurg 76: 689–695
67. North RB, Fowler KR, Nigrin DA, Szymanski RE, Piantadosi S (1992) Automated 'pain drawing' analysis by computer-controlled, patient-interactive neurological stimulation system. Pain 50: 51–58
68. North RB, Kidd DH, Zahurak M, James CS, Long DM (1993) Spinal cord stimulation for chronic, intractable pain: two decades' experience. Neurosurgery 32: 384–395
69. Ohnishi A, O'Brien PC, Okazaki H, Dyck PJ (1976) Morphometry of myelinated fibers of fasciculus gracilis of man. J Neurol Sci 27: 163–172
70. Pineda A (1975) Dorsal column stimulation and its prospects. Surg Neurol 4: 157–163
71. Racz GB, McCarron RF, Talboys P (1989) Percutaneous dorsal column stimulator for chronic pain control. Spine 14 (1): 1–4
72. Ray CD, Burton CV, Lifson A (1982) Neurostimulation as used in a large clinical practice. Appl Neurophysiol 45: 160–206
73. Richardson RR, Siqueira EB, Cerullo LJ (1979) Spinal epidural neurostimulation for treatment of acute and chronic intractable pain: initial and long term results. Neurosurgery 5 (3): 344–348
74. Richardson DE, Shatin D (1991) Results of spinal cord stimulation for pain control: long-term collaborative study Presented at American Pain Society, New Orleans, Louisiana, Poster #91240, program, p 56
75. Robb LG, Robb MP (1990) Practical considerations in spinal cord stimulation. Pain 5: S234
76. Sances A, Swiontek TJ, Larson SJ, Cusick JF, Meyer GA, Millar EA, Hemmy DC, Myklebust J (1975) Innovations in neurologic implant systems. Med Instrum 9 (5): 213–216
77. Sánchez-Ledesma MJ, Garcia-March G, Diaz-Cascajo P, Gómez-Moreta J, Broseta J (1989) Spinal cord stimulation in deafferentation pain. Stereotact Funct Neurosurg 53: 40–55
78. Shatin D, Mullett K, Hults G (1986) Totally implantable spinal cord stimulation for chronic pain: design and efficacy. Pace 9: 577–583
79. Shealy CN, Mortimer JT, Reswick JB (1967) Electrical inhibition of pain by stimulation of the dorsal columns: preliminary clinical report. Anesth Analg 46: 489–491
80. Shealy CN (1975) Dorsal column stimulation: optimization of application. Surg Neurol 4: 142–145

81. Shelden CH, Paul F, Jacques DB, Pudenz RH (1975) Electrical stimulation of the nervous system. Surg Neurol 4: 127–132
82. Siegfried J, Lazorthes Y (1982) Long-term follow-up of dorsal column stimulation for chronic pain syndrome after multiple lumbar operations. Appl Neurophys 45: 201–204
83. Simpson BA (1991) Spinal cord stimulation in 60 cases of intractable pain. J Neurol Neurosurg Psychiat 54: 196–199
84. Spiegelmann R, Friedman WA (1991) Spinal cord stimulation: a contemporary series. Neurosurgery 28: 65–71
85. Sweet W, Wepsic J (1974) Stimulation of the posterior columns of the spinal cord for pain control. Clin Neurosurg 21: 278–310
86. Urban BJ, Nashold B (1978) Percutaneous epidural stimulation of the spinal cord for relief of pain: long term results. J Neurosurg 48: 323–328
87. Vogel HP, Heppner B, Hümbs N, Schramm J, Wagner C (19867 Long-term effects of spinal cord stimulation in chronic pain syndromes. J Neurol 233: 16–18
88. Waddell G, McCulloch JA, Kummel EG, Venner RM (1980) Non-organic physical signs in low back pain. Spine 5: 117–125
89. Waisbrod H, Gerbershagen HU (1985) Spinal cord stimulation in patients with a battered root syndrome. Arch Orthop Trauma Surg 104: 62–64
90. Winkelmüller W (1981) Experience with the control of low back pain by the dorsal column stimulation (DCS) system and by the peridural electrode system (Pisces). In: Hosobuchi Y, Corbin T (eds) Indications for spinal cord stimulation. Excerpta Medica, Amsterdam, pp 34–41
91. Young RF, Shende M (1976) Dorsal column stimulation for relief of chronic intractable pain. Surg Forum 27: 474–476
92. Young RF (1978) Evaluation of dorsal column stimulation in the treatment of chronic pain. Neurosurgery 3: 373–379
93. Zumpano BJ, Saunders RL (1976) Percutaneous epidural dorsal column stimulation. J Neurosurg 45: 459–460

Author's address:
R. B. North, MD
Associate Professor of Neurosurgery
Johns Hopkins University School of Medicine
600 N. Wolfe St., Meyer 7-113
Baltimore, Maryland 21287-7713
USA

How to evaluate the results of neuromodulative procedures in pain?

J. M. Gybels, R. C. Kupers

Department of Neurosurgery, University Hospital Gasthuisberg, K.U.Leuven, Leuven, Belgium

Introduction

Evaluation of pain treatment, be it neuromodulative or some other treatment, is no trivial affair. Already in 1959, Beecher, an anesthesiologist, wrote a remarkable article far in advance of his time, "The measurement of pain" (1). Since this pioneering publication, important progress has been made in the field of pain measurement. It has become recognised that pain is a complex and multi-dimensional experience that is co-determined by affective, motivational and environmental factors. This has led to the development of new instruments for pain assessment that take into account these various aspects. The interested reader can find an extensive overview of the different aspects of pain assessment in some recently published textbooks (3, 16).

Does a gold standard exist for "how to measure pain"? The answer to this question depends on many factors such as the study population, the type of pain, and the aims of the investigator.

Outcome measures in treatment evaluation

In the evaluation of neuromodulative procedures, be it electrical stimulation or an intraspinal drug administration, therapeutic success is often equated with pain reduction. Consequently, many authors limit themselves to the measurement of pain and pain relief. However, therapeutic success is not necessarily synonymous with pain reduction, and certainly not in the treatment of chronic non-cancer pain. Functional improvement, improvement in quality of life, the cost-benefit of a treatment, and the occurrence of side-effects are also important aspects of therapeutic outcome.

Pain and pain relief

Pain can be measured by asking the patient for a verbal report of his pain. In addition, pain patients also show particular pain behaviours by which pain can be assessed. Finally, attempts have been made to measure pain by means of physiological correlates.

Verbal pain report

In the evaluation of pain and relief, the following aspects should be assessed:

Pain as a sensation

The pain experience has an important sensory component. This can be described in terms of intensity, quality, temporal characteristics and anatomical distribution.

1) Pain intensity:

Pain intensity is the most assessed dimension of therapeutic outcome. The visual analogue scale (VAS), verbal category scales, and numerical rating scales are the most commonly used scales. A widely used category scale is the four-point intensity scale (none, mild, moderate, and severe). However, this scale has not enough levels to accurately describe treatment effects. Improved category scales with more descriptors were proposed by Gracely et al. (6). A discussion of the strengths and weaknesses of the different pain intensity measures can be found in Jensen and McFarland (8).

In many clinical pain conditions, pain intensity fluctuates over time. Asking the patient for a mean pain intensity score leaves us ignorant about the actual pain intensity levels. For instance, a patient may suffer a moderate intense background pain on which are superposed regular short pain episodes of an extreme intensity. A solution to this is to ask the patient to rate the percentage of time his pain falls within certain intensity categories (e.g., very intense: 20 %, intense: 30 %, and mild 50 % of the time).

Pain or pain relief? Whereas pain intensity scales focus on the present pain experience, pain relief scores rely on the patient's memory for pain. Since patients tend to overestimate their past pain, the use of pain relief scores may lead to an overestimation of the effects of the treatment, certainly in cases of prolonged follow-up. On the other hand, there is some evidence that pain relief category scales are more sensitive to small reductions in pain (11). In any case, when no baseline pain ratings are available, pain relief scores are the only measures to rely on.

2) Pain quality:

Pain can also be described in qualitative terms. The McGill pain questionnaire offers a list with pain quality descriptors. Assessment of pain quality is important because it may give important information on the underlying etiology.

Pain affect dimension

It has become generally accepted that pain must be described both in terms of sensory-discriminative and affective dimensions. Gracely (5) distinguished three aspects in the pain affect dimension. First, feelings associated with the immediate pain sensation (the unpleasantness). Second, feelings associated with human thought (uncertainty, fear), the way in which pain experiences are cognitively integrated into the patient's life (cognitive-evaluative dimension) and third the effect of pain on psychological health (emotional factors). Pain affect can be measured by a multidimensional scale such as the McGill pain questionnaire. Disadvantages of this scale are its length and the complexity of its vocabulary which makes it unsuitable for very sick and not sufficiently educated patients. However, simpler scales exist that more specifically assess the affective dimension (4, 6). Several studies have shown that the sensory-discriminative and affective dimension of pain can be independently affected (10, 14).

Behaviour and self-reports of behaviour

Pain can also be inferred from overt behaviour. Examples of pain behaviours are guarding, rubbing, grimacing, and sighing. Most protocols for measuring overt pain behaviour have been developed and validated for chronic back pain although there also exist protocols for rheumatoid arthritis, headache, and head and neck cancer pain (9).

Behavioral pattern assessment techniques are rather time-consuming and require a training in behavioural observation techniques. A simpler method to assess pain behaviour is by asking the patient how he behaves. The most commonly assessed pain behaviour is the consumption of analgesic medication. Other frequently scored activities are sitting, walking, lying down and sleeping. The information can be obtained during (structured) interviews, by means of questionnaires or through the use of patient diaries. Although the validity of self-reports of behaviour has been questioned, they may be an alternative when behavioural observation techniques are difficult to perform.

Physiological measures

Numerous physiological correlates of pain have been proposed. However, none of these measures has been shown to co-vary reliably with subjective pain reports. Among the most promising are cortical and brainstem evoked potentials and spinal reflex activity (RIII reflex). Just like pain behaviours, physiological measures do not offer an index of pain intensity, but they may provide an "objective" measure in the assessment of the effectiveness of an intervention.

Assessment of quality of life and health status

Over the last decade, a growing number of clinical trials have included measures of quality of life. In the evaluation of the treatment of chronic diseases such as, e.g., diabetes, they have become an important indicator of whether or not a treatment can be considered as successful. Several measures of daily activities, social adjustment and family functioning have been developed and their validity assessed in different populations (15).

A distinction should be made between generic and disease-specific measures. Generic measures are intended to be applicable to many different impairments, illnesses, and patients. Disease-specific measures on the other hand are those designed to assess specific diagnostic groups, with the goal of measuring "clinically important changes" (13).

Assessment of side-effects

Side-effects can be evaluated by means of a checklist with prespecified events or on the basis of a spontaneous report by the patient. Whereas the checklist may lead to an overreporting of events, the spontaneous report approach may lead to an underestimation of side-effects. It is advisable to score each side-effect for its severity (absent, mild, moderate, severe, and very severe). In addition, the patient can be asked to judge how distressing the side-effects are to him/her.

What is success?

A difficult problem in the evaluation of the efficacy of a treatment is the definition of the outcome criteria for success. Just as there is no gold standard for pain measurement, no universal measure of success exists. The chosen criteria for success depend on different factors, such as the theory on pain relief, the type of pain patients, and the therapeutic goal. For instance, whereas in a neurosurgical context, the primary aim of an intervention is to reduce pain, in a behavioural treatment program the primary aim may be functional improvement.

To allow comparisons between the results of different studies, it is important that the criteria of success are clearly defined and that attempts are undertaken to come to a consensus about which criteria of success should be used.

In studies where multiple outcome measures are assessed, the question arises of which one shall be used to determine the effectiveness of the treatment? There are two possibilities. First, one can designate a particular measure as the primary outcome measure for success. The other measures are then excluded from the definition of success and are designated as secondary outcome measures. Another possibility is to use composite scores and to define success on the basis of the outcome of different measures (e.g., 50 % pain reduction + improved functional capacity).

Design of studies for the evaluation of neuromodulative pain treatment

First, the need of placebo controls must be considered. Improvement in pain subsequent to treatment may be due to specific as well as non-specific treatment effects. Therefore, (placebo) controls are necessary. Beecher already pointed out that surgery may act as a powerful placebo (2). It should be admitted that only few invasive procedures allow a genuine placebo-controlled approach. One of the exceptions is electrical stimulation of pain suppressive systems that do not require paresthesias or other behavioral manifestations (e.g., motor cortex stimulation). Another example is intraspinal drug administration via implantable pumps. In many surgical trials, placebos seem to raise serious ethical problems. To the best of our knowledge, no extensive discussion has been published on this issue.

Future trials should include the following features:

1) Randomised cross-over or parallel group design. Cross-over designs are preferable but are seldomly accomplishable in a neurosurgical context. Exceptions are neurostimulation and spinal drug administration procedures. When cross-over designs are not possible parallel group designs can be used.

2) Management of narcotics before randomising patients. Many candidates for a neuromodulative intervention are taking significant amounts of opioid drugs and other analgesics. There are two possibilities. First, the patient can be allowed to continue taking his analgesics. The reduction in the consumption of analgesics that is expected to occur in case the intervention is successful can then be used as a parameter of success. The second possibility is that narcotics are reduced prior to considering a neuromodulative intervention. Loeser (12) suggests that for pain with an unclear cause of the pain behaviour (e.g., in non-malignant diseases), the patients should be converted from short-duration narcotics to a long-acting drug, and that gradually the dose should be reduced. According to Loeser, in many patients the pain behaviour diminishes as narcotics are reduced and no intervention is required. In others, a more accurate diagnosis can be made as the narcotic-induced mental impairment clears.

3) Assessment by an independent observer. The evaluation of the treatment should ideally be done by a person who is not directly involved with the treatment of the patient. Preferably, the observer should be blind with regard to the treatment condition and he should have sufficient experience in pain evaluation.

4) Homogenous groups of patients. Optimal pain treatment evaluation is hindered by heterogeneous patient samples. What one wants to know is the effectiveness of an intervention for a well described diagnostic category. Therefore, homogenous patient samples should be used. Moreover, the diagnostic categories must be strictly defined using generally accepted classification systems.

5) Multi-dimensional outcome measures. The effect of an intervention should be assessed on a broad range of outcome measures. A taskforce of the IASP (International Association for the Study of Pain) is in the process of establishing such a multidimensional evaluation protocol. It is important that the tests are carefully explained to the patient and the investigator should try to find out whether the patient understood what is meant. In our experience, even such a simple test as the VAS is often not correctly understood by the patient.

6) Multiple assessments and prolonged follow-up. In the assessment of pain it is important to distinguish between current pain and usual pain. Usual pain is the average of an individual's report of pain intensity over a specific period of time. The primary outcome variable of interest in a clinical study is a comparison of the average pain experienced before and after the intervention. Single ratings of pain intensity do not provide a reliable measure of average pain since pain reports may change substantially over time and since many factors influence pain ratings obtained at a single time-point. Therefore, verbal descriptor home "diaries" are advisable; they provide an overall measure that incorporates pain fluctuations. Jensen et al. (8) showed that a composite pain intensity score calculated from an average of 12 ratings across 4 days provides a reliable and valid measure of average pain.

Concluding remarks

Evaluation of results of pain treatment is not trivial, but rather, complex and time consuming. Pain is a complex multi-dimensional experience and adequate pain assessment and treatment evaluation requires that data on these different dimensions are collected. The time that success could be measured with a single rating of pain relief has definitely passed (7). Future studies need to incorporate measures of quality of life and functional and psychological functioning. Only in this way can comparison of results obtained from investigators with a different theoretical orientation be compared.

Methods of pain measurement differ considerably according to the type of pain. Efforts should be undertaken to develop and validate pain pathology-tailored test instruments or batteries which would enable the comparison of results by different authors.

References

1. Beecher T (1959) The measurement of pain. Pharmacol Rev 9: 59–209
2. Beecher T (1961) Surgery as placebo: A quantitative study of bias. J Am Med Ass 176: 1102–1107
3. Chapman CR, Loeser JD (1989) Issues in pain measurement. Adv in Pain Res Ther 12. Raven Press, New York
4. Duncan G, Bushnell MC, Lavigne G (1989) Comparison of verbal and visual analogue scales for measuring intensity and unpleasantness of experimental pain. Pain 37: 295–303
5. Gracely RH (1991) Theoretical and practical issues in pain assessment in central pain syndromes. In: Casey KL (ed.) Pain and Central Nervous: The Central Pain Syndromes. Raven Press, New York, pp 85–101
6. Gracely RH, McGrath P, Dubner R (1978) Validity and sensitivity of ratio scales of sensory and affective verbal descriptors: manipulation of effect of diazepam. Pain 5: 19–29
7. Gybels J, Sweet WH (1989) Neurosurgical treatment of pain. Karger, Basel
8. Jensen MP, McFarland CA (1993) Increasing the reliability and validity of pain intensity measurement in chronic pain patients. Pain 55: 195–203
9. Keefe FJ (1989) Behavioural measurement of pain. Adv Pain Res Ther 13: 405–424
10. Kupers RC, Konings H, Adriaensen H, Gybels J (1991) Morphine differentially affects the sensory and affective pain ratings in neurogenic and idiopathic forms of pain. Pain 47: 5–12
11. Littman GS, Walker BR, Schneider BE (1985) Reassessment of verbal and visual analog ratings in analgesic studies. Clin Pharmacol Ther 38: 16–23
12. Loeser JD (1990) Ablative neurosurgical procedures. In: Bonica JJ (ed) The Management of Pain, 2nd ed., Lea and Febiger, Philadelphia, pp 2040–2043
13. Patrick DL, Deyo RA (1989) Generic and disease-specific measures in assessing health status and quality of life. Med Care 27: S217–S232
14. Price DD, Barrell JJ, Gracely RH (1980) A psychophysical analysis of factors that selectively influence the affective dimension of pain. Pain 8: 137–149
15. Spilker B (1990) Quality of Life Assessments in Clinical Trials. Raven Press, New York
16. Turk D, Melzack R (1992) Handbook of Pain Assessment. Guilford Press, New York

Author's address:
Prof. J. M. Gybels, MD PhD
Dept. of Neurosurgery and
Center for Experimental Surgery and Anesthesiology
Provisorium 1
Minderbroedersstraat 17
B-3000 Leuven
Belgium

Evaluation of the effects of spinal cord stimulation by infrared thermography

J. Devulder, F. Castille, M. De Laat

Department of Anesthesia, Section Pain, Clinic, University Hospital of Ghent, Ghent, Belgium

Introduction

In 1967, Shealy introduced Spinal Cord Stimulation into clinical medicine to treat pain (9). Since its introduction it has been used to treat numerous disorders. Spinal cord stimulation seemed to have beneficial effects in the treatment of pain (5), motor disorders (3), and vascular disease (4). The real physiological mechanisms by which pain is alleviated are not well known yet.

Nevertheless, one criterion should be fulfilled: the pain area should be overlapped by the paresthesia area. Still, only the patient can inform us about the exact localization of pain and stimulation paresthesiae. We do not possess any monitor to evaluate that.

Already in 1981, Meglio proved that Spinal Cord Stimulation also had beneficial effects on peripheral blood flow (7). His findings were confirmed by Augustinsson (1) and Jacobs (6) with the help of capillaroscopy. These authors showed a significant increase in the microcirculation. Spinal Cord Stimulation even has limb-saving properties.

If the microcirculation is improved it is obvious that other monitoring techniques should be investigated and evaluated. Infrared thermography is an instrument that displays skin temperature on an image. It has been used to assess nerve injury (2) and neuromusculoskeletal abnormalities in the spinal column (8). In our pain department we use the technique to visualize pain etiology because pain is mostly accompanied by inflammation or sympathetic reactions. The technique has proven very suitable to visualize skin perfusion alterations. We studied its ability to map spinal cord stimulation in eight chronic pain patients with failed back surgery syndrome. All of them experienced good pain relief after percutaneous implantation of a temporary bipolar electrode.

Methods

The patients were examined on five consecutive days under identical standard conditions. Examinations took place at 8 a.m. The patiens were fasted did not intake fruids or smoke. They were acclimatized at an ambient room air temperature of 24 °C. After 15 min of acclimatization a first thermogram was taken. Then, after 10 min consecutive thermograms were taken up to 55 min. To evaluate 25 identical skin points a metallic object was attached at a standard point in the gluteal region. The patient experienced stimulation paresthesias in that painful area. Depending upon the protocol, the patient acclimatized with or without stimulation. Because a long acclimatization period might induce orthosympathetic reflexes, we studied two groups of measurements. In the first group, we studied the temperature differences between 25 min and 15 min of acclimatization. We determined if starting, stopping, not starting or not stopping the stimulator had any affect on skin temperature measurement. In the second group, we studied the same effects but enlarged the observations to the later events after 35, 45 and 55 min of acclimatization. The Wilcoxon's signed test was used to study statistical significance.

Results

Considering $p < 0.05$ as a statistical significant result, we could prove that:

1) Infrared thermography can visualise starting or stopping Spinal Cord Stimulation.

2) Infrared thermography confirms that the effects of continuous stimulation equal the effects of starting the stimulation. Not starting the stimulation is equal to the effects of halting the stimulator.

3) Starting or maintaining the stimulation seems to lower skin temperature to a statistically significant degree and more so than halting or not starting the stimulator.

These results could be demonstrated in both observation groups.

Discussion

If a drop in skin temperature is equivalent to vasocostriction, these results conflict with earlier observations made by Augustinsson (1) and Jacobs (6).

Nevertheless, we note:

1) We can question if infrared thermography can be compared with capillaroscopy and laser flowmetry.

2) Are the effects of Spinal Cord Stimulation in failed back surgery patients equal to those in ischemic patients? Indeed, the etiopathogenesis of these two diseases might be completely differently. The resulting effects of Spinal Cord Stimulation might also be different.

3) Are sympathetic activity and blood flow measurements in the gluteal region comparable with those in the toes?

To answer these questions, a comparative study between infrared thermography of the feet and capillaroscopy with spinal cord stimulation should be performed.

However, the results of this study should encourage us to evaluate the effects of stimulation in different parts of the body other than the painful gluteal region. Such an evaluation could tell us if infrared thermography could be used as a mapping instrument for spinal cord stimulation.

References

1. Augustinsson L, Holm J, Carl A, Carlsson L (1985) Epidural electrical stimulation in severe limb ischemia. Evidence of pain relief, increased blood flow and a possible limb saving effect. Annals of Surgery 202: 104–111
2. Brelsford KL, Uematsu S (1985) Thermographic presentation of cutaneous sensory and vasomotor activity in the injured peripheral nerve. J Neurosurg 62: 711–715
3. Dimitrijevic M, Larsson L (1981) Neural control of gait: clinical neurophysiological aspects. Appl Neurophysiol 44: 152–159
4. Dooley D, Kasprak M (1976) Modification of blood flow of the extremities by electrical stimulation of the nervous system. Southern Medical Journal 69: 1309–1311
5. Hoppenstein R (1975) Percutaneous implantations of chronic spinal cord electrodes for control of intractable pain. Surg Neurol 4: 195–198
6. Jacobs MJ (1990) Foot salvage and improvement of microcascular blood flow as a result of epidural spinal cord electrical stimulation. J Vasc Surgery 12/3: 354–360
7. Meglio M, Cioni B, Dal Lago A, De Santis M, Pola P, Serrichio M (1981) Pain control and improvement of peripheral blood flow following epidural spinal cord stimulation. J Neurosurgery 54: 821–823
8. Plaugher G (1992) Skin temperature assessment for neuromus culoskeletal abnormalities of the spinal column. J of Manipulative and Physiologic Therapeutics 15: 365–381
9. Shealy C, Mortimer J, Hagfors N (1970) Dorsal Column electroanalgesia. J Neurosurg 32: 560–564

Author's address:
J. Devulder, MD
Dept. of Anesthesia
University Hospital of Ghent
De Pintelaan 185
9000 Ghent
Belgium

Management of Critical Limb Ischemia

Definition, epidemiology and pathophysiology of critical limb ischemia

C. Diehm

Department of Internal Medicine and Angiology, Clinic Karlsbad, FRG

"Man is as old as his arteries and the arteries of men with critical leg ischemia are very old. Treating such patients with severe leg ischemia is unglamorous and ultimately a losing battle."
John Dormandy

The evaluation and treatment of critical leg ischemia has been the concern of doctors from a wide range of traditional medical specialities that includes general and vascular surgery, angiology, diabetology, cardiology, hematology, and radiology, depending on both the local circumstances and national traditions.

Few problems in vascular medicine are as challenging as the management of critical limb ischemia (CLI), which may ultimately end in amputation and death. The author of this overview was a member of the working group that discussed and created a Consensus Document on Critical Limb Ischaemia. The basis for this paper is that document published in Circulation in 1991 (12, 29).

Definition of CLI

The earliest and most widely accepted classification of PAOD is that described by Fontaine et al. in the 1950s; he was, at that time, Head of the Department of Surgery in Strasbourg (13). The Fontaine classification based on signs and symptoms has a long tradition and has clearly been found useful by many clinicians. The common meaning of the various stages involving severe ischemia is as follows:

Stage I

Patients in whom the condition is asymptomatic or oligosymptomatic, causing no or only mild and atypical discomfort in a foot or leg.

Stage II

Patients with intermittent claudication, where pain occurs after walking a certain distance and disappears at rest.

Stage III

Patients who complain of rest pain – severe persitent pain, usually localized in the forefoot, which is characteristically intensified when the limb is horizontal and eased by letting the foot hang down. Rest pain often prevents sleep and forces the patient to sleep in a sitting position. Strong analgesia is typically needed to relieve this pain.

Stage IV

Patients who have skin breakdown, causing ulceration or gangrene; it is generally associated with severe rest pain.

In the United States and United Kingdom the term "Critical limb ischaemia" is becoming more widely used than the corresponding Fontaine stages.

In 1982, Bell defined CLI as persistent and severe pain in the foot, at rest, preventing sleep and requiring repeated analgesia (3). The symptom duration was greater than 4 weeks and superficial skin necroses of the foot or interdigital gangrene was required to make the diagnosis. Ankle systolic blood pressure measures were less than 40 – 60 mmHg.

Both of the above definitions formed the basis for the discussion document from the First European Consensus Meeting on CLI in 1990 (12), now superseded by the Second European Consensus Document on Chronic Critical Leg Ischemia (29).

In this document critical limb ischemia in both diabetic and non-diabetic patients is defined by either of the following two criteria (29):

Persistently recurring ischemic rest pain requiring regular adequate analgesia for more than 2 weeks
plus an ankle systolic pressure $\leq$ 50 mmHg
and/or a toe systolic pressure $\leq$ 30 mmHg
or
Ulceration or gangrene of the foot or toes
plus an ankle systolic pressure $\leq$ 50 mmHg
or a toe systolic pressure $\leq$ 30 mmHg.

Critical limb ischemia is therefore ischemia which endangers the limb or part of the distal limb. Acute ischemia should be distinguished from chronic ischemia. Acute ischemia (e.g., that which results from an embolus) will not be discussed here, although it is recognized that for many patients with chronic ischemia there will be episodes of exacerbation, possibly caused by superimposed thrombosis.

A further recommendation was added in the Consensus Document for published reports or for the design and reporting for clinical trials. In addition to the above definition, further evidence of ischemia has to be obtained by angiography and/or one of the following tests:

- toe systolic blood pressure $<$ 30 mmHg
- transcutaneous oxygen pressure of the ischemic area ($tcPO_2$) $\leq$ 10 mmHg and which does not increase with inhalation of oxygen.

In diabetic patients sensory neuropathy alone can cause pain in the absence of ischemia. In these cases the toe systolic pressure measurements should be performed because a false high ankle systolic pressure is frequently found in diabetic patients due to Möckeberg's sclerosis of the media. A pressure of 30 mmHg is based on the fact that the majority of diabetic patients with a toe systolic pressure of less than 30 mmHg have a very poor prognosis (1).

Epidemiology

In comparison with coronary heart disease there is little information on the epidemiology of PAOD and especially of critical limb ischemia (9, 10, 33).

The true incidence of critical limb ischemia and amputations in the general population cannot be easily estimated. More is known about the incidence of amputation in the population of patients with intermittent claudication (Table 1). Two large epidemiological studies, the Framingham study and the Basle study, showed that only 1.6 % and 1.8 % of patients with claudication came to amputation (17, 27, 32). The early hospital mortality following below-knee and above-knee amputations ranges from 3 % to 10 %. The hospital mortality after an above-knee amputation is nearer 20 %. There are six series where longer-term mortality figures are quoted, ranging from 25 – 30 % 2 years after amputation and 50 – 75 % after 5 years (29).

In an extensive literature survey by Dormandy et al. it was found that even patients with claudication, but not critical ischemia, had a more than doubled mortality rate within 5 years, compared to the general population (9). The life expectancy of the people affected is about 10 years shorter than that of a comparable control population.

From the studies referred to and from other data it can be estimated that the prevalence of peripheral arterial occlusive disease (PAOD) in the whole population is 5 % in men aged over 50 years (14). Progression of early stage PAOD to critical limb ischemia occurs in 20 – 30 % of patients over a 6-year period and is estimated to affect 500 – 1000 patients per million adults (19).

For diabetic patients the incidence is higher; probably there is a five times higher risk for diabetics of developing critical leg ischemia. Ulcers and gangrene occur in 10 % of elderly diabetic patients (18).

Concomitant Diseases

Several prospective epidemiological studies revealed that initially healthy persons developing PAOD had a four to six times higher morbidity from coronary heart disease compared with those remaining free of PAOD (5, 7, 16, 24, 27).

Tabelle 1. Epidemiology: Amputations statistics (29)

Incidence of major lower-limb amputations	Incidence *
UK district hospitals	120
Referral to UK limb-fitting centres	200
Veterans Administration (US)	260
Framingham Study (US)	300
Danish Hospital Survey	320

* million population/year
2nd European Consensus Document on Critical Leg Ischemia

Up to 50 % of patients with intermittent claudication and up to 90 % of patients with critical limb ischemia have coronary heart disease (24). The presence of PAOD also identifies a group of patients with high mortality from myocardial infarction. Therefore, it is now recommended that young and middle-aged patients with symptomatic PAOD, including those with critical limb ischemia, should be investigated by means of exercise ECG (if possible), echocardiography, thallium scanning, and coronary arteriography to identify those at high risk. CLI may be aggravated by emboli from the heart and other sites in some patients. It may more commonly result from the combination of arterial occlusive disease and decreased cardiac output, for example, from dysrhythmias, decreased myocardial contractility or drug-induced hypotension (20, 21).

Patients with PAOD are also at increased risk of cerebrovascular disease (16, 24). The early-detected PAOD group in the Basle study developed signs of cerebrovascular disease three times more frequently than the controls. In PAOD patients, concomitant secondary hypertension due to renal artery stenosis is significantly more prevalent than in subjets without PAOD. Kidney disease caused by microangiopathy and/or pyelonephritis is particularly prevalent in the diabetic PAOD group. Patients with CLI are at a particularly high risk of arterial thromboembolism and, if bedridden for some time, venous thromboembolism.

Prognosis can be quantified by the rates of rehabilitation and mortality. In CLI rehabilitation is generally slow due to wound healing by secondary intention in 15 % of the cases. A further 15 % require re-amputation at a higher level, and frequently amputation of the other leg as well (30).

The fate of the patient with PAOD is, to a large extent, determined by the stage of the disease; even in the stage of intermittent claudication there is a threefold excess mortality mainly due to coronary heart disease and stroke.

Pathophysiology of CLI

In recent years, there has been increasing interest in the pathophysiology of critical limb ischemia because it is hoped that greater understanding of such disturbances may suggest new approaches to prevention and treatment, as much of our present treatment is still very empirical. Nevertheless, the pathophysiology of CLI in man remains to be established.

Pathophysiology of the macrocirculation

CLI occurs when stenosis or obstruction of one or more major arteries increases proximal limb vascular resistance so severely that the blood flow to the limb can no longer meet the nutritive requirements of the resting limb tissues.

Atherosclerosis is the underlying cause of PAOD in more than 90 % of the cases, although inflammatory arteries, which affects medium-sized arteries, or diabetic microangiopathy can also play a central role in this disease. In atherosclerosis, plaques form within the intima of the artery and there is proliferation of the cells in the vessel wall, accompanied by the formation of thrombi. These changes narrow the vessel lumen thus impeding blood flow and perfusion pressure to the more distal circulation, giving a reduced flow to the microcirculation. CLI occurs when arterial stenoses or occlusions impair blood flow to an extent where, despite compensatory mechanisms such as collateral formation, nutritive requirements of the microcirculation cannot be met. This usually results from the presence of multilevel disease or occlusion of critical collaterals.

Platelets and leucocytes (activated as they pass over ulcerated or ruptured atherosclerotic plaques or in poststenotic vortices) and impaired prostacyclin-like and fibrinolytic activity may promote arterial thrombosis.

Pathophysiology of the Microcirculation

The microcirculation comprises the arterioles, capillaries, venules, and initial lymphatic vessels. The importance of the microcirculation in critical limb ischemia is highlighted by the significant overlap between ankle/brachial pressure indices in patients with varying stages of PAOD. This overlap indicates that it is not just the macrocirculation that is responsible for the development of the signs and symptoms of PAOD and ultimately critical limb ischemia, but that changes in the distal microcirculation are of considerable importance in determining skin perfusion (34).

New techniques that have recently improved understanding of the skin microcirculation include capillaroscopy, fluorescence videomicroscopy (4) Laser-Doppler fluxmetry, and $tcPO_2$ measurements (15).

Combinations of these techniques give more information than any of the techniques used alone.

Compensatory responses to a reduced arterial blood flow include reflex dilatation and the development of a collateral circulation. However, the flow rate and the perfusion pressure in the distal circulation ultimately fall. This leads to claudication and later to rest pain and gangrene.

Although the exact sequence of events leading to reduced capillary perfusion in PAOD is unknown, mechanisms involved include the collapse of pre-capillary arterioles because of low transluminal pressure, arteriolar vasospasm, abnormal vasomotion, microthrombosis, collapse of capillaries due to interstitial edema, capillary occlusion by endothelial cell swelling, platelet aggregation, rigid adhesive leucocytes, rigid red cells or blood cell/platelet aggregates and local activation of the immune system. Fibrinogen levels are elevated in CLI, which further increases plasma viscosity and erythrocyte aggregation. Fibrinogen levels are increased by smoking, diabetes, and infection. The activation of platelets and leucocytes and damage of the vascular endothelium may result in vicious cycles between these cells via a range of mechanisms and mediators.

Skin microcirculation and disruption of normal vasomotion

Skin microvessels can be subdivided into thermoregulatory and nutritional vessels. Although the relative distribution of blood flow between the non-nutritional thermoregulatory vascular bed and the nutritional vessels varies considerably between different skin areas, nutritional capillaries usually carry less than 15 % of total blood flow in the foot (4). CLI occurs when a maldistribution of microcirculatory blood flow in the skin reduces the perfusion of the nutritive capillaries, which eventually leads to tissue necrosis (Fig. 1) (4, 29). Total capillary blood flow is not the critical factor – in fact, in CLI total blood flow is often paradoxically increased because of arteriolar vasodilatation (22). Therefore, the ultimate cause of CLI is presumably maldistribution of skin microcirculation in addition to reduced total blood flow.

There is also a circadian rhythm of blood flow to the foot, with the lowest values occuring at night, partly explaining why ischemic rest pain appears to worsen during night (2).

Vasomotion (low frequency waves of blood flow through the capillaries) is a normal phenomenon that occurs as the result of alternate constriction and relaxation of precapillary vessels. This vasomotion helps to distribute blood evenly throughout the microcirculation (31). Laser-Doppler flowmetry of the skin has demonstrated an abnormal pattern on vasomotion in CLI (31). In healthy limbs, vasomotion consists of low frequency waves of about three cycles per minute in the foot. In CLI, high-frequency flow waves of about 21 cycles per minute appear, which are only rarely seen in a normal limb. Loss of vasomotion may contribute to maldistribution of flow in the microcirculation, which causes underperfusion of some capillaries and no perfusion in others (29). Interestingly, the pathological pattern of vasomotion can be corrected by percutaneous catheter procedures.

Impairment of blood rheology

In the healthy limb, the intrinsic flow properties of blood probably have minimal influence on blood flow through the microcirculation. Blood has a low viscosity, and

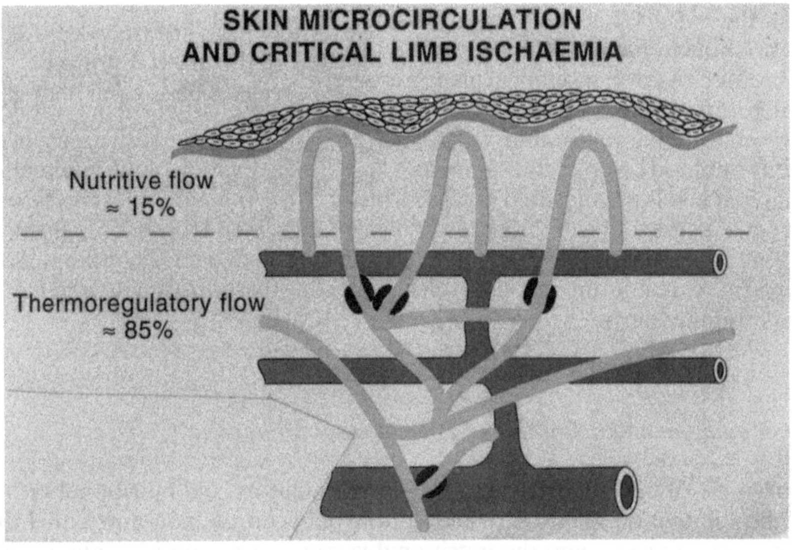

Fig. 1 Skin microcirculation and critical limb ischemia (8).

normal erythrocytes are readily deformed by physiological shear stresses. Erythrocytes and leucocytes must deform to pass through nutritive capillaries, because their diameter is wider than that of the narrower capillaries. In the normal microcirculation they deform easily under high perfusion pressures and high shear stresses, even though leucocytes are much more rigid than erythrocytes (29).

The filterability of blood through micropore filters which mimic nutritive capillaries (pore diameter 5 μm) is decreased in PAOD, with a greater impairment in CLI than in patients with intermittent claudication. This impaired blood filterability in PAOD is thought to reflect the influence of the accompanying leucocytosis, hyperfibrinogenemia and increased plasma viscosity (8, 20, 21). There is no apparent loss of erythrocyte deformability when filtration methods are used to assess leucocytefree, washed erythrocytes from PAOD patients, where the influence of leucocytes and fibrinogen has been excluded.

In PAOD, blood viscosity increases due to an increased hematocrit and raised plasma fibrinogen level, changes that result partly from the influence of cigarette smoking. In critical limb ischemia, a further increase in fibrinogen due to ischemic necrosis, and occasionally infection, causes a more marked increase in plasma viscosity and erythrocyte aggregation. A reduced perfusion pressure and shear stress together cause a reduction in erythrocyte deformation and an increase in aggregation. An increased bulk viscosity then results from this decreased deformation and an increased erythrocyte aggregation (20, 21).

The additional consequences of ischemia such as acidosis, hyperosmolarity and calcium accumulation further impair erythrocyte deformability. It is likely that blood flow in the nutritive microcirculation is adversely affected by the changes in blood rheology seen in PAOD patients (Fig. 2).

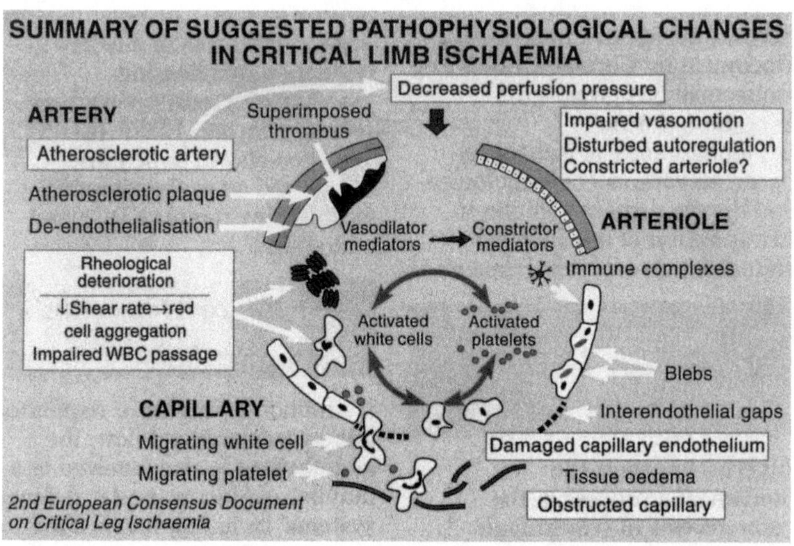

Fig. 2. Factors affecting blood rheology in critical leg ischemia (8).

Platelets in CLI

Peripheral arterial occlusive disease has been shown to cause a number of platelet abnormalities. A combination of both in vitro and in vivo studies using blood from PAOD patients has shown an increased turnover of platelets due to a shortened survival time, an increase in the mean platelet volume, a decreased platelet count, and increased platelet aggregation (6, 11, 20, 25, 28, 35).

Activated platelets express adhesion receptors and produce a variety of release products, which may promote vasoconstriction and fibrin formation and inhibit fibrinolysis (Fig. 3).

Abnormal activation of platelets is thought to be important in the pathogenesis of critical limb ischemia for a number of reasons. Activated platelets may encourage the progression of atherosclerosis by releasing platelet-derived growth factor (PDGF), which has been shown in vitro to stimulate smooth muscle cell proliferation. Activated platelets may aggravate tissue ischemia by releasing chemical mediators such as serotonin (5-HT) and thromboxane A_2 (TX A_2) which cause vasoconstriction of arteries. PAOD also causes a significant elevation in plasma levels of the platelet release product betathromboglobulin (β-TH), which is a marker of in vivo platelet activation.

Finally, the increase in platelet aggregation caused by PAOD is likely to be important in the pathogenesis of critical limb ischemia. Platelet aggregation in PAOD patients is accentuated by exercise that induces ischemia. Increased levels of platelet aggregates in the circulation correlate with the increase in plasma fibrinogen, seen in PAOD.

Fibrin formation plays a major role in arterial thrombosis. There are data showing that in toes of CLI patients up to 90 % of 30 – 50 micrometer precapillary arterioles are occluded by microthrombi (29).

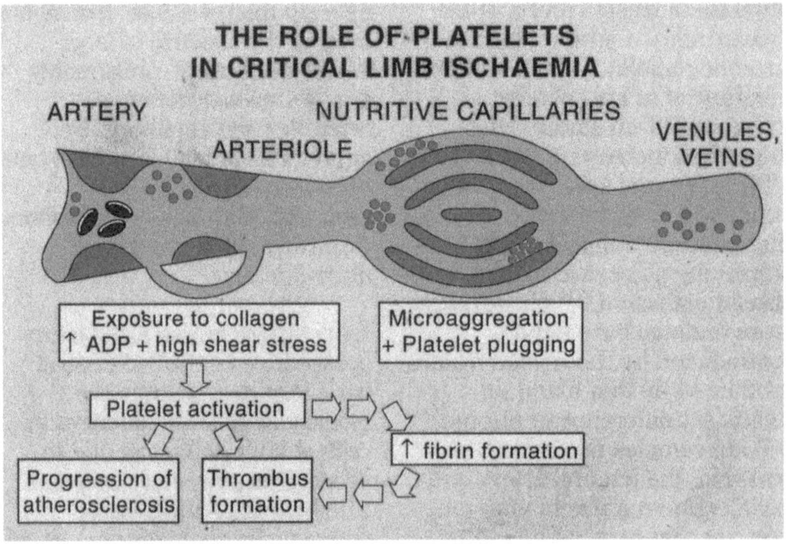

Fig. 3. The role of platelets in critical limb ischemia (8).

The role of leucocytes in critical limb ischemia

There is an increased evidence that white blood cells may play an important role in both the progression of atherosclerosis and in the pathogenesis of critical limb ischemia (20, 21, 26). Patients with CLI have leucocyte activation, as shown by filtration studies, which is normalized after surgery. Leucocyte activation may occur as cells pass over an ulcerated atherosclerotic plaque, partly due to a chemical stimulus from contact with the damaged vessel lining and partly due to a physical stimulus of shear stresses at the site of the arterial stenosis. In vitro studies have demonstrated that leucocytes become activated when they are exposed to high shear forces. The presence of activated platelets has also been shown to activate neutrophil leucocytes.

The reduced filterability of activated leucocytes is likely to lead to plugging of nutritive capillaries within the microcirculation. Activated leucocytes also release a number of chemical mediators, including PAF, leukotrienes, superoxide anions, and proteolytic enzymes (23). Leucocyte activation products have the combined effects of causing platelet aggregation, vasospasm and endothelial damage, all of which may contribute to the pathogenesis of critical limb ischemia. Thus, the leucocyte may be a possible therapeutic target for the treatment of CLI.

The role of the endothelium

PAOD causes a number of changes in the normal function of the endothelium, changes which are thought to be important in both the progression of atherosclerosis and the pathogenesis of critical limb ischemia. Elevated release of von Willebrand

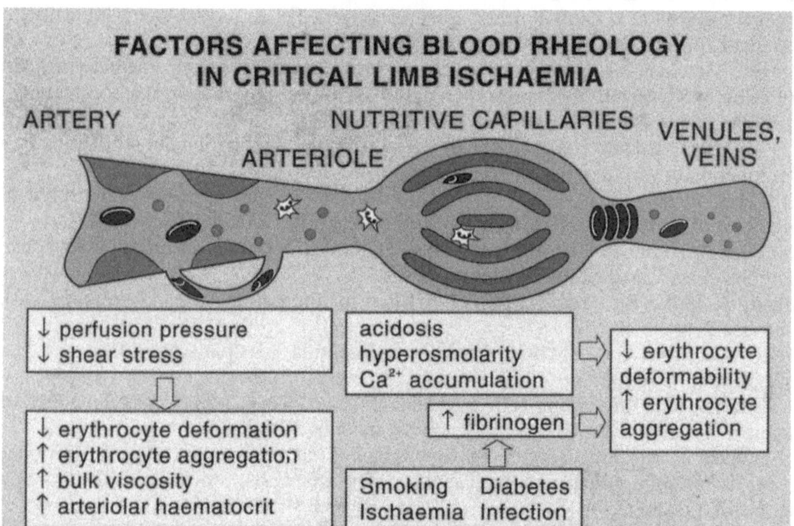

Fig. 4. Summary of suggested pathophysiological changes in critical leg ischemia at different levels of the circulation (WBC, White Blood Cell (29)).

factor (vWF) has been reported in PAOD. This may promote platelet adhesion to the subendothelium and endothelium-derived constricting factor (EDGF) stimulating vasoconstriction. Hypoxic damage to the endothelium is thought to result in an imbalance in the secretion of EDRF and EDGF. A reduced production of EDRF allows leukotrienes released from activated leucocytes to provoke vasospasm, which further might exacerbate CLI (20, 21).

To summarize, the ultimate cause of critical limb ischemia is likely to be the maldistribution of blood to the skin microcirculation in addition to a reduction in total blood flow. The sequence of events leading to a decrease in the capillary perfusion is not yet established totally but several potential causes can presently be suggested (8):

- collapse of precapillary arterioles because of low transmural pressure
- arterial vasospasm
- abnormal vasomotion
- microthrombosis
- collapse of capillaries due to interstitial oedema
- capillary occlusion by endothelial cell swelling, platelet aggregates, rigid and adhesive lucocytes or rigid red cells
- local activation of the immune system.

References

1. Apelquist J, Castenfors J, Larson J, Stenstrom A, Agardh CD (1989) Prognostic value of systolic ankle and toe pressure levels in outcome of diabetic foot ulcer. Diabetes Care 12: 6, 115–120
2. Bartoli V, Dorigo B, Tedeschi E et al. (1970) Circadian periodicity of calf blood flow in subjects with intermittent claudication. Angiology 21: 215
3. Bell PRF (1982) The definition of critical ischemia of a limb. Working Party of the International Vascular Symposium. Br J Surg 69: 52
4. Bollinger A, Fagrell B (1990) Clinical Capillaroscopy: A Guide to its Use in Clinical Research and Practice. Toronto, Hogrefe & Huber
5. Brothing S, Metelitsa VI, Barth W et al. (1976) Prevalence of ischemic heart disease, arterial hypertension and intermittent claudication and distribution of risk factors among middle aged men in Moscow and Berlin. Cor et Vasa 18: 104
6. Cella G, Zahavi J, de Haas HA et al. (1979) Beta-thromboglobulin, platelet production time and platelet function in vascular disease. Br Haematol 43: 127–136
7. Criqui MH, Coughlin SS, Fronek A (1985) Noninvasively diagnosed peripheral arterial disease as a predictor of mortality: results from a prospective study. Circulation 71: 768
8. Critical Limb Ischemia. A Slide Lecture Kit (3), Lowe GDO (ed) Produced by professional Postgraduate Services, Europe Ltd, Worthing UK
9. Dormandy J, Mahir M, Ascady et al. (1989) Fate of the patients with chronic leg ischemia. J Cardiovasc Surg 30: 50–57
10. Dormandy JA, Stock G (eds) (1990) Critical Leg Ischemia – Its pathophysiology and Management. Berlin: Springer Verlag
11. Evans G, Irvine WT (1966) Long-term arterial graft patency in relation to platelet adhesiveness, biochemical factors and anticoagulant therapy. Lancet ii: 353–355
12. First European Consensus Document on Critical Limb Ischemia (1990) In: Critical Leg Ischemia: Its Pathophysiology and Management. (Dormandy JA, Stock G, eds) Berlin: Springer Verlag, pp 1XXLV111
13. Fontaine R, Dubost C (1954) Les greffes vasculaires. Rapport au Congrès de Chirurgie, Paris, 226ff
14. Fowkes FGR (1988) Epidemiology of atherosclerotic arterial disease in the lower limbs. Eur J Vasc Surg 2: 283–291

15. Franzeck UK, Talke P, Bernstein EF, Golbranson FL, Fronek A (1982) Transcutaneous PO_2 measurements in health and peripheral arterial occlusive disease. Surgery 91: 156–163
16. Hertzer NR, Raven EG, Young JR et al. (1984) Coronary artery disease in peripheral vascular patients – a classification of 1000 coronary angiograms and results of surgical management. Ann Surg 199: 223
17. Kannel WB, Skinner JJ, Schwartz MJ, Shurtleff D (1970) Intermittent claudication-incidence in the Framingham Study. Circulation XLI: 875
18. Krolowski AS, Warram JH (1991) Epidemiology of diabetes mellitus, in Marble A, Krall LP, Bradley RS, Christlieb AR, Soulidner JS (eds) Joslin's Diabetes mellitus (ed 12) Philadelphia, Pa, Lea & Ferbiger, pp 12–42
19. Lasila R, Lepäntalo M, Lindfors O (1986) Peripheral arterial disease – natural outcome. Acta med Scand 220: 295–298
20. Lowe GDO, Reavey MM, Johnston RV et al. (1979) Increased platelet aggregates in vascular and nonvascular illness: correlation with plasma fibrinogen and effect of ancrod. Thromb Res 14: 377–386
21. Lowe GDO (1990) Pathophysiology of critical limb ischaemia, in Dormandy J, Stock G (eds) Critical leg ischemia: its Pathophysiology and management. Berlin, Springer-Verlag, pp 17–30
22. Mc Ewan AL, Ledingham IMcA (1971) Blood flow characteristics and tissue nutrition in apparently ischemic feet. Br Med J iii: 220
23. Mehta JL (1989) The role of leucocytes in critical limb ischemia. In: The Pathophysiology of Critical Limb Ischaemia and Pharmacological Intervention with a Stable Prostacyclin Analogue: RMS Services, pp 13–17
24. Müller-Bühl U, Diehm C, Sieben U et al. (1987) Prävalenz und Risikofaktoren von peripherarterieller Verschlußkrankheit und koronarer Herzkrankheit. Vasa, Suppl 21: 1–53
25. Murphy EA, Mustard JF (1962) Coagulation tests and platelet economy in atherosclerotic and control subjects. Circulation 25: 124–125
26. Nash GB, Thomas PRS, Dormandy JA (1969) Abnormal flow properties of white blood cells in patients with severe ischaemia of the leg. Br Med J 296: 1699–1701
27. Nissen C, Schweizer W (1981) Koronare Herzkrankheit (1981) In: Basler Studie. (Widmer LK, Stähelin HB, Nissen C, da Silva A, eds) Bern: Hans Huber
28. O'Brien JR Etherington MD, Jamieson S et al. (1975) Blood changes in atherosclerosis after myocardial infarction and venous thrombosis. Thromb Diath Haem 34: 483–497
29. Second European Consensus Document on Chronic Critical Leg Ischemia (1991) Circulation 84, 4: 1-21
30. Stirnemann P, Nachbur B, Oesch A (1986) In: Angiologie 86 (Widmer LK, Zempf E (eds)) Bern: Hans Huber
31. Seifert H, Jaeger K, Bollinger A (1988) Analysis of flow motion by the laser-Doppler technique in patients with peripheral arterial occlusive desease. Int Microcirc Clin Exp 7: 223–236
32. Widmer LK, Biland L, da Silva A (1985) Risk profile and occlusive peripheral artery disease (OPAD), in Proceedings of the 13th International Congress of Angiology, Athens 9–14 June
33. Wolfe JHN (1986) Defining the outcome of critical ischemia: a one year prospective study. Brit J Surg 73: 321
34. Yao JST (1970) Haemodynamic studies in peripheral arterial disease. Br J Surg 57: 761–766
35. Zahavi J, Zahavi M (1975) Enhanced platelet release reaction, shortened platelet survival time, and increased platelet aggregation and plasma thromboxane B_2 in chronic obstructive arterial disease. Thromb Diath Haem 34: 483–497

Author's address:
Prof. Curt Diehm, MD PhD
Department of Internal Medicine and Angiology
Rehabilitation Clinic Karlsbad
Affiliated Academic Hospital of the University of Heidelberg
D-76307 Karlsbad-Langensteinbach
FRG

Prostanoids in the treatment of critical limb ischemia

J. D. Gruß

Department of Vascular Surgery, Kurhess. Diakonissenhaus Kassel, Germany
(Head: Prof. Dr. J. D. Gruß)

Introduction

Vascular surgery may claim to be one of the first applications in the endless history of prostanoids. When attending a congress in Japan, I remember seeing a number of young male patients with stages III and IV inoperable arterial occlusive disease being treated with prostaglandin E_1 at the University Vascular Surgery Clinic Nagoya (S. Shionoya). Continous intra-arterial therapy was carried out with a timer-controlled roller pump so that the patient received on average 0.2 ng PGE_1/kg body weight/min. I have to admit that I had only heard of this compound once during my studies and without any connection with a therapeutic active constituent. The treatment results reported by Shionoya appeared to me so convincing that I was able, with the assistance of the manufacturer Ono and the support of S. Shionoya himself and Flughafen AG Frankfurt to import the compound into Germany during the following months and years in a continuous refrigeration chain, in order to collect initial experience in inoperable stage III and IV arteriosclerosis patients (30, 42). Attempts to publish our first clinical experience with PGE_1 in a serious German-language journal failed as a result of their absence of credibility, so that a first communication was only possible in 1978 in the form of a reader's letter in the Deutsche Medizinische Wochenschrift and then only on the recommendation of my teacher, G. Schettler (19).

A subsequent literature study, as so often happens, revealed that this was in no sense a new discovery. The presence of prostaglandins in human seminal fluid had already been detected in 1930 by Kurzrock and Lieb (29). The authors were able to show that this compound had a stimulating influence on the smooth muscle and promoted rise to uterine contractions. The same compound was detected in 1933 by Goldblatt (18) and in 1934 by Euler (14, 15) in the seminal vesicle of sheep, goats, and monkeys. The name prostaglandin dates back to Euler himself as he thought it was a secretion from the prostate gland. Euler recognized that prostaglandins were lipids, i.e., fatty acids, which he was able to obtain in pure form by ether extraction. The structural formula of E-prostaglandins has been known since 1976. In the same year, PGI_2 (prostacyclin), a compound formed in the vascular wall, was discovered by Moncada and Vane and described as a physiological antagonist of thromboxane A_2 formed in platelet cells (31 – 34).

Even the intra-arterial treatment of advanced peripheral arterial occlusive disease (pAOD) by the administration of prostaglandins is not a Japanese discovery. All credit is however due to the Japanese authors for having studied the Western literature better than their European colleagues. Two Swedish papers by Carlson and Erikson from 1972 and 1973 had dealt with the intraarterial treatment of advanced pAOD with prostaglandin E_1 (7, 8). A further Scandinavian paper from 1959 had already reported the effect of intravenous PGE_1 infusion in subjects with no vascular damage

(3, 4). Clinical interest was initially concentrated on the compound PGE_1 mainly because the chemical instability of PGI_2 prevented its clinical use on any significant scale. The stable prostacyclin analogues ilomedin and taprosten are no longer subject to this disadvantage, but they do involve serious unwanted side-effects which complicate their clinical use (27, 35, 41, 47).

The following effects of prostanoids (PGE_1 and PGI_2 analogues) can be regarded as having been reliably established. Their effect on the smooth muscles cause dilation of the arterioles and a slackening of the precapillary sphincters (4, 40, 41). Platelet activation is inhibited with a consequent reduction in adhesion and aggregation (13, 41, 45). Thromboxane synthesis is also reduced. In contrast to PGI_2 and its analogues, PGE_1 inhibits neutrophil activation and, in consequence, the release of oxygen radicals and lysosomal enzymes (16, 35). Fibrinolytic activity is increased by stimulation of the plasminogen activator, thus reducing blood plasma viscosity. The inhibition of platelet aggregation and adhesion and the simultaneous inhibition or erythrocyte aggregation, accompanied by an improvement in erythrocyte flexibility, also reduces corpuscular blood viscosity (9, 45). Taken overall, therefore, prostanoids have a favorable effect on the rheological properties of the blood. Oxygen and glucose utilization is increased, thus improving cell metabolism at the periphery (9, 40). In addition to these ad hoc effects prostanoids inhibit proliferation of the smooth muscle cells and reduce lipid deposits in the vascular wall so that it is reasonable to speak of an overall favorable effect on the advancing progress of the basic condition (43–46).

Clinical applications

In light of these introductory comments we first used prostanoids in vascular surgery on patients suffering from a stage III and IV arterial occlusive disease, i.e., what can in fact be described as conservative therapy in the strict sense. The therapeutic results on our first 105 patients who received intra-arterial treatment are shown in Table 1, although this does not of course constitute a prospective, randomized trial (see above).

In the relatively small group of endangiitis patients, 71 % of the stage III or IV patients could be restored to stage IIb (Table 2). Amputation of the thigh was necessary only in 11 % of the patients. In the group of patients with arteriosclerosis accompanied by diabetes mellitus regression to stage IIb was only possible in 30 % of the cases, whereas amputation of the thigh was unavoidable in 34 %. The results obtained in arteriosclerosis patients without diabetes mellitus occupied an intermediate position between those of the first two groups: a regression to stage IIb was obtained in 47 % of cases, while amputation of the thigh was still required in 20 % of patients.

Table 1. Results of a single PGE_1 treatment over a mean 38-day period administered to 105 patients with arterial occlusive disease (stage III/IV) at the time of discharge from hospital

Number of patients	Mortality	Amputation	Limb salvage
105	9	25	71

The overall results were therefore that of 105 patients threatened with amputation of the lower limbs, 71 retained the functional use of those limbs; this applied to 50 % of the patients at the 6-month stage after only a single cycle of intra-arterial treatment (Table 3) (1, 19, 20, 39).

In the meantime, we have been informed that intermittent administration of PGE_1 is more effective than continuous administration. Since then we have administered 10 – 20 μg over an 8-h period, followed by 15000 IU heparin only, administered with an injection pump over the remaining 16 h of the day. Continuous administration had already led to a clearly marked reduction in clinical efficacy as a result of a rise in platelet concentration and a reduction in the number of receptors on the platelet surface.

Authorization of the use of PGE_1 for the treatment of advanced peripheral arterial occlusive disease in stages III and IV was granted by the Federal Health Office in 1984. In addition to a wide range of pharmacological and physiological research results, this authorization was based in the final instance on the uncontrolled clinical trial referred to above. The results of this trial were of course subsequently confirmed by prospective, randomized, intra-arterial and intravenous therapeutic trials. Since 70 – 80 % of the PGE_1 compound undergoes metabolism even during the first passage through the lungs, the initial favorable experience with the intravenous form of administration could not be explained. Only the discovery of the stable metabolite 13,14-dihydro-PGE_1 provided a rational basis for the intravenous form of administration (2, 5, 6, 12, 28, 36, 48, 49).

Table 2. Results of a single PGE_1 treatment of 105 patients suffering from inoperable arterial occlusive disease at the time of discharge from hospital

	Group 1 Endangiitis obliterans	Group 2 Arteriosclerosis with diabetes mellitus	Group 3 Arteriosclerosis without diabetes mellitus
No. of patients	28	47	30
Regression from Stage III/IV to Stage IIb	21 (71 %)	14 (30 %)	14 (47 %)
Amputations (total)	12 (43 %)	25 (53 %)	10 (33 %)
Minor amputations	9 (32 %)	9 (19 %)	4 (13 %)
Major limb amputations	3 (11 %)	16 (34 %)	6 (20 %)

Table 3. Results recorded after 6 months of a single PGE_1 treatment over a mean period of 38 days in patients with inoperable arterial occlusive disease

No. of patients	Mortality	Major limb amputations	Repeated treatment	Limb salvage
71	12	4	5	50

Long-standing acute arterial occlusive disease due to embolism or thrombosis

Vascular surgeons continually find themselves faced with acute arterial vascular disease, necessitating thrombectomy or embolectomy with a need to treat obliteration of the main arteries with no or only minimal reflux. The pulse is no longer palpable on the back of the foot within 2 – 3 h after the operation. Similar failures occur during aspiration embolectomy with or without PTA and lysis. In vascular surgery such cases have come to represent the primary field of action for adjuvant intra-arterial PGE_1 therapy. We have found that after a second thrombectomy, performed a few hours after the first and the insertion of an intra-arterial catheter for PGE_1 therapy, the pulse very often remains palpable and the limb can be saved. As a result of a further improvement in this procedure, it is now our frequent practice to administer an 8-h intra-arterial PGE_1 infusion (20 μg) alternating with a 16-h urokinase infusion (1 million IU) making sure that the fibrinogen level does not fall below 150 mg. This therapeutic regime has on occasion to be continued over an 8 – 10 day period. No prospective randomized trial results on this therapeutic concept are yet available.

Adjuvant PGE_1 treatment in femoro-distal venous bypass

The trend of the reconstructive vascular surgery is moving all the time toward the periphery and in the direction of femoro-pedal bypasses, and bypasses on isolated tibial artery segments are carried out today on a routine basis in clinical practice. Borderline reconstructions on stage III and IV limbs, threatened with amputation, together with a borderline outflow tract, to a large extent involve the risk of immediate and early occlusion, even with the use of vein grafts and with use of the in situ technique. Even after vascular surgical revision the fate of any such long peripheral bypass is statistically inferior to that of a non-revised, primary open transplant. The primary 5-year permeability of femoro-tibial in situ bypasses in our hospital is 64.9 %, whereas the result of transplants after successful revision has been reduced to 39.5 %.

The idea of an additional PGE_1 therapy arose from consideration of its pharmacological mechanism of action. It was thought that maximum vasodilation would reduce peripheral resistance. The effect on the platelets would then prevent aggregation and adhesion of platelets to suture lines, clip suture sites and venous valves. The effect of adjuvant PGE_1 therapy has been examined in a prospective randomized trial on 99 consecutive femoro-tibial, in situ bypass operations. 0.2 ng PGE_1/kg body weight/min together with 15000 IU heparin was administered continuously (i.e., not intermittently) over a 10-day period using a fine plastic catheter which was inserted in a high venous branch, to the 50 patients in the PGE_1 group, while the control group received a similar administration of 15000 IU heparin only. Immediate arterial occlusion occurred in 4 % of the patients in the PGE_1 group as compared with 14.3 % in the control group. The difference was accordingly statistically significant (17, 22, 24).

Adjuvant PGE_1 therapy in femoro-distal alloplastic bypasses

A study was made in a prospective, randomized, multicenter trial on whether a reduction in immediate and early occlusion could be obtained by an adjuvant, intravenous administration of PGE_1 in alloplastic infrapopliteal bypasses. PGE_1 therapy was carried out in this case by central access, 40 μg being infused over a 2-h period at 10-h intervals. The patients of the PGE_1-group received 2 x 40 μg PGE_1 during 24 h over a 10-day period. The patients in the control group received only physiological salt infusions in accordance with the same therapeutic scheme. Both groups were treated in identical fashion with 500 mg ASA and 2 x 7500 IU heparin. Statistical assessment of the results in terms of immediate and early occlusions revealed no significant differences in favor of the study group. It is open to question whether the dose and the duration of the PGE_1 treatment were sufficient in this case.

Adjuvant PGE_1 therapy in three level occlusions

Eighty-three patients suffering from a so-called triple occlusion received PGE_1 treatment during a prospective, randomized and controlled trial. All the patients were clinical stage III and/or IV cases. All the patients presented a fairly clearly marked stenosis or occlusion of the terminal aorta and the pelvic arteries with an open profunda femoris artery and in all cases there was an angiographic finding of extensive occlusion of the femoro-popliteal vascular section. In none of the cases was a completely permeable, freely patent artery present in the lower leg, so that the prior conditions for a peripheral vascular reconstruction were not initially available.

All the patients were treated by means of profundaplasty. In 62 % of patients this was performed as part of an aorto-femoral reconstruction, in most cases involving the use of an 8 mm knitted Dacron prosthesis. In 21 % of cases the profundaplasty operation was carried out exclusively from a high inguinal incision, specifically in those cases where stenoses or occlusions of the iliac arteries were treated by balloon-dilatation preoperatively. Dacron or PTFE patch material was used with equal frequency. All the patients receiving an aorto-femoral bypass simultaneously underwent a lumbar sympathectomy involving the removal of the L2-L5 ganglia. The 42 patients in the prostaglandin group received 60 μg PGE_1 in 250 ml physiological saline solution via a central venous catheter twice daily. An interval of 10 h was allowed to elapse between the two prostaglandin infusions. The 41 patients in the control group received only 250 ml physiological salt solution in accordance with the same therapeutic scheme. Adjuvant therapy was started on the day of the operation and continued for 3 weeks. All the patients also received 0.5 g ASA from the first day after surgery and also 2 x 7500 IU Calciparine from the date of admission. The target parameters for the trial were the disappearance of pain at rest and the healing of the peripheral necroses, i.e., the avoidance of major limb amputations and the retention of a functional limb in stage II.

None of the patients died during the operation or while in hospital. In the PGE_1 group (n = 42) 29 patients received an aorto-femoral bypass and underwent lumbar sympathectomy, while only 13 patients underwent a local profundaplasty operation at the inguinal level. In the control group, 33 patients required an aorto-femoral bypass with lumbar sympathectomy and only eight patients were treated with an inguinal profundaplasty operation. In the PGE_1 group (n = 42) 26 patients (61 %) were restored to stage II. The pain at rest disappeared completely in these patients so that no further analgesics had to be administered. The peripheral necroses also healed completely. An equivalent result in the control group (n = 41) was obtained in only 15 patients (35 %). The difference between the two groups was statistically significant. Major limb amputations were unavoidable in two cases in the PGE_1 group and in two cases in the control group. There was no statistically significant difference between the two groups in this respect. Minor amputations, i.e., amputations which left the foot functional without prosthetic assistance (borderline toe and forefoot amputations) were required in seven cases in the PGE_1 group and in nineteen cases in the control group. This difference was found to be highly statistically significant. There were no differences between the two groups in the numbers of patients receiving inguinal surgery and those requiring an aorto-femoral bypass with sympathectomy (25, 26).

Trash phenomena

Trash phenomena occur in patients will extensive atheromatous changes in the terminal aorta and pelvic arteries, in particular in the case of arteriosclerotic, parietally thrombosed aortic and pelvic artery aneurysms and, here again, most frequently during surgical manipulations. This gives rise, in most cases during surgery but also spontaneously on occasion, to embolization of the atheromatous material (trash) in the peripheral limb arteries and in the mesenteric and lumbar arteries. This embolization can then cause disseminated necroses of the skin and muscles and necrosis of the colon and spinal cord.

Over a 20-year period (1971 – 1991), 1164 patients were operated on in our hospitals for infra-renal abdominal aortic aneurysm. The surgical technique used was broadly standard: the introduction of a peridural catheter, median upper and lower abdominal laparotomy, systemic heparinization with 5000 IU before clamping, in each case the peripheral clamps being applied before the central clamp. 896 patients received a bifurcation bypass and 268 patients a tubular prosthesis. In all cases the outflow tract was controlled with a Fogarty catheter and the peripheral area filled with heparin-saline solution. Low-dose heparinization was continued during the post-operative phase.

During the above observation period we encountered 19 cases of severe trash syndrome, on 17 occasions in patients suffering from aneurysms and only twice in patients with aorto-iliac arterial occlusion disease. All the patients had an exceptionally painful, spotted, livid blue discoloration of the skin of both legs, the buttocks and lower abdomen. The skin was cold, although the pulse on the dorsum of the foot was initially palpable. In all cases blood pressure was high. During the first few hours after surgery the pulse in the foot disappeared, followed later by the popliteal pulse. In five cases an unsuccessful attempt was made at a unilateral or bilateral thrombectomy. The pulse in the dorsum of the foot was again palpable for a few hours, but then disappeared after a further few hours in spite of therapeutic heparinization. All the patients required pain therapy with bupivacaine and/or morphine because of the exceptionally intense pain. Relaporotomy was necessary in eight cases because of severe abdominal pain symptoms. In spite of pulsation of the mesenterial arteries, six patients presented a clearly marked colon necrosis and, as a result, colon resection was unavoidable. Only two patients presented spots of cyanosis of the intestinal wall, thus indicating the possibility of recovery. The histological finding after colon resection revealed the presence of embolized trash material into the small arteries of the bowel.

A paraparesis, caused by embolization in the lumbar and spinal arteries, was present in two patients during the post-operative phase. Both these patients died. The presence of trash material in the spinal arteries was detected during post-mortem examination. No cases of embolism in the renal arteries which might have been caused by the direct application of a clamp in the infrarenal area were observed in our patients.

Seven patients were treated between 1971 and 1980. Treatment consisted of complete heparinization, hemodilution and intravenous administration of vasoactive compounds such as naftidrofuryl and pentoxifylline. Three of the patients died within the first 3 days after surgery. In all three cases a colon resection had previously been carried out, two of the patients were suffering from paraparesis, and one had also undergone thigh amputation. Four of the patients survived, two after colon resection and one after bilateral amputation.

Between 1981 and 1991, we treated 12 patients with a severe trash phenomenon. In these patients high doses of intravenous PGE_1 were administered immediately after the diagnosis had been made. These patients also received 2 x 60 μg systemic PGE_1 over a period of 2 h, followed by heparinization in increasing doses (15000, 25000, 35000 and 40000 IU) again by systemic administration.

All 12 patients survived, three of them after relaporotomy; in one case colon resection was necessary. In addition, one thigh amputation and one knee exarticulation were unavoidable. Both patients, after local thrombectomy, received alternating intra-arterial administrations of PGE_1 and urokinase (see above). A diffuse embolization of trash material was detected in the muscular blood vessels of the amputated limbs. This clinical study report covering two separate intervals of time cannot claim to be a randomized, control trial and cannot therefore justify statistical analysis (23).

Phlegmasia cerulea dolens

There is general agreement today in angiology and vascular surgery that phlegmasia cerulea dolens is an emergency situation in vascular surgery for which immediate thrombectomy is the treatment of choice. It normally affects the lower limbs. Phlegmasia cerulea dolens in the arm is extremely rare. The pathophysiological background of phlegmasia consists of a thrombotic occlusion of the complete venous cross-section. By reflex action and as a result of a rise in pressure in the compartment, this gives rise to involvement of the arterial section of the vascular system and progressive ischaemia. Venous thrombectomy is generally sufficient to interrupt this vicious circle, i.e., by decompression and recovery of the pulses in the foot. There are however cases in which a rapidly advancing so-called venous gangrene develops in spite of a successful thrombectomy and extensive fasciotomy. This so-called venous gangrene, in fact, naturally involves a progressive development of necrosis as a result of an insufficient arterial blood supply.

In six such cases, five affecting the lower and one an upper limb, a fine plastic catheter was introduced into the artery and continuous, intra-arterial PGE_1 perfusion carried out with 0.2 ng/kg/min. Necrosis development in four of the five lower limbs proved to be reversible within a few hours so that a major limb amputation was required in only one case. The patient with the rare phlegmasia cerulea dolens of an upper limb died as a result of a fulminating pulmonary embolism before the outcome of the arm could be assessed (21).

Ergotism

Interruption of the vasospastic reaction in ergotism can be achieved in most cases by discontinuing the ergotamine-containing medication. Ergotism is most frequently observed as a result of long-term migraine therapy with ergot alkaloids. Some measure of iatrogenic ergotism has been reported in recent years. We have reported data on five cases, four of which had previously received several weeks of prophylactic treatment against thrombosis with a DHE-heparin combined preparation. Four of these patients were multiple trauma cases, while the fifth case was a 38-year-old female patient admitted to the medical intensive care unit for endocarditis. In the four multiple trauma cases the ergotism related to a lower limb, and in the endocarditis patient to an upper limb. In all five cases combined intra-arterial and intravenous treatment was administered because of the fulminating course of the condition.

The intra-arterial PGE_1 therapy (0.25 g PGE_1/kg body weight/min) was administered on a continuous basis. This was combined with the systemic administration of intravenous PGE_1 in large doses. After a few hours the angiography revealed an interruption of the vasospasm. However, only too often treatment comes too late when a clearly defined destruction of the tissue has already occurred. In our own group of patients, for example, only two of the lower limbs and one upper limb could be saved by the combined PGE_1 treatment (10, 11, 21).

Arteriovenous and venous ulcers of the leg appear to be a further good indication for the intravenous administration of prostanoids. Initial rewarding experience has been reported by Rudofsky (37) which we have in the meantime been able to confirm in our own patients. The continued administration over a 3-week period of 2 x 40 μg or 2 x 60 μg intravenous PGE_1 was found to be satisfactory, accompanied by the performance during this period of any necessary vascular surgery measures – Babcock operation, crossectomy, perforans interruption and skin grafting after cleaning of the ulcers.

A further indication for low-dose, intravenous PGE_1 therapy (2 x 40 μg) is stages III and IV obliterating angiopathy of the digital type (38). Here again a 3-week course of treatment has proved satisfactory.

Last but not least, reference should be made to the intra-arterial or intravenous treatment of endangiitis obliterans with PGE_1, which at the same time marked the starting point and initial indication for prostanoid therapy in Central Europe (20, 39, 42). In addition to PGE_1 the more stable PGI_2 analogue ilomedin has now also been authorized by the Federal Health Office. Here once again the general rule is to administer a 3-week course of treatment. In our experience roughly equivalent results are achieved by intravenous or intra-arterial administration.

One final point to conclude. We have also administered PGE_1 in special cases, for example with organic digital artery occlusion for pharmaco-angiography of the arm and leg, in which case the compound is injected (20 μg) into the corresponding artery of the limb with a Seldinger catheter immediately before injection of the contrast agent. This list of possible uses for prostanoids in vascular surgery does not however lay any claim to completeness.

References

1. Akaba N (1981) Intra-arterial infusion therapy of prostaglandin E_1 with insulin for diabetic gangrene. Surg Diag Treat (Japan) 23: 122
2. Balzer K, Rogatti W, Ruttgerodt K (1989) Therapeutische Wirksamkeit von Prostaglandin E_1 – intraarterielle und intravenose PGE_1 – Therapie im Stadium III/IV. Therapiewoche 39: 2736–42
3. Bergstrom H, Duner H, von Euler US, Pernow B, Sjovall J (1959) Observations on the effects of infusion of prostaglandin E_1 in man. Acta Physiol Scand 45: 145
4. Bergstrom S, Ryhage R, Samuelsson B, Sjovall J (1963) Prostaglandins and related factors. The structure of prostaglandin E_1, F_{10} and F_{16}. J biol Chem 238: 3555–64
5. Blume J (1987) Klinische Wirksamkeit der intraarteriellen Infusionstherapie mit Prostaglandin E_1 im Stadium IIB der arteriellen Verschlußkrankheit. Therapiewoche 37: 4819–23
6. Böhme JIM, Brülisauer M, Härtel U, Bollinger A (1989) Periphere arterielle Verschlußkrankheit im Stadium III und IV – Kontrollierte Zweizentren-Studie zur Wirksamkeit von intraarteriellen Prostaglandin – E_1 – Infusionen. Med Welt 40: 1501–3
7. Carlson LA, Ericsson M, Erikson U (1972) Prostaglandin E_1 (PGE_1) in peripheral arteriographie. Acta Radiol Diagn (Stockholm) 14: 583
8. Carlson LA, Erikson I (1973) Femoral artery infusion of prostaglandin E_1 in severe peripheral vascular disease. Lancet 1: 155
9. Creutzig A, Creutzig H, Alexander K (1986) Effects of intra-arterial prostaglandin E_1 in patients with peripheral arterial occlusive disease. Europ J Clin Invest 16: 480–5
10. Creutzig A (1992) Aufhebung von Vasospasmen beim Ergotismus unter i.v. PGE_1 Therapie. In: Gruss JD (Hrsg) Angiologie im Bild. Köln, Echo Verlag: 23
11. Creutzig A, Kamin K, Flöge J, Wannske M, Alexander K, Wagner HH (1985) Ergotamininduzierte periphere Durchblutungsstörungen – ein Fallbericht. Röntgenblätter 38: 193–5.
12. Diehm C, Hübsch-Müller C, Stammler E (1988) Intravenöse Prostaglandin-E_1-Therapie bei Patienten mit peripherer arterieller Verschlußkrankheit (AVK) im Stadium III – eine doppelblinde plazebokontrollierte Studie. In: Heidrich K, Böhme H, Rogatti W (Hrsg) Prostaglandin E_1-Wirkungen und therapeutische Wirksamkeit. Berlin Heidelberg New York, Springer: 133–43
13. Emmons PR, Hampton JR, Harrison MJG, Honour AJ, Mitchel JRA (1967) Effect of prostaglandin E_1 on platelet behaviour in vitro and in vivo. Br Med J 2: 468–72
14. von Euler US (1935) Über die spezifische blutdrucksenkende Substanz des menschlichen Prostata- und Samenblasensekretes. Klin Wochenschr 14: 1182
15. von Euler US (1983) History and development of prostaglandins. Gen Pharmac 14: 3
16. Fantone JC, Kunkel SL, Ward PA, Zuner RB (1981) Suppression of human polymorphonuclear leukocyte function after intervenous infusion of prostaglandin E_1 – Prostaglandins Med 2: 195–8
17. Fietze-Fischer B, Gruss JD, Bartels D, Vargas-Montano H, Stritter W (1987) Prostaglandin E_1 as an adjuvant therapy in the event of femoro-popliteal and crural saphenous vein in situ bypass surgery. Vasa (Suppl) 17: 23–5
18. Goldblatt MW (1935) Properties of human seminal plasma. J Physiol (London) 84: 208
19. Gruß JD, Kawai S, Karadedos C, Bartels D (1978) Erste Erfahrungen mit der intraarteriellen Langzeitperfusion von Prostaglandin E_1 bei fortgeschrittener arterieller Verschlußkrankheit der unteren Extremitäten im Stadium IV, Dtsch Med Wochenschr 41: 1624
20. Gruß JD, Vargas-Montano H, Bartels D, Simmenroth HW, Sakurai T, Schafer G, Fietze-Fischer B (1984) Use of prostaglandins in arterial occlusive diseases. Int Angio Suppl 3: 7
21. Gruß JD (1986) Experiences with PGE_1 in patients with phlegmasia cerulea dolens and in ergotism. In: Sinzinger H, Rogatti W (eds) Prostaglandin E_1 in Atherosclerosis. Berlin Heidelberg New York, Springer: 99–105
22. Gruß JD, Fietze-Fischer B (1988) Die adjuvante PGE_1-Therapie bei femoro-distalen Rekonstruktionen. In: Heidrich H, Rogatti W (Hrsg) Prostaglandin E_1 Wirkungen und therapeutische Wirksamkeit. Berlin Heidelberg New York, Springer: 151–9
23. Gruß JD (1989) Experiences with PGE_1 in patients with post-operative trash-foot. Vasa (Suppl) 28: 57–60
24. Gruß JD (1991) Adjuvante Therapie bei femoro-distaler Bypasschirurgie. In: Landgrat H (Hrsg) Aktuelle Therapieprinzipien bei der peripheren arteriellen Verschlußkrankheit. Braunschweig, Vieweg: 43–56

25. Gruß JD (1991) Adjuvant intravenous PGE_1 treatment after profundaplasty for limb salvage. In: Diehm C, Sinzinger H, Rogatti W (eds) Prostaglandin E_1. New Aspects on Pharmacology, Metabolism and Clinical Efficacy. Berlin Heidelberg, Springer: 109–13
26. Gruß JD (1992) Gliedmaßenerhaltung bei peripherer arterieller Verschlußkrankheit im Stadium IV. Der Bay Int 12: 35–8
27. Heidrich H, Breddin HK, Rudotsky G, Scheffler P (1992) Kardiopulmonale Wirkungen von Prostaglandin E_1. Med Klin 87: 123–30
28. Heidrich H, Ranft J, Peters A, Rummel S (1987) Früh- und Spätergebnisse nach intravenoser Prostavasm-Therapie bei peripher-arteriellen Durchblutungsstörungen mit Ruheschmerz und Nekrose. Vasa (Suppl) 20: 202
29. Kurzrock L, Lieb CC (1930) Biochemical studies of human semen. II. The action of semen on the human uterus. Proc Soc Exp Biol Med 28: 268
30. Mishima Y (1975) Peripheral vascular disorders. Metabolism and disease. Japan 12: 1727
31. Moncada S, Gryglowski RJ, Bunting S, Vane JR (1976) An enzyme isolated from arteries transforms prostaglandin endoperoxides to an unstable substance that inhibits platelet aggregation. Nature 263: 663
32. Moncada S, Vane JR (1979) Pharmacology and endogenous roles of prostaglandin endoperoxides, thromboxane A_2 and prostacyclin. Pharmacol Rev 30: 292
33. Moncada S, Vane JR (1981) Discovery, biological significance and therapeutic potential of prostacyclin. In: Lewis PJ, O'Grady J (eds) Clinical Pharmacology of Prostacyclin. New York. Raven: 1
34. Moncada S (1982) Biological importance of prostacyclin. VII Gaddum Memorial Lecture. Br J Pharmacol 76: 3
35. Ney P, Schrör K (1989) E-type prostaglandins but not doprost inhibit platelet activating factor-induced generation of leukotriene B_4 by human polymorphnuclear leukocytes. Br J Pharmacol 96: 186–92
36. Peskar BA, Hesse WH, Rogatti W, Diehm C, Rudofsky G, Schweer H, Scyberth HW (1991) Formations of 13, 14 dihydro-prostaglandin E_1 during intravenous infusions of prostaglandin E_1 in patients with peripheral arterial occlusive disease. Prostaglandins 41: 225–8
37. Rudofsky G (1989) Intravenous prostaglandin E_1 in the treatment of venous ulcers – a double blind, placebo-controlled trial. Vasa (Suppl) 28: 39–43
38. Rustin MHA, Kovacs JB, Cooke ED, Dowd PM, Bawcoks SA, Kirby JDT (1984) Experience with PGE_1 and PGI_2 infusions in patients with systemic sclerosis and Raynaud's phenomenon. Int Angiol 3: 43
39. Sakagushi S, Kusaba, Mischima Y, Kamiya K, Nashimura A, Furukawa K, Shionoya S, Kawashima M, Katsumura T, Sakuma A (1978) A multi-clinical double blind study with PGE_1 (a cyclodextrin clathrate) in patients with ischemic ulcer of the extremities. Vasa 7: 263
40. Scheffler P, de la Hamette D, Leiprinz G (1989) Therapeutic efficacy of intravenously applied prostaglandin E_1. Vasa 28 (Suppl): 19–25
41. Schrör K (1984) Prostaglandine und verwandte Verbindungen. Stuttgart, Thieme: 101–25
42. Shionoya S, Matsubara J, Hirai M, Kawai S (1976) Dauerperfusion mit Prostaglandin E_1 bei peripheren arteriellen Verschlußkrankheiten. Gekachiryo 213: 34
43. Sinzinger H (1986) Inhibition of mitotic and proliferative activity of smooth muscle cells by prostaglandin E_1. In: Sinzinger H, Rogatti W (eds) Prostaglandin E_1 in Atherosclerosis. Berlin Heidelberg New York, Springer: 39–48
44. Sinzinger H, Fitscha P, Wagner O, Kaliman J, Rogatti W (1986) Prostacyclin E_1 decreases activation of arterial smooth-muscle cells, Lancet I: 156–7
45. Sinzinger H, Fitscha P (1987) Influence of PGE_1 on invivo accumulation of radiolabelled platelets and LDL on human arteries. Vasa 17 (Suppl): 5–10
46. Sinzinger H, Virgolini J, Lupatelli G, Hanyai M (1991) PGE_1 and 13, 14 dihydro PGE_1 increase low-density lipoprotein receptors and improve arterial wall lipid metabolism. In: Diehm C, Sinzinger H, Rogatti W (eds) Prostaglandin E_1. Berlin Heidelberg New York, Springer: 39–48
47. Spiecker M, Buereke M, Darius H, Meyer J (1992) Antithrombotische und hämodynamische Effekte der Prostacyclin-Analoga Hoprest und Taprosten in vivo. Perfusion 11: 326–30
48. Trübestein G, Ludwig M, Diehm C, Gruß JD, Horsch S (1987) Prostaglandin E_1 bei arterieller Verschlußkrankheit im Stadium III und IV. Dtsch Med Wochenschr 112: 995

49. Trübestein G, v. Bary S, Breddin K, Diehm C, Gruß JD, Heidrich H, Horsch S, Kriessmann A, Maass U, Marin N, Scheifler P (1989) Intravenous prostaglandin E_1 versus pentoxifylline therapy in chronic arterial occlusive disease – a controlled randomized multicentre study. Vasa (Suppl) 28: 44–49

Author's address:
Prof. Dr. J. D. Gruß
Kurhess. Diakonissenhaus
Dept. of Vascular Surgery
Goethestraße 85
D-34119 Kassel
FRG

Arterial vascular reconstruction in critical ischemia of the lower extremities

A. Branchereau, P. E. Magnan

Dept. of Vascular Surgery, Hôpital Sainte-Marguerite, Marseille, France

The diagnosis of critical limb ischemia according to precise criteria acknowledges an unavoidable short or long term risk of amputation. This risk lies at 80 % after 1 year without treatment and at 25 % after percutaneous or surgical revascularisation (12). Due to the complexity of vascular alterations found in these patients, only a small proportion can receive endovascular treatment. The larger part of these patients can be surgically treated, since even complex reconstructive surgery is possible due to new technological developments in recent years.

General

The diagnosis of critical limb ischemia is based upon a meticulous examination of the vascular patient. Clinically there should be rest pain present and/or trophic changes, the doppler index at the ankle must be less than 50 mmHg and the $tcPO_2$ less than 30 mmHg and clinical symptoms are resistant to medical therapy and should be present for at least 2 weeks in order to differentiate symptoms from an acute ischemia (12). The pre-operative diagnosis should include a complete medical work-up in order to judge risk factors and to attempt therapeutic optimalisation of coexisting diseases: diabetes; coronary heart disease, hypertension general condition etc. Vessels should be visualized from the renal arteries down to the foot angiographically. Some times it is difficult to adequately document peripheral vessels making necessary intra-arterial angiography with the ipsilateral femoral artery as the puncture site. The two methods of demonstrating vessels are very interesting and complementary (3). If the ischemia is very severe, intra-operative angiography can additionally be used. Ultrasound as well as CT-scanning can document vascular sclerosis or aneurysma formation in the aorto-iliac region and play an important role in choosing an optimal treatment for each individual patient.

Extra-anatomical Bypass Graft

This is an interesting alternative for occlusive aorto iliac disease if this cannot be corrected using PTA and the surgical risk of a major abdominal intervention is to high for patients with major risk factors. Due to improvements in anaesthetics and postoperative intensive care medicine, the latter reason is becoming increasingly rare for not operating intra-abdominally. The femoro-femoro cross-over bypass, however, show interesting results despite a decreased long-term permeability rate compared to anatomical bypasses, as they are minimally aggressive towards the general health state of older patients (23). Unfortunately an indication for such surgery is rare, as it is seldom, that one of the iliac vessels is with so little atherosclerotic change to warrant this type of surgery. In unilateral vessel occlusion with contralateral iliac artery stenosis it would, however, be possible to do a cross-over bypass with an intra-operative PTA of the stenosed side (Fig. 1). Axillofemoral or axillobifemoral bypasses are for more seldom performed these days compared to the 70's due to the poor permeability and high complication rates (Tab. 1). They still remain the only solution for

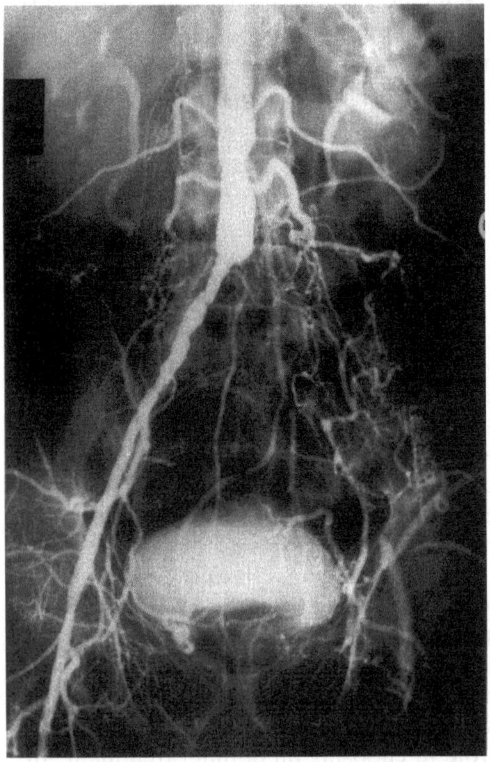

Fig. 1. Stenosis of the right iliac artery associated with an occlusion of the left iliac axis. These lesions may be treated by balloon dilatation and cross-over bypass

Table 1. Results of the axillo-femoral bypasses

Author	Year	N cases	Postoperative mortality	Permeability after 5 years
Courbier R	1982 (5)	220	3.6	64
Allison HF	1985 (6)	109	6.4	16
Donaldson MC	1986 (7)	100	8	48
Christenson JT	1986 (3)	85	3.6	68
Bergeron P	1989 (9)	182	2.7	89

patients in a catastrophical general health state and if endovascular reconstruction is impossible.

Aortobifemoral Bypass Graft

They are the technique of choice to treat aortoiliac occlusive disease. The postoperative mortality and morbidity is less than 25 % in all studies published to date (Tab. 2). The mortality is slightly higher in critical ischemia due to the poor general health state of patients, but still remains in acceptable ranges especially when assessing the 3 and 6 months mortality figures compared to primary amputation follow-up (21, 24). The long-term results of these bypasses are satisfying with patency rates of more than 70 % after 10 and 15 years (Tab. 2). Most late occlusions can be ascribed to a deterioration of the peripheral vessels. These deteriorations should be timeously recognised in order to react accordingly and avoid occlusions. The limb salvage rate after 5 years following aortobifemoral bypass surgery lies between 75 an 98 % (6). Roughly 80 % of patients with critical ischemia due to aortoiliac occlusion have changes in the femoropopliteal region. About one third will require bypass lengthening to more distal levels in the course of the disease so that one can generalise and say that 25 % of patients with critical ischemia in the presence of iliac occlusion are candidates for a femoropopliteal bypass graft which could possibly be implanted in the same operation (Fig. 2). The advantages of a simultaneous two stage operation are an immediate improvement with better haemodynamic results and renewed surgery with exposure of the initial bypass graft in the inguinal region is avoided (5). A disadvantage is prolonged surgery and thereby increasing the surgical aggression to the general health. In the presence of extensive trophic lesions, a poor popliteal segment and a fair general health state support the two stage surgery in one sitting. Only proximal reconstruction should be applied in the presence of severe gangrene or very localised lesions, good representation of the popliteal artery at above knee level or for patients of poor general health.

Lesions of the inguinal vessels

Although the situation is rare, an occlusion or high grade stenosis of the common femoral the superficial femoral and the deep femoral artery can cause a critical ischemia (Fig. 3). Percutaneous transluminal angioplasty is possible, but has 2 disad-

Table 2. Results of the aorto-bifemoral bypasses

Author	Year	N Cases	Postoperative mortality	Permeability 5 years	10 years	15 years
Crawford ES	1981 (10)	949	3.6	87	79	70
Poulias GE	1985 (11)	500	3.2	87	78	–
Szilagyi DE	1986 (12)	1748	4.9	77	76	73
Nevelsteen A	1991 (13)	869	4.2	82	74	70

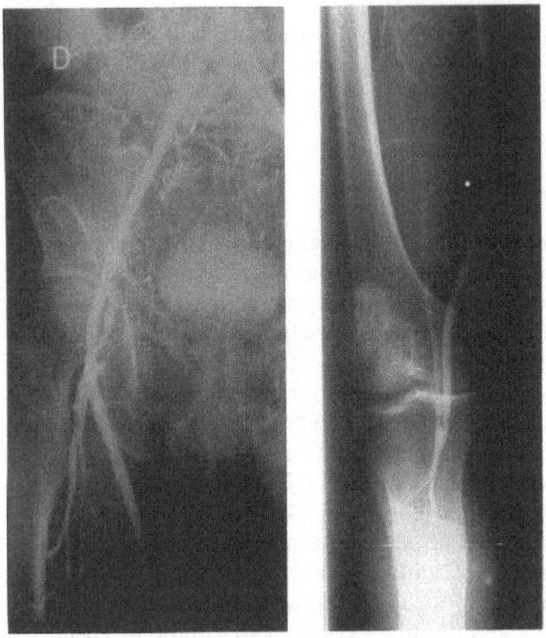

a b

Fig. 2. Postoperative angiography of a two-stage reconstruction consisting of an aorto-bifemoral bypass (A) and a femoro-popliteal bypass (B)

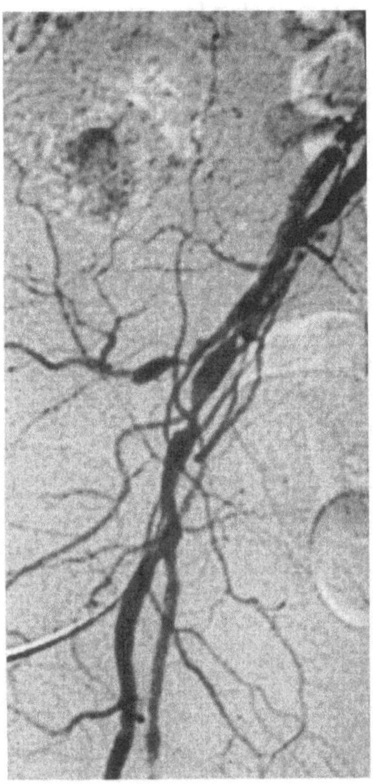

Fig. 3. Tight stenosis of the left common femoral artery

vantages: it requires a contralateral arterial puncture and if the procedure proves to be unsuccessful, there is the risk of acute ischemia. Surgical angioplasty of inguinal vessels is a small surgical procedure which can even be performed under local or regional anaesthesia with permeability rates of 97 % after 1 year and 94 % after a 4 year follow-up (20).

Femoropopliteal crural Bypass Graft

These bypasses are the most frequently applied surgery for the described sinaria. In our experience 85 % of patients with critical ischemia of the lower extremities receive such surgery. Mortality rates after this form of reconstruction are almost zero in patients suffering from intermittent claudication, and 2 to 7 % in patients with critical ischemia due to the poor general state (Tab. 3). Above-knee bypasses should not be considered here, as they are never solely indicated in critial ischemia. Below-knee bypasses, regularly applied in critical ischemia, show several difficulties and results, depending on the availability of a saphenous vein as bypass material and whether the below knee anastomosis is at the trifurcation or crural. The in situ vein bypass is the method of choice nowadays. It is the prefered method by most surgeons (27). One advantage is, that the diameter corresponds to that of the arteries at all levels of the leg (Fig. 4). This is particularly important for crural bypasses. Long-term results and limb salvage rates are very good and show no major difference between below-knee and crural bypasses (Tab. 4). The reversed vein bypass also show good long-term results (Tab. 5). It does, however, seem, that the patency rates for crural bypasses using the reverse technique are poorer than for the below-knee technique, which could be explained by problems of congruence.

Prosthetic bypass grafts have markedly worse results (Tab. 6). There is a large difference between patency rates of below-knee bypasses, which still have acceptable

Table 3. Postoperative mortality for inguinal bypass surgery

Autor	Year	N cases	Mortality %
Veith FJ	1986 (17)	845	5.3
Bandyk DF	1987 (18)	192	3
Leather RP	1988 (19)	1038	6.7
Kent KC	1989 (20)	266	1.4

Table 4. Results of in situ saphenous vein bypasses. Collected results from the literature according to Dalman and Taylor (10)

Type of bypass	Permeability			Limb salvage		
	1 month	2 years	4 years	1 month	2 years	4 years
Femoro-popliteal (below the knee)	95	75	68	97	84	83
Leg artery	94	76	68	96	88	83

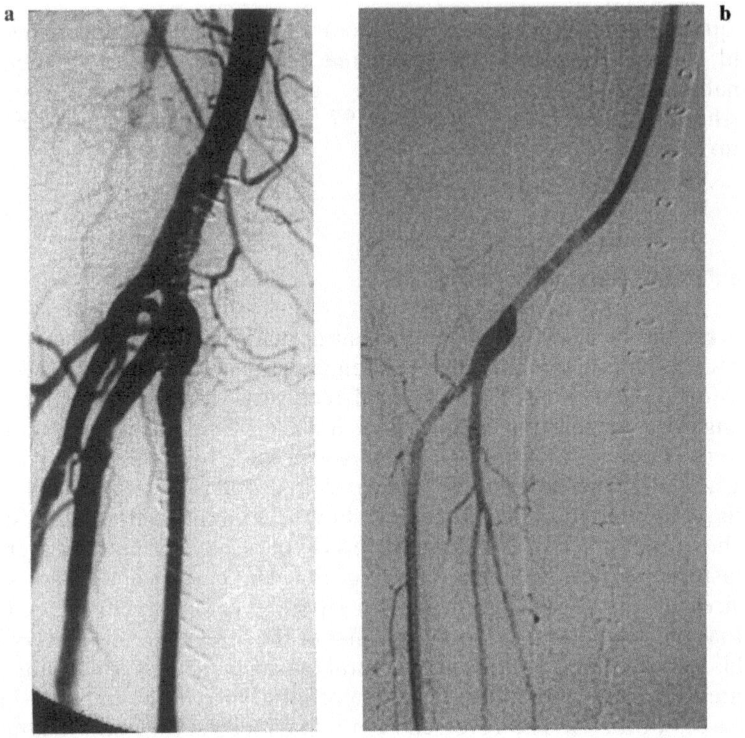

Fig. 4. Control angiography of a low femoro-popliteal bypass with in situ saphenous vein. A: Upper anastomosis. B: Lower anastomosis

Table 5. Results of reversed saphenous vein bypasses. Collected results from the literature according to Dalman and Taylor

Type of bypass	Permeability			Limb salvage		
	1 month	2 years	4 years	1 month	2 years	4 years
Femoro-popliteal (below the knee)	98	79	77	100	88	75
leg artery	92	70	62	95	83	82

Table 6. Permeability of posthetic grafts. Collected results from the literature according to Dalman and Taylor (10)

Type of bypass	Permeability		
	1 month	2 years	4 years
Femoropolitead (below the knee)	96	61	40
lag artery	89	32	21

results, and crural bypasses with prosthetic material. The latter have such poor outcome, that many surgeons no longer want to perform these procedures. Permeability of these prosthetic bypasses onto the lower leg arteries can and must be improved with improved techniques of constructing the distal anastomosis. This can be done by using composite grafts with a small venous interposition or constructing a graft according to Miller's technique. This technique makes an anastomosis possible without directly suturing the graft to the arterial wall (19). The success using this technique is said to have been proven (25).

Bypasses to Ankle or Foot Arteries

In the last 10 years vascular surgeons have attempted reconstructions down to the ankle joint or foot in order to preserve a limb. This was due to improved experience and technical improvements, especially of the in situ vein bypasses (Fig. 5). In this way, bypasses onto the pedal artery, posterior tibial and plantar artery can be per-

a

b

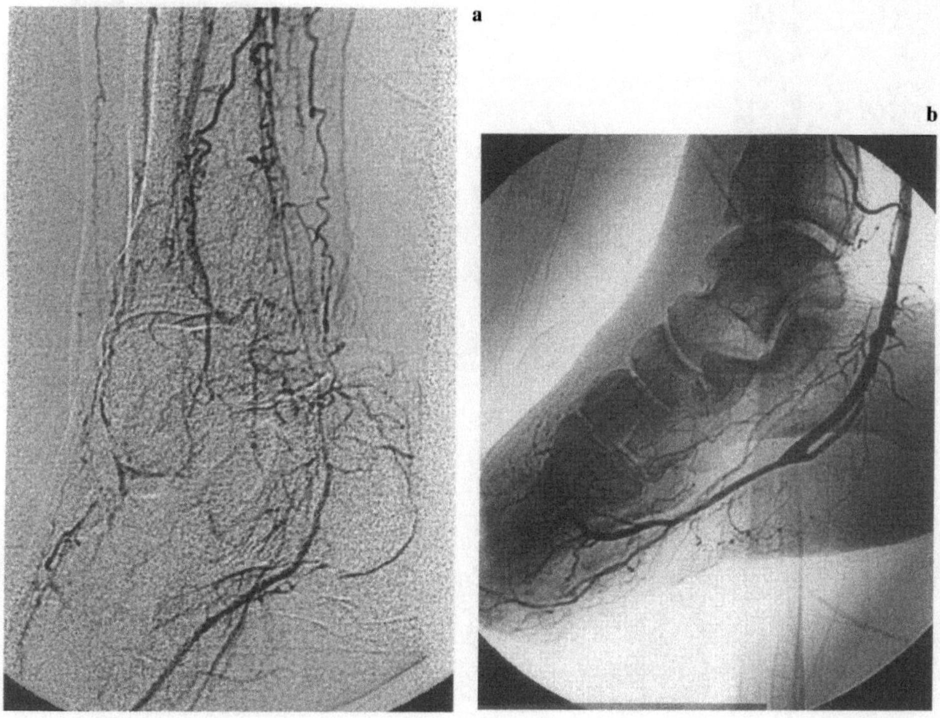

Fig. 5. Vein bypass on the lateral plantar artery. A: Preoperative angiography. B: Postoperative angiography of the lower anastomosis

formed (16). It does however require a usable saphenous vein and microsurgical techniques. Results in table 7 are comparable to these achieved with vein bypasses on the crural arteries.

Table 7. Results of hyperdistal bypass surgery. Collected results from the literature according to Dalman and Taylor (10)

	1 month	1 year	3 years
Secondar. permeability	93	92	72
Foot salvage	99	93	84

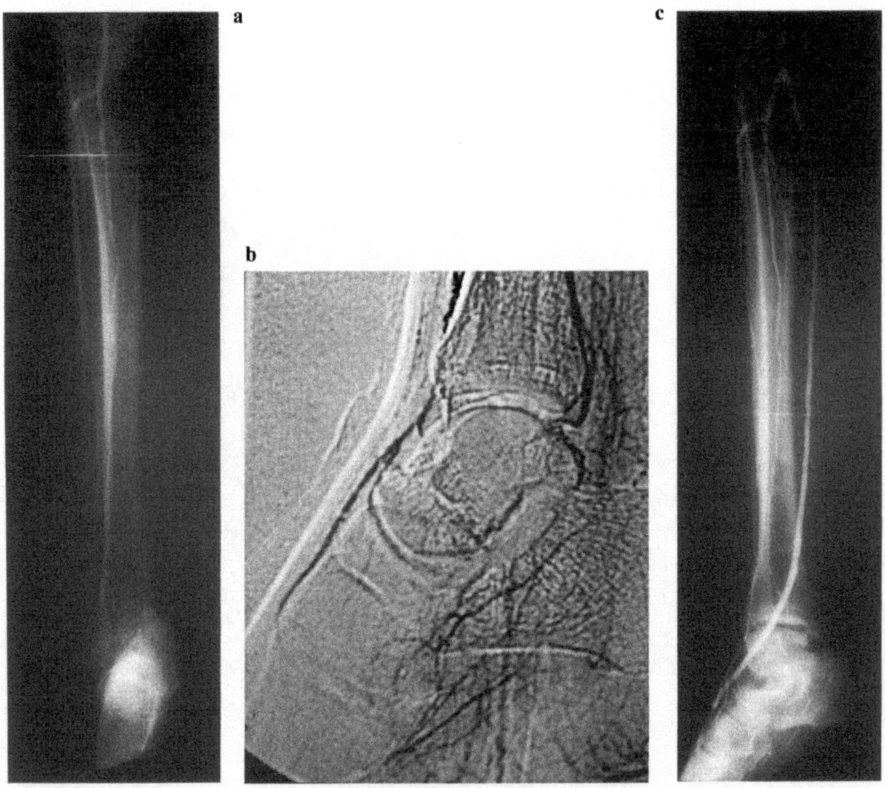

Fig. 6. Conventional angiography of the lower right limb showing a poor distal arterial network. B: Digital angiography showing the artery of the foot. C: Saphenous vein bypass between the lower popliteal artery and the artery of the foot

Arterial Transplantation

Vascular reconstruction cannot be applied despite critical ischemia in the absence of a usable saphenous vein in a desolate peripheral arterial situation where no prosthetic graft can be used. With regards to a poor peripheral arterial situation the possibilities for vascular reconstruction have been markedly and regularly improved for 3 reasons:

1) Better pre- and intra-operative diagnostic availability which can even document arteries which are hardly perfused.

2) Pedal bypasses have made vascular reconstructions in patients with severe ischemia and absent lower leg arteries possible.

3) The classical contraindications to reconstructions have been frequently adjusted so that a surgeon will nowadays even attempt a reconstruction onto only a few centimeters of demonstrable vessel which appears relatively free of atherosclerotic change (Fig. 6). In fact, these situations are often non-reconstructable in the absence of adequate vein. The use of arterial transplants in recent years has also changed this situation (15). These arteries are salvaged from coma patients during multi-organ-donations. They are stored in cryopreservation and left in quarantine for 3 months to

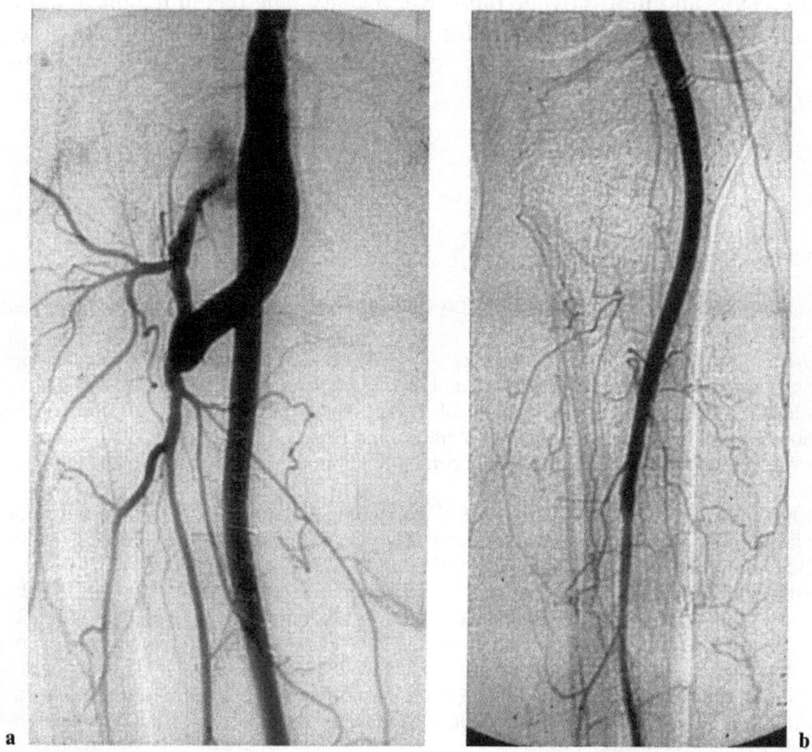

Fig. 7. Angiography of a deep iliofemoral (A) and femoroperoneal bypass (B) using an arterial allograft

avoid viral infections. These arteries are of a high quality since they usually are healthy arteries and a number can be stored at a time. The same artery as the one required can then be used for surgery (Fig. 7). Between November 1991 and April 1993 we have performed 23 such bypasses to crural levels in 23 patients with critical ischemia. The average doppler index was 25 ± 21 mmHg in these patients. 15 had no saphenous vein and 8 had a saphenous vein of poor quality. In 17 a crural reconstruction had already been attempted and ended with graft infection. The distal anastomosis was applied to lower leg arteries in 20 cases and to arteries of the ankle and dorsal foot in 3 cases. Complications were one thrombosis and 4 amputations during follow-up, where 1 amputation had to be performed despite pedent bypass. The permeability rate was 63 % after 2 years. These results are promising, and we have caused us to continue this method. To document final results, more patients have to be monitored over a larger time period.

Summary

Below-knee bypasses are the most frequently used technique for critical ischemia of the lower extremities. The in-situ vein bypass is the technique of choice with the best long-term results and limb-salvage rates over 5 years. The recent technical improvements and the possibility of an arterial transplantation have made it possible to perform always some form of vascular reconstruction to improve the peripheral haemodynamic situation.

References

1. Allison HF, Terblance J, Immelman EJ (1985) Axillofemoral bypass: a 2-decade experience. S Alfr Med J 68: 559–562
2. Bandyk DF, Kaebnick HW, Stewart SW et col. (1987) Durability of the in situ saphenous vein arterial bypass: A comparison of primary and secondary patency. J Vasc Surg 5: 256–268
3. Bartoli JM, Kuredjian S, Espinoza H et col. (1990) Apport de l'angiographie numérisée dans l'exploration des ischémies critiques des membres inférieurs. Ann Radiol 33: 250–254
4. Bergeron P, Mangialardi N, Sarradon P et col. (1989) Pontages axillo-fémoraux: résultats à long terme. J Chir 126: 575–582
5. Branchereau A, Rosset E, Di Mauro P (1992) Restauration combinée aorto-iliaque et fémorale superficielle. In: Branchereau A, Jausseran JM, eds. Traitement des lésions obstructives de l'artère fémorale superficielle. Marseille, CVN, pp 157–170
6. Brewster DC, Cooke JC (1993) Longevity of aortofemoral bypass grafts. In: Yao JST, Pearce WH, eds. Long-term results in vascular surgery. Norwalk, Appleton & Lange, pp 149–162
7. Christenson JT, Broome A, Norgren L et col. (1986) The late results after axillo-femoral bypass grafts in patients with leg ischemia. J Cardiovasc Surg 27: 131–135
8. Courbier R, Jausseran JM, Bergeron P (1992) Axillo-femoral bypass material of choice. In: Greenhalgh RM, ed. Extra-anatomic secondary arterial reconstruction. Bath, Pitman press, pp 122–130
9. Crawford ES, Bomberger RA, Glaeser DH et col. (1981) Aortoiliac occlusive disease: factors influencing survival and function following reconstructive operation over a twenty-five year period. Surgery 90: 1055–1067

10. Dalman RL, Taylor LM Jr (1990) Basic data related to infrainguinal revascularization procedures. Ann Vasc Surg 4: 309–312
11. Donaldson MC, Louras JC, Buckham CA (1986) Axillofemoral bypass: a tool with a limited role. J Vasc Surg 3: 757–763
12. European working group on critical leg ischemia (1991) Second European consensus document on chronic critical leg ischemia. Circulation 84: IV1–IV26
13. Fichelle JM, Marzelle J, Colacchio G et col. (1995) Pontages infrapoplités en PTFE et pontages composites: facteurs influençant les résultats. Ann Chir Vasc 9: 187–196
14. Flanigan DP (1987) Pre-bypass operative arteriography. In: Flanigan DP (ed) Perioperative surgery. New York, Marcel Dekker, pp 189–201
15. Gournier JP, Adham M, Faure JP et col. (1993) Cryopreserved arterial homografts: preliminary study. Ann Vasc Surg 7: 503–511
16. Jacobs M (1995) Artères de la cheville et du pied. In: Branchereau A, Magnan PE, Rosset E, eds. Voies d'abord des vaisseaux. Paris, Arnette Blackwell, p 291–298
17. Kent KC, Whittemore AD, Mannick JA (1989) Short-term and mid-term results of an all-autogenous tissue policy for infrainguinal reconstruction. J Vasc Surg 9: 107–114
18. Leather RP, Shah DM, Chang BB et col. (1988) Resurection of the in situ saphenous vein bypass. Ann Surg 208: 435–442
19. Miller JM, Foreman RK, Ferguson L et col. (1984) Interposition vein cuff for anastomosis of prosthesis to small artery. Aust NZ J Surg 54: 283–285
20. Mukherjee D, Inahara T (1989) Endarterectomy as the procedure of choice for atheresclerotic occlusive lesions of the common femoral artery. Am J Surg 157: 498–500
21. Nevelsteen A, Wouters L, Suy R (1991) Aortofemoral dacron reconstruction for aortoiliac occlusive disease: a 25 year survey. Eur J Vasc Surg 5: 179–186
22. Poulias GE, Poletsis L, Skoutas B et col. (1985) Bilateral aorto-femoral bypass in the presence of aorto-iliac occlusive disease and factors determining results: experience and long-term follow-up with 500 consecutive cases. J Cardiovasc Surg 26: 527–538
23. Ricco JB, AURC (1992) Unilateral iliac artery occlusive disease: A randomized multicenter trial examining direct revascularization versus cross-over bypass. Ann Vasc Surg 6: 209–19
24. Szilargyi DE, Elliot JP JR, Smith RF et col. (1986) A thirty-year survey of the reconstructive surgical treatment of aortoiliac occlusive disease. J Vasc Surg 3: 421–436
25. Tyrrel MR, Chester J, Vipond MN et col. (1990) Experimental evidence to support the use of interposition vein collar patches in distal PTFE anastomoses. Eur J Vasc Surg 4: 95–109
26. Veith FJ, Gupta SK, Ascer E et col. (1986) Six-year prospective multicenter randomized comparison of autologous saphenous vein and expanded polytetrafluoroethylene grafts in infrainguinal arterial reconstructions. J Vasc Surg 3: 104–114
27. Watelet J, Cheysson E, Poels D et col. (1986) In situ versus reversed saphenous vein for femoropopliteal bypass: A prospective randomized study of 100 cases. Ann Vasc Surg 1: 441–452

Author's address:
Prof. Alain Branchereau MD PhD
Dept. of Vascular Surgery
Hospital Sainte-Marguerite
University of Marseille
BP 29, 13274 Marseille Cedex 9
France

Results of pedal bypass surgery for critical limb ischemia

H.-H. Eckstein, J.-R. Allenberg

Chrirurgische Universitätsklinik Heidelberg, Sektion Gefäßchirurgie

Introduction

The incidence of critical limb ischemia is estimated to be about 500 – 1000 per 1 million population in Western Europe. Today, 25 % of patients are treated conservatively including PTA-techniques, 25 % have primary amputation, and 50 % receive arterial reconstruction (1, 22). Particularly limbs with infrapopliteal occlusive disease in the preoperative angiogram are frequently considered unreconstructible. Perioperative mortality after major amputation is about 10 % and the prognosis is also poor in those patients who cannot walk with a prosthesis and are confined to bed or a wheelchair (12). In the last decade the lower limit of distal revascularization has been further extended to the arteries of the ankle and the foot and several reports documented long-term patency- and limb salvage-rates between 60 and 90 %, even in diabetics and multimorbid patients (2–4, 8, 9, 11, 14, 15, 21, 23, 24, 26–29). In addition, it has been shown that femoro-distal revascularization to the foot vessels decreases the number of major lower limb amputation in 25 to 50 %. These number, however, have been achieved in few hospitals and still await validation in nationwide or large area statistics (13, 14, 17, 25).

To update our own data (16) and reevaluate the criteria for pedal bypass grafting, we analyzed all patients who underwent arterial reconstruction with a venous graft to the foot vessels for severe limb-threatening ischemia in the period 1984–1994.

Patients and methods

Between April 1984 and September 1994, we performed 50 pedal vein bypasses in 34 men and 16 women. The mean age was 68.3 years (34–88). Thirty-six patients were diabetics, 35 suffered from hypertension, and 23 had coronary heart disease with previous myocardial infarction in 10 cases. Thirty-two patients were cigarette smokers and 14 had a previous arterial reconstruction (thrombendarterectomy of femoral artery three times, femoro-popliteal and femoro-crural bypasses five and six times). Three patients had major amputation on the contralateral side. Five mono-prosthetic grafts from the beginning of this series were not taken into account. All pedal reconstructions were done for limb salvage. Chronic critical leg ischemia was defined as gangrene, non-healing ischemic ulcer or rest pain for at least 2 weeks with an ankle Doppler < 50 mm Hg in the non-diabetic patients and with severe signs of an advanced peripheral arterial occlusive disease in the angiogram (occlusion of the femoral artery and/or the tibial vessels). The indication for pedal reconstruction was ischemic rest pain in 13 patients (26 %) including four patients with acute ischemia by thrombosis and known advanced peripheral arterial occlusive disease (non-available lysis-therapy). The majority (74 %) were operated on for tissue loss by gangrene or non-healing ulcers. No procedures were done for intermittent claudication (Table 1).

The *preoperative noninvasive evaluation* included medical history, physical examination, Doppler ultrasonography, x-ray of the foot and bacterial cultures examination in cases of necrosis. Patients with gangrene or non-healing ulcer received a broad-spectrum antibiotic as appropriate.

All patients underwent *transfemoral angiography.* A selective "needle-arteriogram" of the limb with x-ray films of the foot in anterio-posterior and in lateral position was obtained if no distal vessel was detected by conventional angiography. Patients with aorto-iliac disease or a patent popliteal or crural artery were not considered candidates for pedal bypass. Primary amputation was only considered when no distal vessel could be detected by Doppler or by angiogram and if the patient was multimorbid and had been confined to bed for other diseases.

The *operative procedures* and the site of the distal anastomosis are shown in Table 2 and Fig. 1. The level for the proximal anastomosis was located based on the preoperative angiogram, whereas the site of the distal anastomosis was determined intraoperatively after exposing and opening of the artery. Criteria for performing the bypass procedure were a smooth injection of heparin solution in the distal outflow and a distal diameter of at least 2–3 mm. Calcification was not a contraindication, although the procedure became more difficult. In 34 cases distal anastomosis were located at the dorsal pedal artery and in 16 patients at the posterior tibial artery below the ankle as end-to-end-anastomosis in 35 cases and end-to-side-anastomosis in 15 cases. All distal anastomoses were performed under loupe-amplification. Whenever possible, we used autologous vein of the same limb (n = 33) with the proximal anastomosis above knee-level in 15 cases. The proximal anastomosis was performed below knee in case of adequate inflow to the popliteal or to a crural artery (n = 18). When the length of saphenous vein was inadequate, a composite ("jump") graft was done with a first segment of a polytetrafluorethylene graft (PTFE/6 mm) to the popliteal artery and a second segment of reversed saphenous vein from the distal portion of the PTFE graft to a pedal artery (n = 17). In this series no prosthetic monograft was done. To assess the technical adequacy of the distal anastomosis and the presence of any residual arteriovenous fistulas in the patient with an *in situ* bypass (n = 4) intraopera-

Table 1. Clinical characteristics of patients receiving a pedal vein bypass (n = 50)

Sex (male: female)		34:16
Age (year, range)		68.3 (34–88)
Follow-up (months)		0–112 (median 29)
Diabetes mellitus		36 (72 %)
Hypertension		35 (70 %)
Coronary heart disease		23 (46 %)
Cigarette smokers		32 (64 %)
Indications for surgery:	ischemic rest pain	13 (26 %)
	tissue loss/gangrene	37 (74 %)
Previous arterial reconstruction		14 (28 %)

Table 2. Operative procedures/site of anastomoses and type of pedal graft implanted (n = 50)

Graft type/distal anastomosis	Dorsal pedal artery (n = 31)	Post. tibial artery (n = 17)	Med. plantar artery (n = 2)
Long vein (above knee, n = 15)	7	7	1
Short vein (below knee, n = 18)	10	7	1
Composite ("Jump") graft (n = 17)	14	3	

Saphenous vein as reversed graft in 21 cases, orthograde bypass in seven and *in situ* bypass in five cases

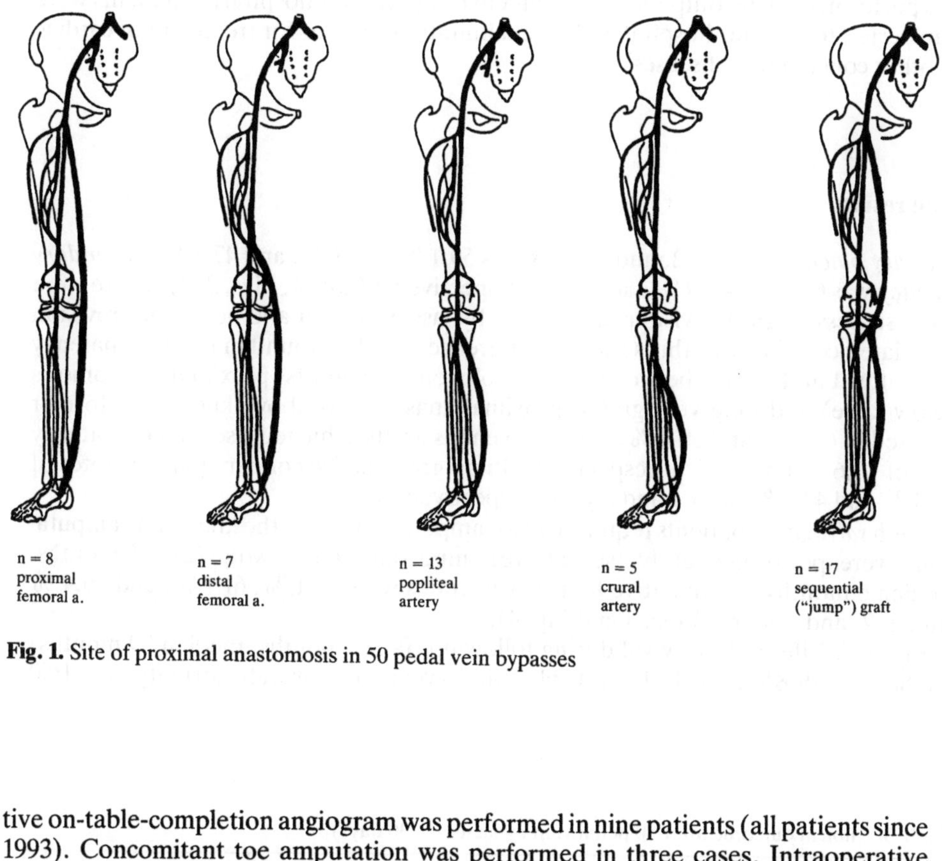

Fig. 1. Site of proximal anastomosis in 50 pedal vein bypasses

tive on-table-completion angiogram was performed in nine patients (all patients since 1993). Concomitant toe amputation was performed in three cases. Intraoperative systemic heparinization was performed routinely, postoperative anticoagulation consisted of anticoagulant-therapy (Marcumar).

Follow-up was obtained from outpatient records (physical examination, Doppler pressure) and telephone interviews. Three patients were lost to follow-up 22–28 months. Follow-up angiograms were only performed if graft failure was suspected. Patient survival, primary and secondary graft patencies were calculated by the use of the Kaplan-Meier method.

Early results

One death occurred in the perioperative period (30 days) secondary to a bowel perforation. Eleven grafts (22 %) occluded within the first week, but only three graft revisions (thrombectomy, local lysis and correction of the distal anastomosis) were successful. In two cases major amputation could be postponed by conservative treatment, whereas in two other patients persistent ischemia required amputation inspite of a patent bypass. Altogether, early major amputation became necessary in 8/50 patients (16 %). In 41 of 50 (82 %) patients survival and/or limb salvage on the basis of a functioning bypass could be achieved (Table 3).

Wound infections (incisions, vein harvesting area) were observed in three cases and were treated conservatively. No graft infection occurred and no graft was lost by a wound infection. The mean hospital stay was 24 days. After discharge wound care was performed by the outpatient department or by another hospital (15 patients were transferred to another hospital with a rehabilitation ward or for treatment of cardiac or other concomitant diseases).

Late results

Primary patency after 1, 2, and 4 years was 59.1 %, 47.8 %, and 47.8 %, *secondary patency* was 65.4 %, 47.9 % and 47.9 % respectively (Table 4, Figs. 2, 3). There were three successful graft revisions after early bypass occlusion and no further revision after late occlusions. In this series no difference could be found in terms of patency rates after 1 and 2 years between short autologous vein grafts (proximal anastomosis below knee) and long vein grafts (proximal anastomosis above knee): the former resulted in 63.2 % and 50.1 %, and long venous grafts achieved a secondary patency rate of 70.6 % and 45.4 % respectively. Jump grafts had secondary patency rates of 53.4 % and 44.5 % after 1 and 2 years respectively (n.s.).

Limb salvage: 18 patients required major amputation above the knee, nine amputations were performed early (see above), nine during follow-up (21–47 months, median 6 months). Cumulative limb salvage rates were 71.1 %, 61.1 %, and 56.4 % after 1, 2, and 4 years (Table 4 and Fig. 4).

Survival: Life-table survival during follow-up (0–112 months, median 29 months) was 88.7 %, 79.8 %, and 47.1 % after 1, 2, and 4 years. The overall mortality was 21/50

Table 3. Clinical outcome after 50 pedal vein bypasses (< 30 days)

Result	No.	%
Bypass patent	39	78
Early graft thrombosis	11	22
Early major amputation	8	16
Successful graft revision	3	6
Operative mortality	1	2
Life-and-limb salvage	41	82

Table 4. Patency and limb salvage rates after pedal vein bypass grafting (n = 50, Kaplan-Meier)

Interval	No. at risk	No. failed	Cum. patency	Standard error
		Primary patency rates		
1 month	36	12	75.9	6
6 months	23	18	62.2	7.1
1 year	19	19	59.1	7.4
2 years	11	22	47.8	8.4
4 years	5	22	47.8	8.4
		Secondary patency rates		
1 month	39	9	81.9	5.5
6 months	26	16	68.3	6.8
1 year	20	17	65.4	7.1
2 years	11	21	47.9	8.6
4 years	5	21	47.9	8.6
		Limb salvage rates		
1 month	39	10	80	5.6
6 months	28	14	71.1	6.6
1 year	23	14	71.1	6.6
2 years	15	17	61.1	7.8
4 years	7	18	56.4	8.5

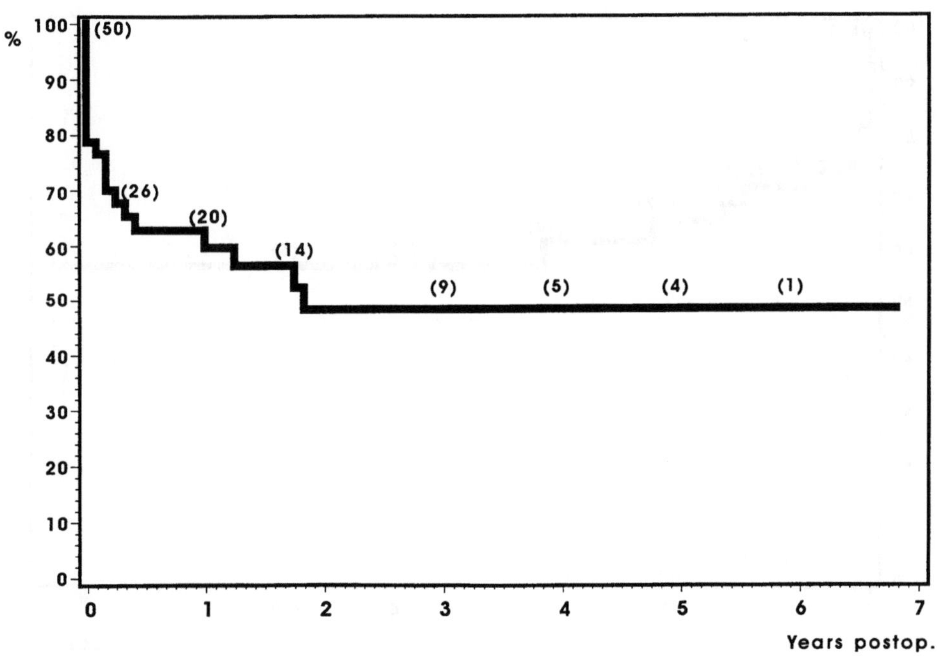

Fig. 2. Primary patency rate in 50 pedal vein bypasses (Kaplan-Meier)

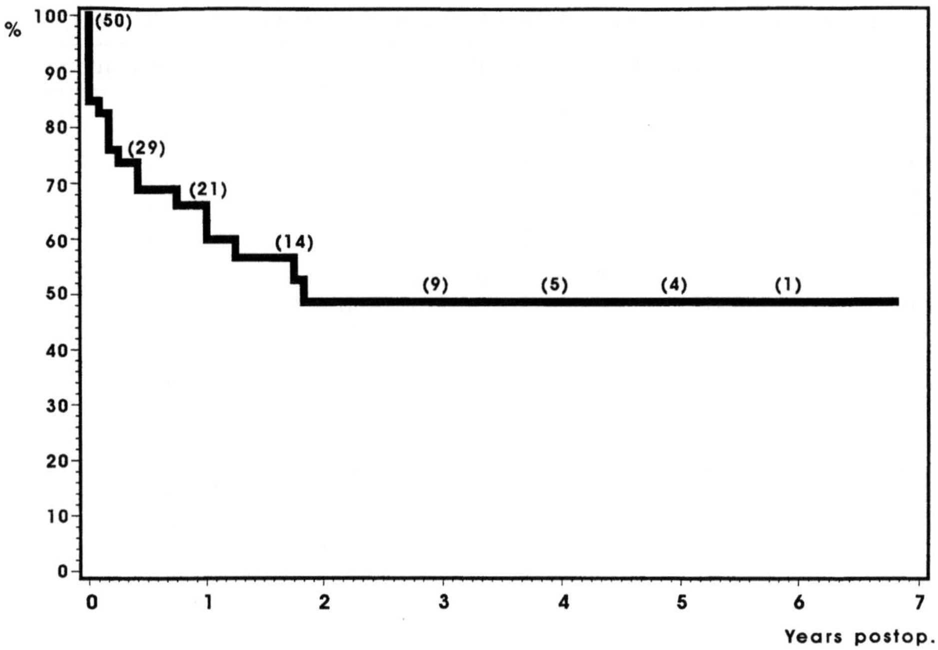

Fig. 3. Secondary patency in 50 pedal vein bypasses (Kaplan-Meier)

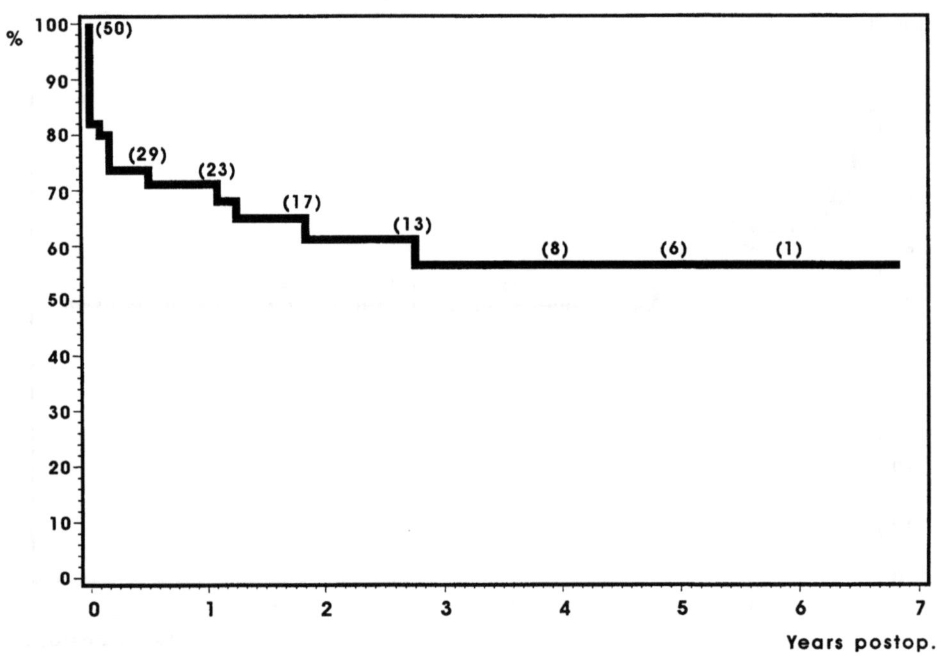

Fig. 4. Limb salvage in 50 pedal vein bypasses (Kaplan-Meier)

Table 5. Mortality during follow-up after pedal vein bypass (n = 50)

	All patients (n = 50)	Primary successfully treated patients (n = 41)
Number	21/50 (42 %)	18/41 (43.9 %)
Major amputation before death	6/21 (38.1 %)	5/18 (27.8 %)
Death with preserved legs	13/21 (61.9 %)	13/18 (72.2 %)

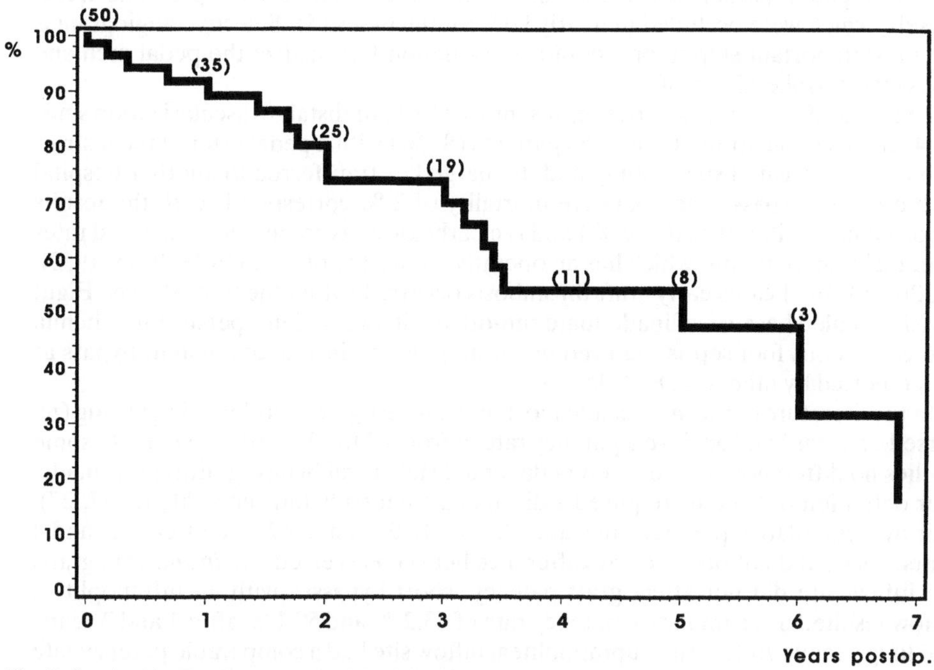

Fig. 5. Survival in 50 pedal vein bypasses (Kaplan-Meier)

patients (cardiac disease n = 13, stroke n = 4, bronchial cancer n = 2, acute limb ischemia following graft occlusion n = 1, perioperative death n = 1, median survival 34 months). Of these 21 patients 13 did not suffer a major amputation before death (61.9 %, median survival 21 months).

In the subgroup of the primary successfully treated patients 18/41 died (median survival 36 months): In addition to the patient who died following graft occlusion, four patients were amputated above the knee because of graft occlusion. In conclusion 13/18 patients (72.2 %) with patent bypasses at discharge died with preserved legs after 2–82 months (median survival 21 months). The bypass was still patent in 11 patients and occluded in two patients after 9 and 12 months without limb-threatening ischemia.

Discussion

Primary amputation is offered as an alternative to many patients with limb-threatening ischemia and a distal pattern of peripheral arterial occlusive disease for the following reasons: advanced age, multiple risk factors, increased cost and prolonged hospitalization, increased morbidity after failed revascularization, and general pessimism about inframalleolar reconstructions. However, several specialized centers have reported feasibility and remarkable long-term patency and limb salvage rates up to 90 % in bypass grafting to the distal arteries beyond and below the ankle (2–4, 8, 9, 11, 14, 15, 20, 21, 23, 24, 26–29).

In a post-mortem study of 140 legs amputated for severe ischemia, Dible reported 65– 70 % patent paramalleolar and foot vessels as compared to the proximal crural vessels, which were occluded in nearly 90 % of the bases (5). Selective angiogram is the most important step in preoperative evaluation to visualize the pedal arch and assess the peripheral run-off.

Venous grafts to pedal arteries represent 7.8 % of our distal revascularization since 1984. In this population 41 out of 50 patients (82 %) with a pedal arterial reconstruction could be treated successfully and discharged or transferred to another hospital with a patent bypass. The operative mortality of 2 % corresponds with the results reported in the literature (0 – 9 %) and is clearly lower as compared to survival rates after major amputation, which has an operative mortality of 7 – 15 % (8, 9, 15, 19, 21, 23, 26, 29). In 11 cases early graft thrombosis occurred within the first 30 days. Eight revisions failed because of inadequate run-off and in two patients persistent ischemia and continuous foot sepsis required major amputation inspite of a patent bypass as also reported by others (2, 8, 9, 15, 29).

In the literature of the last decade most of the investigators prefer vein grafting (reversed or *in situ*) and achieve a patency rate of from 42 to 97 % after 2 years. In some studies no differentiation between pedal and distal crural bypass grafting was made. Our definition of "pedal" required a distal anastomosis below the ankle (6, 17, 27). Our own cumulative patency rates are 59.2 %, 47.9 %, and 47.9 % after 1, 2, and 4 years. As we did not observe any difference between reversed and *in situ* vein grafts the inflow site did not affect graft patency: short bypasses with an infrapopliteal inflow resulted in a cumulative patency rate of 63.2 % and 50.1 % after 1 and 2 years, and long venous graft with a suprapopliteal inflow site had a comparable patency rate of 70.6 % and 45.4 %, respectively. Inspite of similar findings by Schneider et al. in 256 tibial/pedal bypasses, we always use the most distal inflow site possible (distal superficial femoral, popliteal or even a crural artery), providing there is no relevant narrowing in the proximal arterial tree. In agreement with several other investigators, the short bypass facilitates the operation in terms of getting a suitable vein with a proper caliber and it reduces the length of incisions (2, 3, 19, 21, 26, 29). If there is no appropriate vein for the whole distance we will perform a composite ("jump") graft (Dacron of PTFE 6 mm/vein) with end-to-side anastomosis between the two components of the bypass (7). Mono-prosthetic pedal bypass grafting should be avoided because the results in the literature and in our own experience in five earlier cases were not acceptable (26.6 % cumulative patency rate after 2 years).

Limb salvage and survival. In our patient population the cumulative limb salvage rate was 71.1 %, 61.1 %, and 56.4 % after 1, 2, and 4 years, which is about 5 % – 15 % higher than the corresponding patency rates. This agrees with recent data in the literature (8, 9, 11, 18, 21). As explanation for this phenomenon, it has been suggested that not every graft occlusion causes a new limb-threatening emergency, because tissue lesions have healed during the time when the bypass was patent with development of collateral vessels. In addition, it has to be recognized that the definition of "critical limb ischemia" does not mean that major amputation must be performed in every case if therapy – conservative or surgical – is not successful. Sometimes ischemic legs can be preserved for a long time without any medical or surgical treatment – inspite of the presence of all the criterias of chronic critical limb ischemia (30). Although the individual course is not predictable, in every case a therapy for limb salvage has to be chosen. In summary, it could be that the difference between limb salvage and patency rate is also caused by this fact. In contrast, Woelfle et al. reported a limb salvage rate 4 % lower than the corresponding secondary patency rate in six patients with below-knee amputation following spreading plantar infection inspite of a functioning bypass (29).

Twenty-one of our patients died during follow-up which reflects the multimorbidity of pour patient population. Thirteen patients (61.9 %), however, did not suffer a major amputation during the remainder of their lives (median survival 34 and 21 months, respectively). In the subgroup of the primary successfully treated patients with a patent bypass at discharge from hospital, a definite limb salvage was possible in 13 of the 18 who died (72.2 %) during follow-up.

Conclusions

Our results suggest that pedal vein bypasses provide limb salvage in about two-thirds of patients with crural arterial occlusive disease and critical limb ischemia. We therefore conclude that aggressive surgical management including selective angiography is necessary even in the presence of a popliteal pulse and even if revascularization of pedal arteries with poor blood flow and small caliber is necessary. Primary major amputation should be performed in patients who are confined to bed and should also be considered in patients with severe foot infections and no patent distal vessels angiographically.

References

1. Amputation or arterial reconstruction? (1992) Lancet (editorial) 339: 900–901
2. Andros G, Harris RW, Salles-Cunha SX, Dulawa LB, Oblath RW, Apyan RL (1988) Bypass grafts to the ankle and the foot. J Vasc Surg 8: 434–441
3. Ascer E, Veith FJ, Gupta SK et al. (1988) Short vein grafts: a superior option for arterial reconstructions to poor or compromised outflow tracts? J Vasc Surg 7: 370–378
4. Buchbinder D, Pasch AR, Rollins DL, Dillon BC, Douglas DJ, Schuler JJ, Flanigan DP (1986) Results of arterial reconstruction to the foot. Arch Surg 121: 673–677
5. Dible JH (1966) The pathology of limb ischemia. In: Cameron R, Wright GP (eds) Pathological monographs, Oliver & Boyd, Edinburgh, pp 39–53
6. Doerrler J, Mix C, Maurer PC, Pickl U, Holzman T (1986) Extended femoro-distal bypasses for limb salvage: are they worthwile? Int Angiol 5: 131–135
7. van Dongen RJM, Kromhout JG (1986) Femoro-crurale und pedale Rekonstruktionen. Alternative Materialien und Methoden. Angio Archiv 11: 79–82
8. Glovicki P, Morris SM, Bower TC, Toomey BJ, Naessens JM, Stanson AW (1991) Microvascular pedal bypass for salvage of the severly ischemic limb, Mayo Clin Proc 66: 243–253
9. Harrington EB, Harrington ME, Schanzer H, Jacobson JH, Haimov MH (1992) The dorsalis pedis bypass-moderate success in difficult situations. J Vasc Surg 15: 409–416

10. Jacobs MJ, Reul GJ, Gregoric ID et al. (1993) Creation of a distal arteriovenous fistula improves microcirculatory hemodynamics of prosthetic graft bypass in secondary limb salvage procedures. J Vasc Surg 18: 1–8
11. Labbe R, Douville Y, Noel HP (1989) Arterial reconstruction to the foot vessels: Is it worth the trouble? Can J Surg 32: 424–427
12. Lalka SG, Malone JM (1989) Patient evaluation and preparation for amputation. In: Rutherford RB (ed) Vascular surgery, Saunders, London, pp 1680–1685
13. Lindholt JS, Bøvling S, Fasting H, Henneberg EW (1994) Vascular surgery reduces the frequency of lower limb major amputations. Eur J Vasc Surg 8: 31–35
14. LoGerfo FW, Gibbons GW, Pomposelli FB Jr, Campbell DR, Miller A, Freeman DV, Quist WC (1992) Trends in the care of the diabetic foot. Expanded role of arterial reconstruction. Arch Surg 127: 617–620
15. Marks J, King TA, Baele H, Rubin J, Marmen C (1992) Popliteal-to-distal bypass for limb-threatening ischemia. J Vasc Surg 15: 755–760
16. Paetz B, Maeder N, Meybier H, Allenberg JR (1991) Pedal reconstructions for limb salvage. Eur J Vasc Surg 5: 621–625
17. Pedersen AE, Bornefeldt Olsen B, Krasnik M (1994) Halving the number of leg amputations: the influence of infrapopliteal bypass. Eur J Vasc Surg 8: 26–39
18. Pomposelli FB Jr, Jepsen SJ, Gibbons GW, Campbell DR, Freeman DV, Miller A, LoGerfo FW (1990) Efficacy of the dorsal pedal bypass for limb salvage in diabetic patients: short-term observations. J Vasc Surg 11: 745–751
19. Pomposelli FB, Jepsen SJ, Gibbons GW, Campbell DR, Freeman DV, Gaughan BM, Miller A, LoFerfo FW (1991) A flexible approach to infrapopliteal vein grafts in patients with diabetes mellitus. Arch Surg 126: 724–729
20. Procter CD (1991) Inframalleolar arterial reconstruction for limb salvage (editorial), Mayo Clin Proc 66: 322–324
21. Schneider JR, Walsh DB, McDaniel MD, Zwolak RM, Besso SR, Cronenwett JL (1993) Pedal bypass versus tibial bypass with autogenous vein: A comparison of outcome and hemodynamic results. J Vasc Surg 17: 1029–104
22. Second European Consensus Document on critical limb ischemia (1991) Circulation 84 (suppl)
23. Shah DM, Darling RC, Chang BB, Kaufman JL, Fitzgerald KM, Leather RP (1992) Is long vein bypass from groin to ankle a durable procedure? An analysis of a ten-year-experience. J Vasc Surg 15: 402–408
24. Tannenbaum GA, Pomposelli FB, Marcaccio EJ, Gibbons GW, Campbell DR, Freeman DV, Miller A, LoGerfo FW (1992) Safety of vein bypass grafting to the dorsal pedal artery in diabetic patients with foot infections. J Vasc Surg 15: 982–990
25. Veith JF, Gupta SK, Wengerter KR (1990) Changing arteriosclerotic disease patterns and management strategies in lower limb threatening ischemia. Ann Surg 212: 402–413
26. Veith FJ, Ascer E, Gupta SK, White SA, Wengerter KR (1988) In: Greenhalgh RM, Jamieson CW, Nicolaids AN (eds), Limb salvage and amputation for vascular disease, WB Saunders & Co, Philadelphia, pp 189–200
27. Verta MJ (1984) Composite sequential bypasses to the ankle and beyond for limb salvage. J Vasc Surg 1: 381–386
28. Wengerter KR, Yang PM, Veith FJ, Gupta SK, Panetta TF (1992) A twelve-year experience with popliteal-to-distal artery bypass: The significance and management of proximal disease. J Vasc Surg 15: 145–151
29. Woelfle KD, Lange G, Mayer H, Bruijnen H, Leoprecht H (1993) Distal vein graft reconstruction for isolated tibioperoneal vessel occlusive disease in diabetics with critical foot ischemia – does it work? Eur J Vasc Surg 7: 409–413
30. Wolfe JHN for the Joint Vascular Research Group (1986) Defining the outcome of critical ischemia: a one year prospective study. Br J Surg 73: 321

Author's address:
Hans-Henning Eckstein, MD
Dept. of Surgery, Division of Vascular Surgery, University of Heidelberg
Im Neuenheimer Feld 110
D-69120 Heidelberg
FRG

Value of intraoperative techniques in improving bypass patency

K. Balzer

Dept. of Vascular Surgery, Evangelisches Krankenhaus Mülheim an der Ruhr, Mülheim, Germany (Head: K. Balzer, MD)

Introduction

To save a useful leg despite arteriosclerotic changes is an old medical challenge. One legend is that the saints Kosmas and Damian transplanted the entire leg of a dead black man to a white man with extended gangrene. In the story the patient was able to walk after the operation and praised the Lord for that.

That kind of operation will remain a dream, but vascular surgery has made a lot of progress, especially in recent years. The patency rate of bifurcated grafts 5 years after implantation is more than 80 %.

The results for autologous venous bypass in femoral artery occlusions are with 70 % almost as good. The use of alloplastic grafts reduces the patency rates by 10 % in the first popliteal position.

Crural reconstructions show tendency towards worse results; an even worse outcome can be seen in the pedal area (Fig. 1).

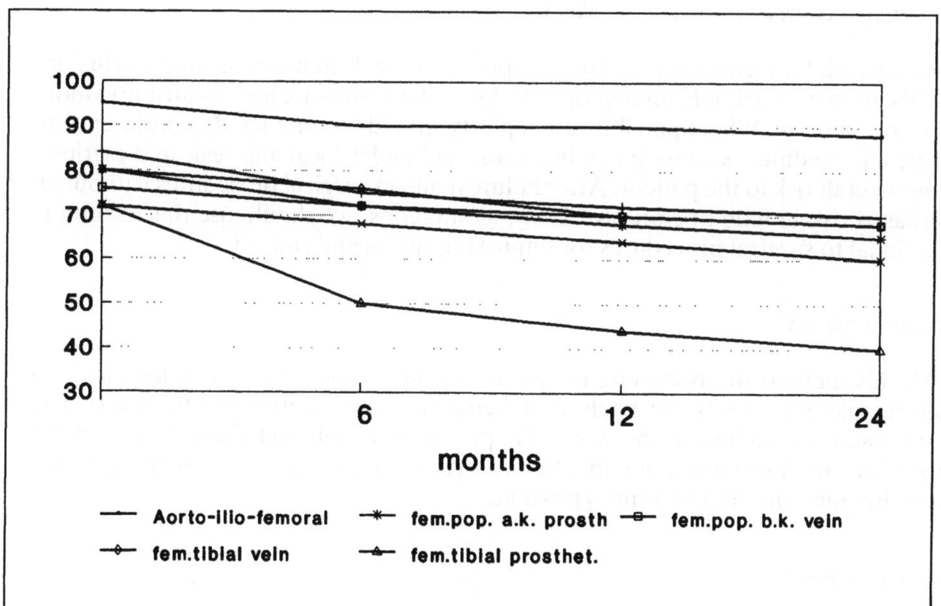

Fig. 1. Patency rates of vascular surgical procedures

Indication for operation

I want to point out that vascular surgery or interventional techniques are the methods of first choice in any patient with critical limb ischemia. But also a successful operation does not solve the problem of the progressive basic disease. A number of patients cannot be operated successfully because of multiple peripheral occlusions, especially in case of diabetes. Of course there are patients who, because of extended gangrene or unhealed limited amputations, can be considered hopeless for any further treatment. In these cases therapy with prostaglandins or spinal cord stimulation may be discussed.

Recommendation 25 of the critical ischaemia consencus document state that "primary amputation should only be undertaken if the possibility of revascularisation procedures has been excluded". In practice, revascularization might be rejected because it is deemed to be inappropriate, unsafe, impossible or inadvisable.

How can we improve the results of peripheral bypass surgery?

Possibility and risk of reconstructive surgery

Until the advent of angioplasty and other reopening procedures surgical reconstruction was the only method available for directly treating the underlying arteriosclerosis in the large vessels. It is still the most commonly used form of treatment for critical ischemia. The aim of such surgery is to bypass or remove the stenosed or occluded artery segment. The main methods employed by the vascular surgeon are as follows:

Percutaneous transluminal angioplasty

Patients with localized disease, for example, those with stenoses or short occlusions (< 10 cm) may be suitable for angioplasty, but so far results are less promising in more extensive disease. Where possible, angioplasty should be conducted in preference to surgical procedures because it can be performed under local anestesic and carries a lower overall risk to the patient. After failure it allows surgical procedures without an increased risk in redo operations. Today, as surgeons, we should use this technique additional to surgical procedures for improving run-in and run-off.

Endarterectomy

With this method the occluding plaque is cut out of the artery. In some cases an autologous vein or synthetic patch is stitched in to widen the lumen of the artery. The more distal the occlusion, the worse the prognosis of this technique. This method should be employed when possible before bypass surgery in spite of worse patency rates, because after it a grafting is possible.

Bypass-surgery

This operation involves bridging of the stenosed or occluded vascular segment with a venous transplant from the patient or using synthetic prostheses if no autologous material is available. Critical leg ischemia is often caused by disease occurring at several levels, and this often requires combined procedures. Frequent assessment of graft patency and immediate treatment of potential problems is preferable to trying to rectify a graft failure. More than 20 % of autologous vein grafts fail because of strictores within the first year. These stenoses should be treated by angioplasty or surgery and not be allowed to progress to complete occlusion. Various objective measurements are available to detect stenoses which could progress to occlusions such as post exercise ankle pressure measurement, Duplex-Scanning, digital subtraction angiography, and impedance-measurement (Table 1).

Value of intraoperative techniques and bypass-patency

Above-knee procedures

In femoral artery occlusions the results of all reconstructive techniques are similar. The use of autologous vein in this position has better patency rates, but this means only a small advantage as in redo operations after occlusions of the first popliteal segment a below-knee venous grafting is not possible anymore. For that, in our opinion, interventional techniques or thrombendarterectomy are methods of first choice and if they are not possible in above – knee procedures a synthetic bypass is preferable to autologous venous material. It is important that the incisions for above-knee bypass grafting do not injure the saphenous vein, so that it can be used in its full length for the redo procedure.

Below-knee procedures

The management for occlusions in the below-knee area is completely different. In the third popliteal segment patency rates of venous bypass are much better than the results for synthetic grafts. For the bridging of the knee joint no other expectation is possible. Thus the recommendation is necessary that, if available, the autologous vein is preferable to any synthetic material. This is especially true if the arteriosclerotic disease extends into the crural vessels. Although bypass grafts to the ankle and

Table 1. Reasons for graft failure

Early graft failure (< 30 days)	– incorrect choice of operation – operative technique – poor distal run off – low flow through the graft – thrombogenicity of the graft
Late graft failure (> 30 days)	– thrombosis – intimal hyperplasia – progressive atherosclerosis – graft structure abnormalities

foot are now commonplace, some of these operations are approaching the limits of surgical efficacy. If a long bypass is indicated and there is no sufficient autologous vein, the bridging of the above-knee occlusion could be done by synthetic grafts additionally, the means for example, a composite or a jump graft from groin to ankle. But the results using this technique fall considerably short with patency rates of only 40 % after 1 year. But they are better than using synthetic grafts alone.

Performing a venous graft in reversed, in situ or ex situ technique is without importance for long-term results. In the literature the best results for the orthotopic ex situ bypass are reported, but it has to be stated that this method was performed only in a few vascular centers. The comparision of the in situ and the reversed technique shows, in principal, only very little difference concerning patency and limb salvage rates. Thus, these methods are of the same value. A small advantage for the distal in situ reconstruction can be detected, probably because of the mismatch using the reversed bypass. So the in situ technique for crural and pedal reconstructions is preferable (Fig. 2).

Synthetic, homologous and heterologous material

There are currently two types of synthetic protheses in femoral and below-knee reconstructions:

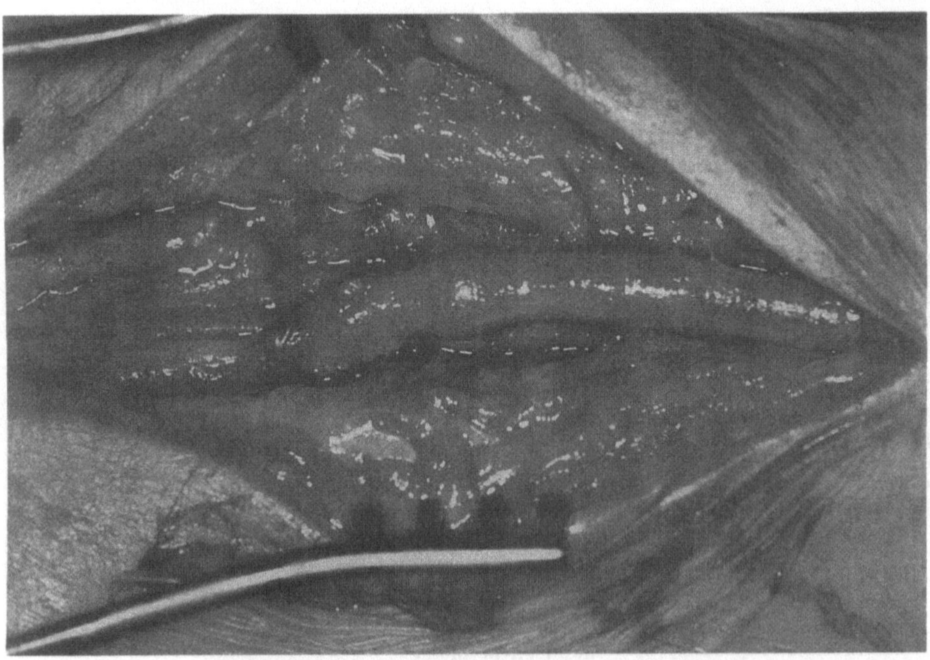

Fig. 2. Pedal anastomosis with a reversed bypass, the mismatch in the diameter of the vein and the artery is evident

1) Knitted or woven Dacron with or without collagene or gelatine coating.
2) PTFE-grafts with or without rings or spiral reinforcement.

In many trials better results for the PTFE-prostheses than for the Dacron grafts were reported. This is true for below-knee reconstructions and especially for the type with ring or spiral reinforcement because of neointimal hyperpoplasia at the distal anastomosis of knitted or woven Dacron prostheses, which worsen the long-term results. But in our opinion, for above-knee reconstruction, the patency rate for PTFE and Dacron is nearly the same, as is also reported in some literature. Therefore, these materials in above-knee use are of the same value. At the moment some trials are underway for proving the advantages of Dacron or PTFE and of collagene coating. We have to wait for the results.

Other synthetic materials, e.g., polyurethane or heterologous grafts such as bovine or ovine prostheses could not be established in the market because of rather poor results and high complication rates, especially aneurysmatic changes of the bovine grafts. Polyurethane seemed to be a better synthetic material because of its physiological compliance in animal experiments, but in clinical trials it proved a failure.

Beside synthetic materials only the umbilical vein could be established. The results are similar as compared with PTFE. In our experience there is no advantage for this type of vascular graft.

Intraoperative Techniques

Angiography

The possibility and efficacy of a surgical reconstruction must be confirmed by angiography. The success of surgery depends as outlined before, on the level of the obstruction. In general, the more distal the obstruction the worse the prognosis. In case of doubt an angiogram should be performed during operation after exposure of the below-knee arteries. Digital substraction angiography in combination with the possibility of "road mapping" leads to excellent x-ray documents and makes the surgeon able to use additional interventional techniques or to decide whether to attempt reconstruction or to advise amputation. The working group for critical limb ischemia made the observation that "in some cases primary amputation may be better than subjecting the patient to repeated surgical procedures with little chance of success and increasing mortality and morbidity". This can be a very difficult decision and a team approach may be useful. Each case should therefore be assessed on its individual merit and every patient should have a chance for vascular surgical reconstruction. The most difficult situation to judge is that in which surgical reconstruction may be technically possible, but with poor chance of lasting success.

Angioscopy

Though angioscopy was described more than 20 years ago, it could be established in routine use only in the last 10 years because of small flexible instruments provided with rinse channels and excellent optical systems. With today's angioscopes inspection of the vessel is possible in an adequate matter. For thrombendarterectomy this method proved to be a better control than angiography, but also for screening the anastomotic sites of the vessel this technique stood the test in detection of technical faults, induced strictures, intimal flaps or thrombotic formations at the arterial wall of the anastomotic or bypass formation. The performance of an in situ-bypass is better possible with angioscopic control because the incoming veins are visible and persistent a-v-fistulas can be avoided, as often seen by x-ray-control only (Fig. 3). Angioscopy is also important for proving patency after percutaneous transluminal angioplasty, especially after reopening of long distance occlusions. Damage to the vessel is substantial and we wonder about the rather good results (Fig. 4). Probably the sufficient patency rates are possible because, in spite of the intimal trauma, the endothelium stays in its place, while after surgical reconstruction it is removed and the vessel has more thrombogenicity.

Cell seeding

Many experimental trials were performed for improving the disappointing results after reconstruction of the arterial vessels using synthetic grafting material by seeding it with physiological endothelium. Several techniques for this are described. The most commonly used is the seeding process by harvesting the cells out of an autologous venous segment. A prospective randomized trial with a large number of patients

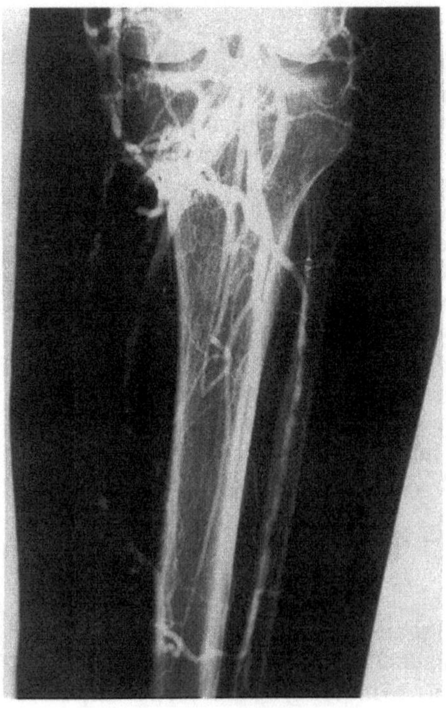

Fig. 3. Persistent a-v fistulas after in situ – bypass without angioscopic control

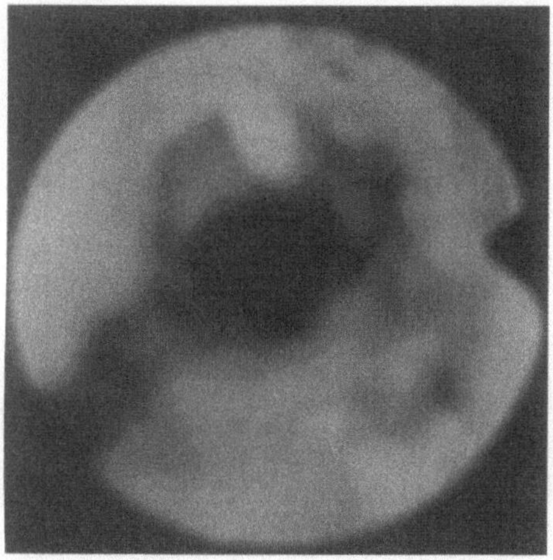

Fig. 4. Angioscopic control after PTA; damage to the arterial wall can be demonstrated

could not prove a beneficial effect for the cellseeding procedure; in contrast, the group with cellseeding had worse patency rates than the patients without, so that only a few centers are still using this technique in some modification.

Technical modifications of the distal anastomosis for improving bypass patency

For infrapopliteal bypass with PTFE-grafts anastomotic hyperplasia was responsible for approximately 25 % of late failures and was second only to progression of distal disease. Therefore, some concepts for better patency were developed. The problem might be helped by the planned insertion of a vein patch across the anastomosis. Indead, the employment of veinpatches has lead to reduction in the incidence of anastomotic hyperplasia but the so-called Linton-Patch cannot fully explain the improved results, and it is proposed that the main advantage may be directly related to the intrinsic property of the vein. In 1979, Siegman described the use of a venous cuff. This technique has been developed further by Miller, who reported encouraging early clinical results. An improved technique for PTFE-bypass grafting with using anastomotic vein-patches was described by Taylor. This technique allows a narrow angle between the graft and the artery. A vein-patch, which should be as large as possible, is used to close the eleptical defect in the anastomosis. Taylor reported a 65 % 5-year patency rate and a 88 % limb salvage rate. That means a significant advantage for this technique in comparison to the normal anastomosis. In a randomized multicenter trial the advantages of this technique are being investigated. We have to wait for further results (Fig. 5).

A-V Fistula

For improving the run-off it was suggested to perform an a-v fistula at the distal anastomotic site. Consequently, the vein receives a part of the arterial blood flow which leads to a higher flow rate through the graft. A graft failure may be related to the flow

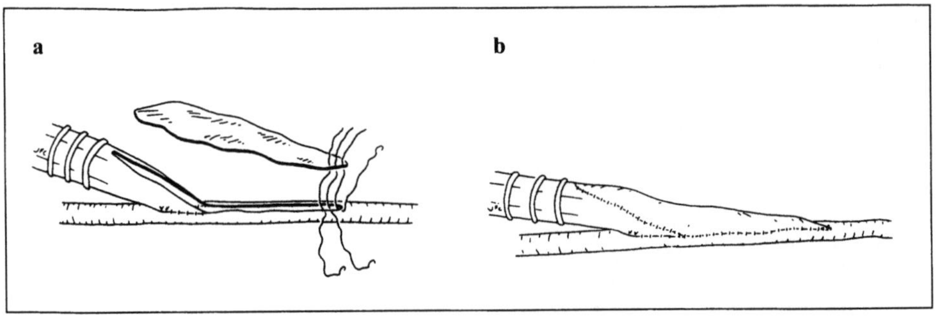

Fig. 5. a) The PTFE-graft is sutured to the below-knee vessel in this form; **b)** a vein patch is stitched in which allows a gradual reduction in diameter (from Taylor RS et al.: Long-term results of PTFE bypass grafting)

properties of blood through the vessel. Greater graft length increases the occlusion rate, increased diameter decreases the flow velocity and increases the occlusion rate. Therefore, theoretically an a-v fistula may be helpful. But it could not be proved by prospective randomized trials than an a-v fistula improves bypass patency or limb salvage. In contrast, a steal effect may reduce the arterial circulation and the nutrition of the dependent tissue. A few cases with salvage of a leg with critical ischemia by arterialization of a peripheral venous segment were described. We could not observe a beneficial effect of an a-v fistula and, for the same reason, we never use an arterial bypass to a peripheral vein for limb salvage.

Adjuvant medication

Streptokinase or rTPA can be used if peripheral vessels are occluded. With either the run-off can be improved if the microcirculation is not completely destroyed. Regional or local thrombolysis is possible during operation without an increased risk of bleeding complications if lysis of the thrombotic material can be achieved (Fig. 6 a, b).

After completion of the distal anastomosis the perfusion with a heparinized saline solution by an implanted small catheter for 48 h (PIDDAcatheter after Stockmann) could probably improve early patency.

A vasospasm after vascular surgical reconstruction can be observed quite often. It can be treated successfully by prostaglandins. We have to consider using this medication in the peripheral vessels during and after reconstructive procedures.

A postoperative application of anticoagulants makes sense and is very often necessary. Heparinization for several days after surgery is mandatory. Certainly a technical fault is always disastrous, even when using heparin. For below-knee reconstruction the postoperative anticoagulation with warfarine is imperative if there are no contraindications. There were some excellent prospective trials which showed improved patency for the below-knee venous bypass procedures using warfarine.

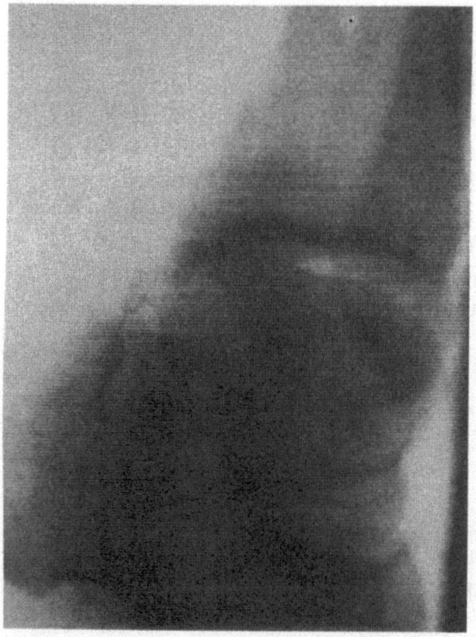

Fig. 6a. Occlusion of a femoro-pedal bypass

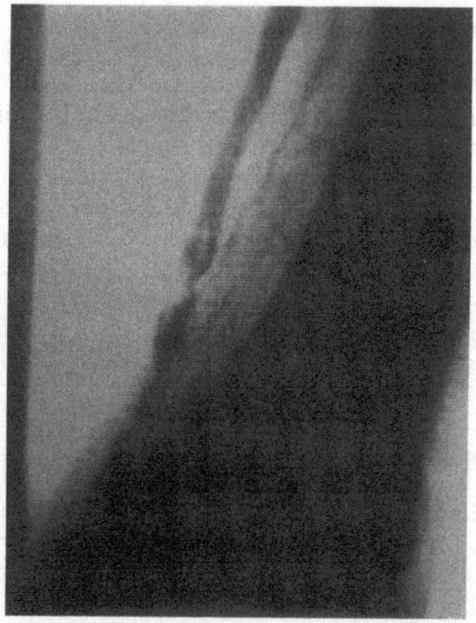

Fig. 6b. The bypass could be reopened by local application of streptokinase. The stenosis of the distal anastomosis after that was treated by angioplasty

Antiplatelet drugs are generally used in all types of arteriosclerotic disease. They are preferable to anticoagulation after thrombendarterectomy. In patients with gastrointestinal disorders, as an alternative, the use of ticlopidine may be discussed.

Vasoactive drugs such as naftidrofuryl, pentoxyphyllin or buflomedile may improve walking distance, but have no influence on patency rates and late results of peripheral bypass procedures.

Most important is an adequate prophylactic management of the underlying arteriosclerotic disease by observing the risk factors such as hypertension, diabetes, cholesterine, etc. Smoking must be stopped because this is the most harmful risk factor to the patient with POAD.

Measurements for improving postoperative results

It remain impossible to predict the possibility of vascular reconstruction or patency rates using different kinds of measurements such as TPO2, thermography, laser-Doppler, peripheral resistance, radio-isotope measurements and, of course, angiography. As described above, only duplex-scanning is able to detect strictures early and leads to an indication for a "service operation" before complete occlusion of the bypass.

Importance of operative experience

For bypass procedures to small vessels the employment of a meticulous surgical technique is mandatory for success. Even a minor error can be disastrous. That means that only a well skilled and experienced surgeon should perform vascular surgical reconstructions to the below-knee arteries. While an aggressive policy towards limb salvage is always justified, some discretion is needed, particularly in patients with poor life expectancy or with hopeless legs. But for the poor prognosis of amputations the consensus document on critical limb ischemia says in its recommendation 21:

"A reconstructive procedure should be attempted so long as there is a reasonable chance of saving a useful limb in a patient with evidence of sufficient run-off and is fit for surgery" (Fig. 7 a, b).

Amputations

Patients requiring below-knee and above-knee amputations are not diectly comparable. The difference in mortality cannot be attributed solely to the level of the amputation. The main advantage of the below-knee procedure is the preservation of the natural knee joint (Fig. 8). If limb salvage or minor amputation is not possible the below-knee or through-knee amputation is to be considered as a success of the vascular surgical procedure as compared to the primary above knee amputation. Shifting the amputation wounds distally as well as a better healing process following amputation is caused by the improved arterial circulation, so the aim of a redo operation may be a below-knee amputation (Table 2).

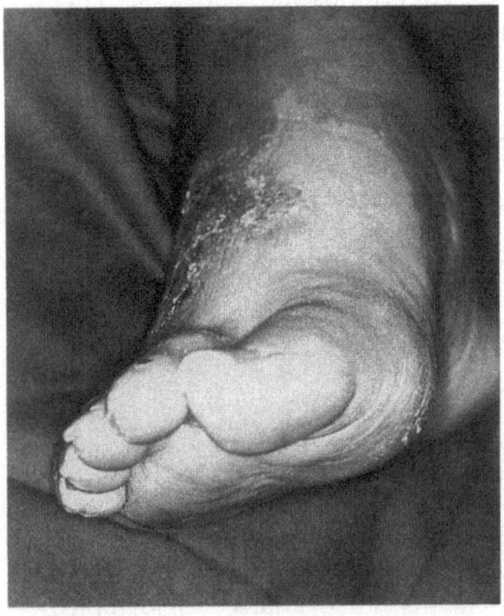

Fig. 7a. Chronic ischemic gangrene with acute occlusion of all below knee arteries

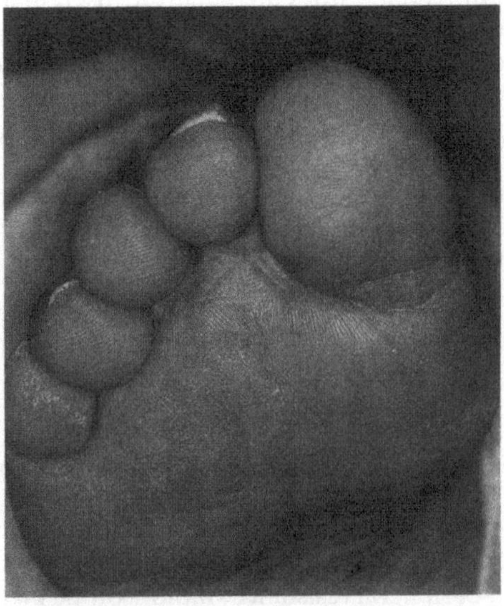

Fig. 7b. Result after reconstruction with femoral distal composite bypass

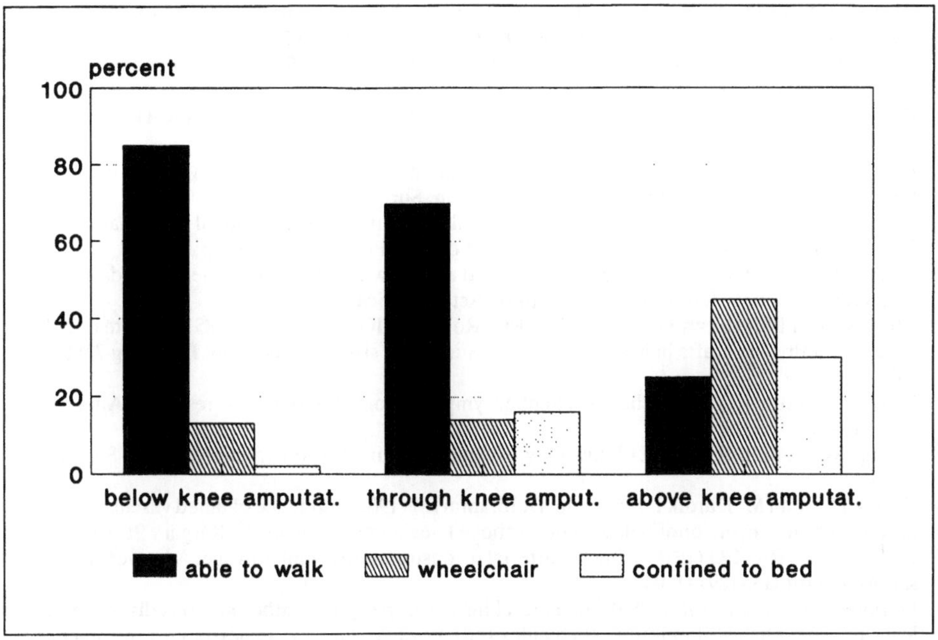

Fig. 8. Degree of rehabilitation according to site of amputation (after Stirnemann)

Table 2. Risk of amputation

	below knee	above knee
Hospital-mortality	4%	8%
1 year mortality	8%	18%
primary healing	70%	85%
secondary healing	15%	12%
further amputation	15%	3%
full mobility	50%	25%

References

1. Abbott WM, Megerman J, Hasson JE, L'Italien G, Warnock DF (1987) Effect of compliance mismatch on vascular graft patency. J Vasc Surg 5: 376–382
2. Adamek L, Balzer K (1988) Stellenwert und Ergebnisse peripherer gefäßchirurgisch-rekonstruktiver Maßnahmen in der Behandlung der AVK beim Diabetiker, angio 10, 5: 227–231
3. Ascer E, Veuth FJ, Morris L, Lesser ML, Gupta SK, Samson RH, Scher VA, White Flores SA (1984) Components of outlow resistance and their correlation with graft patency of lower extremity arterial reconstuctions, J Vasc Surg 1: 817–828
4. Balzer K (1994) Limb salvage, vascular procedures versus primary amputation. In: Horsch S, Claeys L (ed): Spinal Cord Stimulation, Steinkopff Darmstadt

5. Beard JD, Scott DJ, Evans JM, Skidmore R, Horrocks M (1988) Pulse generated run-off, a new method of determining calf vessel patency, Br J Surg 74 (4): 361–363
6. Beard JD, Benveniste GL, Miller JH, Baird RN, Horrocks M (1986) Haemodynamics of the interposition vein cuff. Br J Surg 73: 823–825
7. Bell PRF, Charlesworth D, De Palma R, Jamieson C (1982) The definition of critical ischaemia of a limb, Br J Surg 69: 52, 1
8. Bergan JJ, Veith FJ, Bernhard VM et al. (1983) Randomization of autogenous vein and polytetrafluoroethylene grafts in femorodistal reconstruction. Surg 92: 921–930
9. Bernhard VM (1981) Technical manoeuves to facilitate bypass to the popliteal and tibial vessels. In: Greenhalgh RM (ed) Femorodistal Bypass, London, Pitman Medical, pp 198–210
10. Charles D (1987) Problems related to run in and run off with reference to the profundafemoris artery and secondary femoropopliteal bypass. Acta Chir Scand 538–543
11. Charlesworth PM, Brewster DC, Darling RC, Robinson JG, Hallet JW (1985) The fate of polytetrafluoroethylene grafts in lower limb bypass surgery: a six-year follow-up. Br J Surg 72: 896–899
12. Cross FW, Cotton LT (1985) Chemical lumbar sympathectomy for ischaemic rest pain. Am J Surg 150: 341–345
13. Daling RC, Linton RR (1972) Durability of femoropopliteal reconstructions, Am J Surg 123: 472–447
14. Dardik H, Kahn M, Dardik I, Sussmann B, Ibrahim IM (1982) Influence of failed vascular bypass procedures on vonversionof below knee to above knee amputation levels. Surgery 91: 64–69
15. De Weese JA, Rob CG (1978) Effect of arterial reconstruction on limb salvage: A ten year appraisal. Arch Surg 113: 1297–1304
16. Dormandy JA, Mahir MS (1986) The natural history of peripheral atheromatous disease of the legs. In: Greenhalgh, Jamieson, Nicolaides (ed) Vascular surgery: issues in current practice, Grune and Stratton, London, pp 3–19
17. Dormandy A, Stock G (1990) Critical leg ischaemia, Springer Berlin Heidelberg New York
18. Dormandy JA, Thomas PRS (1988) What is the natural history of critically ischaemic patient with and without his leg? In: Greenhalgh RM, Jamieson CW, Nicolaides AN (ed): Limb salvage and amputation for vascular disease. Publ Saunders, pp 11–26
19. Erasmi H, Walter M, Schmidt R, Prokop A (1993) Peripherer Gefäßverschluß – Bypass oder Amputation? Langenbecks Arch Chir Suppl Kongreßbericht, 591–593
20. Evans LE, Webster MW, Brooks DH, Bahnson HT (1980) Peripheralarterial surgery. N Engl J Med 302: 491–503
21. Gardener GA Jr, Harrington DP, Kolrun W, Whittemore A, Mannick JA, Levin DC (1987) Salvage of occluded arterial bypass grafts by means of thrombolysis, J Vasc Surg 9: 426–432
22. Gupta SK, Veith FJ (1980) Below-knee bypass for limb salvage: Comparison of autogeneous saphenous vein, polytetrafluorethylene and composite Dacron-autogenous-vein grafts. Arch Surg 115: 833–837
23. Gupta SK, Veith FJ, Ascer E, White Flores SA, Gleedmann ML (1988) Cost factors inlimb threatening ischaemia due to infrainguinal artherosclerosis. European J Vasc Surg 2: 151–155
24. Harris PL, Read F, Eardley A, Charlesworth D, Wakefield J, Sellwood RA (1974) The fate of elderly amputees, Br J Surg 61: 665–668
25. Harris PL, Campbell H (1986) Femoro-distal bypass for critical ischaemia: is the use of prosthetic grafts justified? Ann Vasc Surg 1: 66–72
26. Harris P, Moody P (1990) Amputations. In: Dormandy A, Stock G: Critical leg ischaemia, Springer Berlin Heidelberg New York
27. Hertzer NR (1980) Three years experience with expanded polytetrafluorethylene artrial grafts for limb salvage. Amer J Surg 104: 214
28. Hobson RW, O'Donnell JA, Jamil Z, Mehta K (1981) Why do reported graft patency rates vary so wide? In: Greenhalgh RM (ed) Femoro-distal bypass. Pittmann, London
29. Hobson RW II, Lynch TG, Jamil Z et al. (1985) Results of revascularization and amputation in severe lower extremity ischemia: a five-year clinical experience. J Vasc Surg 2: 174–185
30. Holstein P (1985) Skin perfusion pressure measured by radioisotope washout for predicting wound healing in lower limb amputation for arterial occlusive disease. Thesis Acta Orthop Scand Suppl 213
31. Johnson WC (1977) Autogenous venous grafts ten years later, Surgery 82: 775–784

32. Kunlin J (1949) Le traitement de l'arterite obliterante par la greffe veineuse. Arch mal Coeur, 42, 371–372
33. Londrey GL, Ramsey DE, Hodgson KJ, Barkmeier LD, Sumner DS (1991) Infrapopliteal bypass for severe ischemia: comparison of autogenous vein, composite and prosthetic grafts. J Vasc Surg 13: 631–636
34. Miller JH, Foremann RK, Ferguson L, Faris I (1984) Interposition vein cuff for anastomosis of prosthesis to small artery. Aust N Z J Surg 54: 283–285
35. Oblath RW, Buckley FO, Green RM, Schwartz, SL, De Weese JA (1987) Prevention of platelet aggregation and adherence to vascular grafts by aspirin and dipyridamole. Surgery 84: 37–44
36. Parvin SD, Evans DH, Bell PRF (1985) Peripheral resistance measurement in the assessment of severe peripheral vascular disease, Br J Surg 72: 751–753
37. Rafferty TD, Avellone JC, Farrell CJ et al. (1987) A metropolitan experience with infrainguinal revascularization. Operative risk and late results in northeastern Ohio. J Vasc Surg 6: 365–371
38. Ratcliff DA, Clyne CAC, Chant ADB, Webster JHH (1989) Prediction of amputation wound healing: the role of transcutaneous oxygen tension in the selection of amputation level. Am J Surg 147: 510–517
39. Sclenker JD, Wolkoff JS (1975) Major amputations after femoropopliteal bypass procedures. Am J Surg 129: 495–499
40. Seibel RMM, Carstensen G, Balzer K, Grönemeyer DHW, Sehnert C (1989) CT-gesteuerte lumbale Sympathikusausschaltung bei der Behandlung der peripheren arteriellen Verschlußkrankheit (AVK). In: Gröbemeyer DHW, Seibel RMM: Interventionelle Computertomographie, Ueberreuter Wissenschaft, Wien Berlin
41. Siegmann FA (1979) Use of the venous cuff for grafts anastomosis. Surg Gynecol Obstet 148: 930
42. Simms MH (1988) Is pedal arch patency a pre-requisite for successful reconstruction? In: Greenhalgh RM, Jamieson CW, Nicolaides AN (ed) Limb salvage and amputation for vascular disease. Publ Saunders, London, pp 49–62
43. Spence VA, Walker WF, Troup IM, Murdoch G (1981) Amputation of the ischaemic limb: selection of the optimum site by thermography. Angiology 32: 155–169
44. Szilagyi DE, Hagemann JA, Smith RF, Elliott JP (1985) Femoropoplitealer Bypass: Autologe Vene oder PTFE-Prothese? Angio 7, 1: 13–20
45. Stirnemann P (1986) 10 Jahre Erfahrung mit den großen Amputationen beim vasculär-chirurgischen Patienten. In: Widmer LK, Zemp E (eds) Angiologie 86, Hans Huber Bern, 63–64
46. Stockel M, Oresen J, Bröchner-Mortensen J, Emnius H (1982) Standardised photoelectric technique as routine method for selection of amputation level. Acta Orthop Scand 53: 875
47. Stockmann U (1983) Pidda – ein Novum in der cruralen Gefäßchirurgie, Angio 5, 2: 67–71
48. Taylor RS, Loh A, McFarland RJ, Cox M, Chester JF (1992) Improved technique for polytetrafluoroethylene bypass grafting: long-term results using anastomotic vein patches. Br J Surg 348–354
49. Taylor RS (1981) The use of PTFE in Great Britain. In: Greenhalgh RM (ed) Femoro-distal Bypass. London, Pitman Medical, 211–217
50. Taylor RS, McFarland RJ, Cox MI (1987) An investigation into the causes of failure of PTFE grafts. Eur J Vasc Surg 1: 335–343
51. Tilanus HW, Obertop H, Van Urk H (1985) Saphenous vein of PTFE for femoropopliteal bypass. A prospective randomized trial. Ann Surg 202: 780–782
52. Tuchmann A, Strasser K, Axenkopf G (1972) Obliterationsgrad proximaler Unterschenkelarterien in Beziehung zum Ergebnis femoro-poplitealer Thrombendarteriektomien, Vasa 1: 256
53. Veith FJ, Moss CM, Fell SC, Rhodes BA, Haimovici H (1981) Femoropopliteal bypass to the isolated popliteal segment: is PTFE graft acceptable? Surgery 89: 296
54. Veith FJ, Moss CM, Fell SC, Montefusco C, Rhodes BA, Haimovici H (1978) Comparison of expanded polytetrafluoroethylene and autogenous saphenous vein grafts in high risk arterial reconstructions for limb salvage. Surg Gynecol Obstet 147, 749–752
55. Veith FJ, Gupta SK, Ascer E et al. (1986) Six-year prospective multicenter randomized comparison of autologous saphenous vein and expanded polytetrafluoroethylene grafts in infrainguinal arterial reconstructions. J Vasc Surg 3: 104-114
56. Veith FJ, Gupta SK, Daly V (1980) Management of early and late thrombosis of expanded polytetrafluoroethylene (PTFE) femoropopliteal bypass grafts. Favorable prognosis with appropriate reoperation. Surgery 87: 581–587

57. Veterans' Administration Cooperative Study Group 141 (1988) Comparative evaluation of prosthetic, reversed and in situ vein bypass grafts in distal popliteal and tibial-peroneal revascularization. Arch Surg 123: 434–438
58. Wilson SE, Wolf GL, Cross A (1989) Percutaneous transluminal angioplasty versus operation for peripheral arteriosclerosis. Report of a randomised trial in a selected group of patients. J Vasc Surg 9: 1–9
59. Wolfe JHN (1988) Critical ischaemia – is this concept of value? In: Greenhalgh RW, Jamieson CW, Nicolaides AN (ed) Limb salvage and amputation for vascular disease, WB Saunders, London, 3–10

Author's address:
Klaus Balzer, MD
Head of the Dept. of Vascular Surgery
Evangelisches Krankenhaus
Wertgasse 30
D-45468 Mülheim an der Ruhr
FRG

Value of spinal cord stimulation for limb salvage in patients with graft failure

J. P. Favre, A. Richard, J. P. Gournier, X. Barral

Dept. of Cardiovascular Surgery, University of Saint-Étienne, France

Introduction

Direct surgical revascularisation remains the best treatment for critical ischemia. However, for certain patients this is not possible because of poor run-off. In these cases there are three alternatives before amputation: medical treatment with a possible focus on prostaglandins; lumbar sympathectomy, and spinal cord stimulation. The latter has been chosen for evaluation.

Patients and methods

Between October 1989 and September 1992, 425 distal bypasses were performed in our institution on patients with critical ischemia. During this same period, a distal bypass for limb salvage was considered technically impossible in 28 patients who were subsequently offered epidural spinal cord stimulation (ESCS).

Selection criteria

ESCS was only proposed to patients who had a critical ischemia with rest pain or gangrene. The therapeutic decision was based on an angiogram. Conventional or digital angiography was performed in order to visualise the complete limb vascularisation. None of the included patients had a proximal or distal lesion accessible to surgery or angioplasty. All occlusive diseases were taken into account (atherosclerosis, diabetes and Buerger disease). Furthermore, in order for the patient to be included in the study, two criteria were mandatory : their complete understanding and cooperation in that they had to communicate clearly the level of pain experienced; and long-term follow-up had to be possible with a fixed consultation every 6 months. There was no age limit as such, but unstable patients with low life expectency were not included. The presence of a neurological or rachis pathology contra-indicated ESCS.

Patient status

These criteria were filled by 28 patients (20 men and 8 women) with an average age of 68 (41 – 83 years). Six patients had rest pain for more than 3 weeks; 12 had ischemic ulcers and 10 had distal gangrene. Eleven patients were diabetic and two had Buerger's disease. A prior lumbar sympathectomy had been carried out on 11 patients and 10 patients already had a patent distal bypass. Fourteen patients had been amputated of one or several toes. Finally, at least one distal bypass had been performed on every patient, with an average of 2.4 bypasses per patient (Fig. 1).

The pain level was recorded on a scale from 0 to 4 (0: no pain, 1: slight pain easy to forget, 2: continuous moderate pain, 3: significant pain, 4: unbearable pain). Over a 24-h period, the highest pain level was recorded. "0" pain level was not observed in this study. For the entire series, the average pain level before installation of the SCS was 2.82. Morphine was necessary for 11 patients and the remaining 17 were treated with non morphinic drug. The analgesic treatment was recorded from 0 to 2 (0: no drugs, 1: non-morphinic, 2: morphinic).

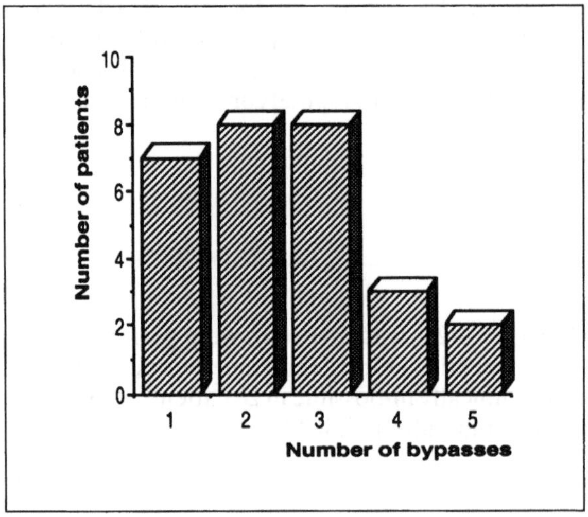

Fig. 1. Number of previous distal bypass graft failure.

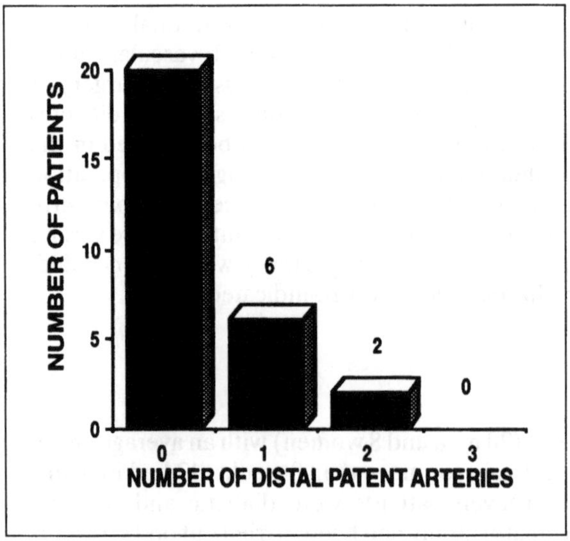

Fig. 2. Angiographic findings: number of patent distal arteries.

In the case of 20 patients, the angiography did not show any patent arteries above knee level, rendering distal revascularisation impossible; However, 8 patients had one or more patent distal arteries (Fig. 2). In these cases a distal bypass was theoretically possible, but a lack of saphenous veins or the thrombosis of prior prosthetic graft contraindicated any such further operation.

Patient evaluation

All patients underwent the following investigations before ESCS:
- a double-view x-ray of the rachis to evaluate technical possibilities for implantation of the lead.
- ankle/brachial index pressure with an average of 0.41 (± 0.21) before ESCS (0.70 in the case of diabetics)
- digital plethysmography which was pulsed in 8 patients out of the 26 in which this investigation was possible (two patients had Parkinson's disease)
- analysis of blood flow at calf level with an electromagnetic flow meter. In 26 patients, the average flow recorded was 31.5 ml/mn (± 23 ml/mn) for a norm of 100 – 120 ml/mn.
- transcutaneous measurement of oxygen pressure (TCPO2) at foot level. This was performed in two positions during the same examination in decubitus and in sitting position. The average TcPO2 was 9 mmHg (± 10) decubitus and 28 mmHg (± 17) in sitting position.

ESCS technique: Implantation of the lead.

In all cases the lead was a Quad type (Medtronic, Minneapolis, MN, USA) with four stimulation poles situated 2 mm apart. The electrode implantation was performed under local anesthesia with a light sedative preparation, with the patient lying on his stomach. The position of the catheter was controlled by x-ray and its efficiency tested by an external stimulator. Paresthesia had to be felt by the patient reaching to the foot. When the electrode was well positionned (generally between D12 and L1) the wires were tunneled under the skin of the left flank and linked to a temporary external stimulator.

ESCS Period:

Continuous stimulation with the external stimulator was carried out for an average of 8 days. During this trial period, various criteria allowed the evaluation of the efficiency of the treatment:
- pain level evolution (recorded on the scale from 0 to 4).
- Antalgic drug prescription (recorded from 0 to 4).
- Level and perception of paresthesia in relation to the position of the patient along with any necessary modifications to the stimulation
- Trophic lesion evolution.
- Repeated non-invasive vascular investigation (Doppler, plethysmography, electromagnetic flow, TCPO2) (Fig. 3)
- a further spinal x-ray to control the position of the lead.

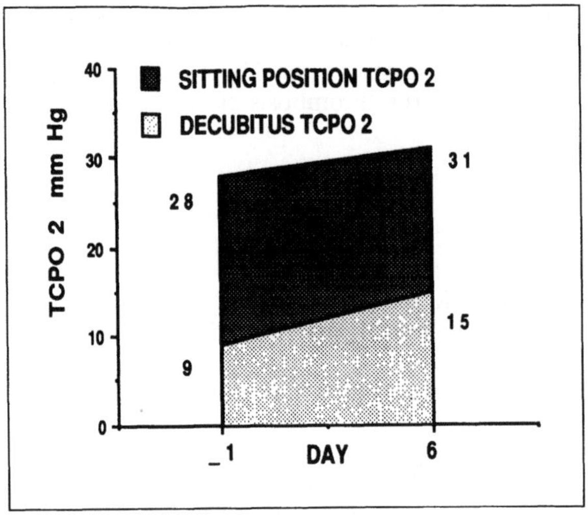

Fig. 3. TcPO2 evolution during trial week (TcPO2 in decubitus and in sitting position).

If the results and clinical evolution were good, the permanent stimulator was inserted under local anesthesia on the right flank and linked to the initial electrode, and the temporary wires were subsequently removed. The average amplitude was 4 volts, pulse width 0.3 micro-seconds and stimulation frequency 95 Hz.

Analysis method

The patients had regular consultations after 1 month, 3 months, and then every 6 months with a non-invasive test (Doppler, TCPO2, plethysmography, electro-magnetic flow meter) performed at each consultation. The evolution and condition of the limb were recorded along with the pain intensity and the use of analgesics. The simulator was also verified to make sure it was in proper working order.

The statistical analysis was carried out with Student's *t*-test.

Results

Twelve patients did not receive permanent ESCS. Eleven patients did not experience any clinical improvement and as a result the permanent stimulator was not implanted. Of these eleven patients, 10 were amputated during follow-up and one was asymptomatic after new femoro-distal by-pass carried out with a prosthesis. These 10 amputations (six below knee and four above knee) were performed after failure of ESCS (mean 2 months). The 12th patient had an infection of the wires which subsequently had to be removed. This patient's ulcer healed 6 months after lumbar sympathectomy. Of the 12 patients, two died during follow-up.

A permanent stimulator was implanted in the remaining 16 patients, of which 11 experienced a great improvement with loss of pain during the trial period. These 11 patients had good results during a mean follow-up of 36 months. The ischemic ulcers and gangrene which were present in nine patients healed after 3 months in seven cases, and after 5 months in the two other cases. During the follow-up, two recurrences of trophic lesions occurred; four generators discharged, but none of them were changed. Two of these 11 patients died after 6 and 18 months.

For the remaining five patients the improvement was less significant, but the stimulator was installed in the hope that the improvement would continue. Among these five patients, four had to be amputated less than 1 month after implantation, the last patient had an infected generator which was removed 15 days after implantation. In this latter case the patient had good results after medical treatment.

In order to find which are the good and poor indications of ESCS, we decided to compare the patients with failure and the patients with success of the technique: 15 patients had failure (11 during the trial period and four after permanent implantation), 11 had good and long-term results. Two patients with sepsis were excluded of this comparison. There was no difference between the two groups concerning the preoperative symptomatology, the number of diabetics, the number of previous bypasses or the ankle/brachial index. But the preoperative TcP02, the plethysmography, and the quality of distal arteries were better when the patient obtained a good evolution (Table 1).

During the trial period, the most important parameters were the evolution of pain level, drug prescription and TcPO2. In the group of poor results there was no evolution of pain level during trial period (Fig. 4). The mean preoperative TcPO2 was better in the group with good evolution and there was an improvement of this TcPO2 during the trial period (Fig. 5). Results of preoperative arteriography seemed also important: patients with one or two patent distal arteries had good evolution, patients with no artery below knee had generally poor results.

Discussion

The use of posterior spinal cord stimulation to obtain an analgesic effect was first proposed in 1967 by Shealy (1). Since this time, ESCS has been considered to be a safe and efficient alternative in the treatment of continuous chronic pain from chronic

Table 1. Comparative study between failed and improved patients. (Two patients with Sepsis were excluded).

	All patients	Good results	Poor results	Comparison
Number of patients	28	11	15	
Diabetics	11	4	6	N.S.
Sympathectomy	11	8	2	$p<0{,}001$
Stage III	6	3	3	N.S.
Gangrene < 3 cm	12	3	8	N.S.
Gangrene > 3 cm	10	5	4	N.S.
A/B index pressure	0,41	0,45	0,39	N.S.
Decubitus TcPO2	10	14,5	5,8	$p<0{,}01$
Sitting position TcPO2	30	39	21,5	$p<0{,}005$
Pulsed plethysmography	8	7	1	$p<0{,}001$
Patent distal artery	8	7	0	

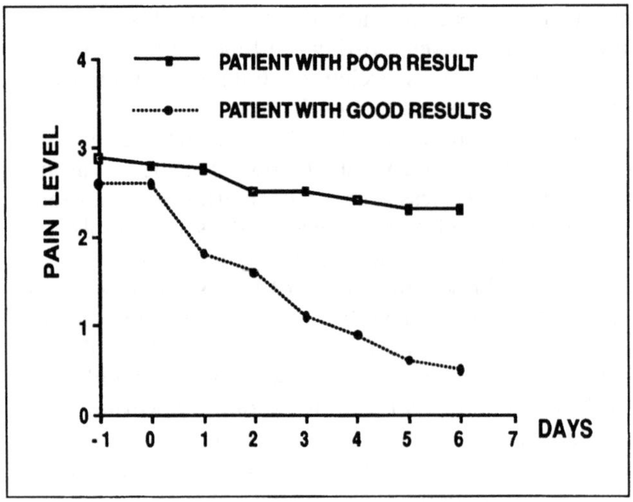

Fig. 4. Pain evolution during trial week: Comparison of patient with good result and patient with poor result. (Two patients with sepsis were excluded)

nerve injury. In 1976, Cook and Dooley (2) noticed an improvement in the condition of the distal vascularisation in the lower limbs of patients with peripheral arterial disease.

Experimental data indicates that ESCS increases peripheral microcirculatory flow by the inhibition of vaso-constriction of the sympathic nerve. Therefore, ESCS is used today in cases of critical ischemia with rest pain, ischemic ulcers or gangrene. Several authors have postulated that the principal factor in the relief of ischemic pain is the inhibition of the pain signal leading to a decrease in sympathetic activity and improved skin circulation (3,4). Pain relief may also result in attenuation of sympathetic activity with vasodilatation, leading to further pain relief. Another hypothesis is that ESCS depresses autonomic sympathetic activity (5). However, many authors, including us, have reported success even after sympathectomy (3, 6).

The affected limb needs hemodynamic and arteriographic investigations to eliminate any possibility of distal bypass before ESCS is considered. Furthermore, the angiogram must be of excellent quality. The contrast agent must be injected into the common femoral artery with appropriate timing to clearly visualise the distal vessels. When all the surgical possibilities are eliminated, the main problem of this technique is to determine the predictive criteria for a good result.

The objective quantitative criteria do not have the same value. The analysis of the ankle / brachial index, by Doppler study, is not reliable because the ESCS does not involve any increase in the distal blood pressure. The electro-magnetic flow meter is also unreliable. In our experience, in the case of critical ischemia, the variation of calf blood flow, before and after ESCS, is insignificant and does not allow for a good result. In our opinion, only two exams are useful for deciding if ESCS will be beneficial or not:

- TCPO2, which is the most reliable flow indicator for tissue metabolism. The TCPO2 is normal over 60 mm Hg. Critical ischemia is defined by a TCPO2 of below 30 mm Hg. The TCPO2 does not increase in patients with no clinical improvement.

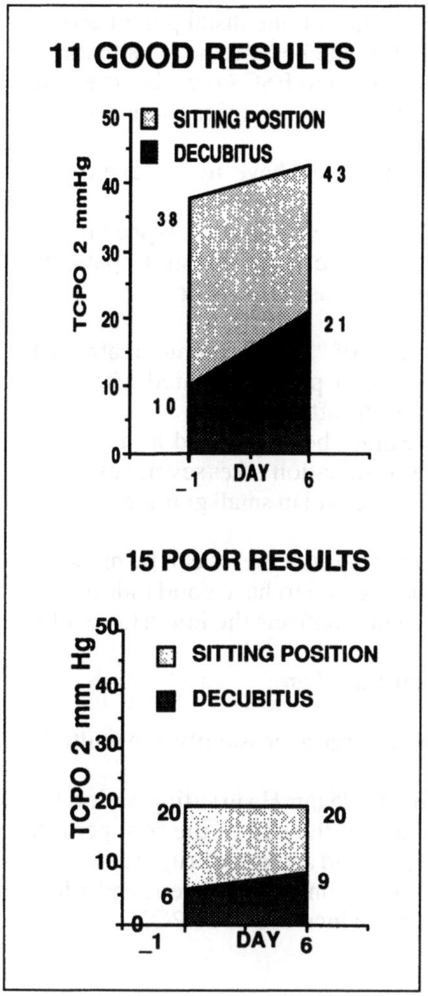

Fig. 5. TcPO2 evolution during trial week: Comparison of patient with good result and patient with poor result. (Two patients with sepsis were excluded)

In this study, before ESCS, there was a significant difference in TCPO2 between the patients with good results (14.5 lying – 39 sitting) and those without (6 lying – 21.5 sitting). We also noted an increase in TCPO2 after 10 days of stimulation both in decubitus and seated position, but only in patients with clinical improvement. This effect takes place rapidly just before the end of the trial period and then continues at a constant level. Our results are similar to those previously published (7 – 9).

- Pulse plethysmography is also a good predictive exam. In our study it was pulsed in seven cases. All of these patients had good long-lasting results after ESCS. It is important to take into account the fact that these patients had at least one patent distal artery visible on the angiogram. They could have had a distal bypass if their saphenous vein had been avaliable. In the absence of patient distal arteries this method is probably less reliable. Boccalon (10) stated that the increase of pulsatility is insignificant after ESCS. Therefore, the presence of one distal patent artery associated with a pulse plethysmography is certainly the best predictive situation. However, in these cases surgery is the best alternative and ESCS must be reserved for certain cases (multi-operated patients, patients in poor condition, patients with no saphenous vein . . .)

Two further criteria, even although they are subjective, have to be taken into account:

- the disappearance of ischemic pain after ESCS. This effect must take place rapidly during the trial period for it to be classed as a good criteria. In this study, patients who were rapidly sedated with either no use or a decreased use of drugs had good follow-up results.
- similarly, patients with an analgesic treatment level of "2" (morphinic treatment) had little chance of good follow-up results. Out of 11 patients treated with morphine before implantation, only two had good results after ESCS.

The improvement of eventual trophic lesions cannot be considered as a criteria because the trial period is too short. The complete cicatrisation takes several months. As shown by Jacobs (6), this cicatrisation is more successful in small grangrenes with a diameter of less than 3 cm.

To sum up, according to our experience, the following statements can be made:

1) out of the 28 patients with critical ischemia who seemed to have good indications for ESCS, only 16 received permanent ESCS. This confirms the importance of a 1-week trial period to avoid rushed implantations.
2) the criteria used for patient selection in the trial period are:
   - critical ischemia without extended lesion.
   - a patent distal artery on the angiogram without surgical possibility or a multiple graft failure.
   - a TCPO2 > 10 mmHg in decubitus increasing to >25 mmHg in sitting position.
3) the decision to implant a pulse generator is made at the end of the trial period: when there is a rapid and complete decrease of pain and analgesic drug intake, and with only the complete understanding and cooperation of the patient and when this clinical improvement has been confirmed by an increase of TCPO2.

Conclusion

In conclusion, the indications for ESCS are rare, but in certain cases of limb salvage it can be useful. The cost of the material results in rigorous patient selection but, in our experience, this can help reduce the number of amputations. In this study, out of 28 patients with critical ischemia, 11 did not undergo amputation.

References

1. Shealy CN, Mortimer JT, Reswick JB (1967) Electrical inhibition of pain by stimulation of the dorsal columns: preleminary clinical report. Anesth Analg 46: 489–491
2. Cook AW, Oygar A, Baggenstos P et al. (1976) Vascular disease of the extremities: Electrical stimulation of the spinal cord and the posterior roots. NY State J Med 76: 366–368

3. Broseta J, Barbera J, De Vera JA (1986) Spinal cord stimulation in peripheral arterial diseases. J Neurosurg 64: 71–80
4. Foreman RD, Chandler MJ, Brennan TJ et al. (1989) Does dorsal column stimulation reduce the activity of spinothalamic tract cells that respond to cardiac input? Circulation 80 (Suppl II): 552
5. Augustinsson LI, Carlsson CA, Fall M (1982) Autonomic effects of electrostimulation. Appl Neurophysiol 45: 185–189
6. Jacobs MJHM, Jorning PJG, Beckers RCY et al. (1990) Foot salvage and improvement of microvascular blood flow as a result of epidural spinal cord electrical stimulation. J Vasc Surg 12: 354–360
7. Claeys L, Ktenidis K, Horsch S (1994) Transcutaneous oxygen tension in patients with critical limb ischemia treated by spinal cord stimulation. In Spinal cord stimulation; Horsch S and Claeys L; ed. Springer International p 145–152
8. Galley D, Elharrar C, Scheffer J, Jeangeorges B, Serena G (1989) Neurostimulation et pathologie vasculaire: intérêt thérapeutique à propos de 49 cas. Cœur 20: 35–44
9. Meglio M, Cioni B, Rossi GF (1989) Spinal cord stimulation in management of chronic pain. A 9 years experience. J Neurosurg 70: 519–524
10. Boccalon H (1992) Les tests d'exploration vasculaires. Intérêt pour les indications et la surveillance de la neuro-stimulation medullaire épidurale. J Mal Vasc 17: 131–137

Authors' adress:
Docteur J. P. Favre
C.H.U. De St-Étienne
Hopital Nord
Chirurgie Vasculaire
42055 Saint-Étienne Cédex 2

Epidural spinal cord stimulation following intravenous prostaglandin E1 therapy in non-reconstructible peripheral arterial occlusive disease stage IV

L. G. Y. Claeys, S. Horsch

Dept. of Vascular Surgery, General Hospital Cologne-Porz
Academic Teaching Hospital of the University of Cologne, Germany

Introduction

Spinal cord stimulation is a medically accepted therapeutic modality for the control of chronic pain (21, 25). For the past two decades, spinal cord stimulation has been advocated as a method of pain relief for therapeutic refractory ischemic pain (8). Strikingly, in vascular patients not only pain relief could be achieved but also healing of ischemic ulcers (2, 7, 10, 11, 12, 13, 24). This suggests that spinal cord stimulation improves the nutritional skin blood flow. This was confirmed in recent studies (15). However, there is a lack of prospective randomized studies, evaluating the effect of spinal cord stimulation on wound healing and limb salvage. Therefore we evaluated the efficacy of spinal cord stimulation on ulcer healing and limb salvage in a randomized-control study in patients with non-reconstructible PAOD undergoing 3 weeks i.v. PG E1. There is enough evidence that prostaglandins are valuable drugs for patients with rest pain and ischemic ulcers. There are no significant differences between the prostacyclin analogue iloprost and PGE1. In several studies it appeared that up to 60 % of patients given iloprost experienced significant pain relief and healing of ischemic ulcers and that during follow-up significantly more patients on iloprost than on placebo were alive without a major amputation (1, 3, 4, 5, 6, 9, 14, 23, 26).

Materials and methods

Study design

A randomized control study was made in patients undergoing 21-day i.v. prostaglandin E1 therapy for non-healing ischemic foot ulcers. Twenty-six patients received adjunctive spinal cord stimulation and 22 only optimal medical therapy. Intra-arterial arteriograms were obtained from all patients and showed occluded crural vessels unsuitable for an angioplasty or a distal bypass procedure. Failed distal bypass procedures were noted in 40 patients. Primary endpoints were Fontaine stage, ulcer healing, and limb salvage. Secondary endpoints were pain-relieving effect and changes in macro- and microcirculatory parameters. All patients received optimum medical therapy (OMT). The patient group receiving spinal cord stimulation in addition to OMT, shall be referred to as the SCS-group.

Baseline data

At baseline, there were no statistically significant diffferences between the two groups in any of the following data: patients with ASO: 15 in the SCS group vs. 10 in the control group; patients with ASO and DM: 5 vs. 5; hypertension: 19 vs. 19; necrotic toe(s) or ulcer > 20 mm diameter: 10 vs. 4; presence of two or more foot lesions: 4 vs. 6; smoking: 17 vs. 16. There was a slight trend toward a poorer physiological status in the SCS group as shown by the mean foot TcPO2: 9.7 vs. 12.0 mmHg and the mean ankle brachial index: 0.266 vs. 0.362. These were only trends due to patient variability and were not significant.

Methods of analysis

Outcomes were measured by Fontaine stage, ulcer size and number, level of amputations, changes in foot oxygen, and changes in ankle brachial index. If an ulcer healed completely and the patient was left with rest pain, they were classified as Fontaine stage III. If they did not even have rest pain, and only pain with exercise, they were classified as Fontaine stage II. Patients that still had lesions, even if the reduction in size was 50 % or greater, were defined as partial success. Patients with unchanged lesions, or larger lesions, or patients with a below-knee or above-knee amputation were considered to have failed.

Statistical methods

$P < 0.05$ was chosen as the level for statistical significance. For 2×2 contingency tables, a Fisher's exact test was used. For comparison of group means, ANOVA was used, and a two-tailed *t*-test.

Results

Outcomes by Fontaine stage

There was a significant difference between both groups concerning healing of ulcers. Seventeen of the 26 patients (65 %) of the SCS group achieved complete healing by 12 months vs. only 6 of the 22 patients (27 %) of the OMT group. In addition, all four of the SCS patients who remained in stage IV had substantial healing of ulcers, more than 50 %, vs. only 2/11 (22 %) of the OMT group, where in four patients the ulcers worsened.

There was no significant difference in the two groups in either minor or major amputations. Both groups had five major amputations, and both had two patients requiring minor amputations of necrotic toes or forefoot. This data does not support the theory that SCS may lead to a lower level of amputation. Indeed, there were more above-knee amputations (AKA) than below-knee amputations (BKA) in the SCS group, which was not true for the OMT group.

Amputations

The rates of minor and major amputations were similar between the SCS and the OMT groups. Of the patients who achieved Fontaine stages II or III, minor amputations were occasionally required. One SCS-patient at stage II required a toe amputation. One SCS-patient was able to heal the ulcers half-way, but only after two necrotic toes were amputated. Two OMT-patients achieved stage III outcomes: one required a toe amputation and one a forefoot amputation. The minor amputations occurred at 2.5 months average, range 1.0 to 7.0 mo., following enrollment in the study.

Major amputations occurred at 3.0 months average, range 1.0 to 6.0 mo., following enrollment in the study. The SCS group had 5 major amputations at a mean of 3.9 mo., two were BKA, three were AKA. The OMT group also had five major amputations at a mean of 2.2 months, not significantly earlier in time in this series. Four were BKA and one was AKA.

Outcomes by risk factors

Whether or not success is defined as complete ulcer healing or as partial ulcer healing, the SCS-group does significantly better than the OMT-group. This is true also for the nondiabetic subgroup of patients, and for diabetic patients also, although, due to sample size, it is a trend only.

Effects on the macrocirculation

Ankle systolic pressures did increase significantly for one subgroup of SCS-patients, those with complete ulcer healing ($n = 17$). The mean increase was 14 ± 21 mmHg, equivalent to 34 % of the baseline mean value ($p < 0.05$). Mean ABI for this group, however, only showed a strong trend ($p < 0.06$).

The entire SCS group, $n = 26$, had an increase in mean ankle systolic pressure of 10% on average, and an increase in mean ABI of 6 %, but high variability made these differences non-significant.

No statistically significant change in ankle systolic pressure or ABI was observed in any outcome subgroup of the OMT-patients. For the entire group of 22 patients, however, mean ankle pressure decreased by 13 % on average, and the ABI decreased significantly by -0.069 (-19 %) of the mean value at baseline.

Effects on the microcirculation

TcPO2 was chosen as parameter of the microcirculation. There were no significant differences between the SCS and the OMT groups at baseline. The mean initial value for all SCS patients was 9.7 ± 7.4 mmHg. The mean value for all patients at 1 year was 18.8 ± 12.7 mmHg. The mean baseline value for all OMT patients was 12.0 ± 7.6 mmHg. Final TcPO2 for these patients at 1 year ranged from 0 to 30 mmHg. The mean value for all patients was 10.7 ± 10.9 mmHg. At 1 year, for the entire population, the mean TcPO2 dropped by -1.3 ± 7.9 mmHg (10.6 %), which is consistent with the concept of a control group for endstage PAOD.

Discussion

Neurosurgeons became interested in stimulation of the nervous system in the late 1960s. Since that time stimulation was performed for different pain indications. This has also led to the use of ESCS to treat chronic ischemic pain. Several published reports confirmed pain relief under ESCS, suggesting an improvement of the nutritional blood flow (2, 7, 10, 11, 12, 13, 15, 24). The theoretical background for pain relief under stimulation is based on the Gate Control Theory which provided a model for the modulation of the nociceptive input to the dorsal horns of the spinal cord (22) and on Reynolds' discovery that electrical stimulation could provoke profound analgesia (22). The exact mechanisms underlying the effect of ESCS on ischemic pain and peripheral blood flow still remain uncertain. Presently, the mechanisms proposed to be responsible for the modulation of ischemic pain are neurophysiological and neurohumoral in nature (16). The neurophysiology varies from simple blocking of impulse traffic in the spinothalamic tract, activation of supraspinal loops relayed via brainstem or thalamocortical system, and activation of descending pain controlling pathways in the spinal cord. SCS might also induce the release of neurotransmitters involved in pain transmission (18). Gamma-aminobutyric acid (GABA), serotonin and substance P are transmitters mediating inhibition of nociceptive transmission in the spinal dorsal horn are released in the dorsal horn by ESCS (17, 19). These substances might contribute to the analgesic effects of neurostimulation. The background for the therapeutic effects may also be an inhibition of sympathetically maintained peripheral vasoconstriction (20).

Several studies have shown that prostaglandins are valuable drugs for patients with rest pain and ischemic ulcers (1, 3–6, 9, 14, 23, 26). In this study we found significant improvement in ulcer healing in the group of patients receiving adjunctive SCS with a concomitant increase in quality of life. These observations are due to an improvement of the nutritional blood flow and a modulation of the transmission of pain impulses. There was no significant difference in the two groups in either minor or major amputations. To evaluate a limb-saving effect we have to include more patients in this study and to reevaluate limb survival at 2 and 3 years. Our data supports the belief that patients with diabetes can do equally well as those without. There is also the converse proposition that hypertensive patients do not benefit from SCS in terms of foot salvage. Our study data supports the opposite theory of the foot salvage studies. Indeed, SCS promotes healing even in hypertensive patients. No statistically significant changes in ABI were observed in the SCS or OMT patients. Subgroup analysis showed a significant increase for the SCS-patients with complete ulcer healing. Mean ABI for this group only showed a strong trend. Neither systolic pressures nor ABI changed significantly for any other SCS subgroup.

Conclusion

This randomized study demonstrates that spinal cord stimulation added to PG E1 infusion therapy for non-reconstructible stage IV patients is an effective treatment. During long-term follow-up of 1 year, both ulcer healing and quality of life remained significantly improved compared with the control group. Ulcer healing is correlated to increase in TcPO2. At 1 year significant differences in limb salvage do not appear. Inclusion of more patients and follow-up studies at 2 and 3 years are necessary.

References

1. Altstaedt HO, Berzewski B, Breddin K et al. (1993) Treatment of patients with peripheral arterial occlusive disease Fontaine stage IV with intravenous iloprost and PGE1: a randomised open controlled study. Prostaglandins, Leukot Essen Fatty Acids 49: 573–578
2. Augustinsson LE, Holm J, Carlsson CA et al. (1985) Epidural electrical stimulation in severe ischemia. Evidence of pain relief, increased blood flow and a possible limb saving effect. Ann Surg 202: 104–111
3. Balzer K, Bechara G, Bisler H et al. (1987) Placebokontrollierte doppel-blinde Multizenterstudie zur Wirksamkeit von Iloprost bei der Behandlung ischämischer Ruheschmerzen von Patienten mit peripheren arteriellen Durchblutungsstörungen. Vasa, Suppl 20: 379–381
4. Balzer K, Rogatti W, Rüttergodt K (1989) Efficacy and tolerability of intra-arterial and intravenous prostaglandin E1 infusions in occlusive arterial disease stage III/IV. Vasa, Suppl 28: 31–38
5. Bliss B, Wilkins D, Campbell WB et al. (1991) Treatment of limb threatening ischemia with intravenous iloprost: a randomised double blind, placebo controlled study. Eur J Vasc Surg 5: 511–516
6. Brock FE, Abri O, Aitsch G et al. (1990) Iloprost in der Behandlung ischämischer Gewebsläsionen bei Diabetikern. Schweiz Med Wochenschr 120: 1477–1482
7. Broseta J, Barbera J, De Vera JA et al. (1986) Spinal cord stimulation in peripheral arterial disease. A cooperative study. J Neurosurg 64: 71–80
8. Cook AW, Oygar A, Baggenstos P et al. (1976) Vascular disease of the extremities: electrical stimulation of the spinal cord and the posterior roots. NY State J Med 76: 366–368
9. Diehm C, Abri O, Baitsch G et al. (1989) Iloprost, ein stabiles Prostacyclinderivat bei arterieller Verschlußkrankheit im Stadium IV. Dtsch Med Wochenschr 114: 783–788
10. Dooley D, Kasprak M (1976) Modification of blood flow to the extremities by electrical stimulation of the nervous system. South Med J 69: 1309–11
11. Fiume D (1983) Spinal cord stimulation in peripheral vascular pain. Appl Neurophysiol 46: 290–294
12. Galley D, Elharrer C, Scheffer J et al. (1989) Neurostimulation et pathologie vasculaire: intéret thérapeutique a propos de 49 patients. Coeur 20: 35–44
13. Groth KE (1985) Spinal cord stimulation for the treatment of peripheral vascular disease. European multicenter study. In: Advances in Pain Research and Therapy, ed. by Fields H. New York Raven Press: 861–870
14. Guilmot J-L, Diot E (1991) Treatment of limb ischemia due to atherosclerosis in diabetic and non diabetic patients with Iloprost, a stable analogue of prostacycline; results of the French multicenter trial. Drug Invest 3: 351–359
15. Jacobs MJ, Jorning PJG, Beckers RCY et al. (1990) Foot salvage and improvement of microvascular blood flow as a result of epidural spinal cord stimulation. J Vasc Surg 212: 354–360
16. Linderoth B (1992) Dorsal column stimulation and pain: Experimental studies of putative neurochemical and neurophysiological mechanisms. Thesis. Stockholm: 11–19
17. Linderoth B, Gazelius B, Franck J et al. (1992) Dorsal column stimulation induces release of serotonin and substance P in the cat dorsal horn. Neurosurgery 31: 289–297
18. Linderoth B, Stiller C-O, Gunasekera L et al. (1993) Release of Neurotransmitters in the CNS by Spinal Cord Stimulation: Survey of Present State of Knowledge and Recent Experimental Studies. Stereotactic Funct Neurosurg 61: 157–170
19. Linderoth B, Stiller C-O, Gunasekera L et al. (1994) Gamma-aminobutyric acid is released in the dorsal horn by electrical spinal cord stimulation: an in vivo microdialysis study in the rat. Neurosurgery 34: 484–489
20. Linderoth B, Herregodts P, Meyerson BA (1994) Sympathetic mediation of peripheral vasodilation induced by spinal cord stimulation: animal studies of the role of cholinergic and adrenergic receptor subtypes. Neurosurgery 35: 711–719

21. Long DM, Erickson DE (1975) Stimulation of the posterior columns of the spinal cord for relief of intractable pain. Surg Neurol 4: 134–141
22. Melzack R, Wall PD (1965) Pain mechanisms: a new theory. Science 150: 971–9
23. Norgren L, Alwmark A, Ängkvist KA et al. (1990) A stable prostacyclin analogue (iloprost) in the treatment of ischemic ulcers of the lower limb. A Scandinavian-Polish placebo controlled randomised multicenter study. Eur J Vasc Surg 4: 463–467
24. Robaina FJ, Dominguez M, Diaz M et al. (1989) SCS for relief of chronic pain in vasospastic disorders of the upper limbs. Neurosurgery 24: 63–67
25. Shealy CN, Mortimer JT, Reswick JB (1978) Electrical inhibition of pain by stimulation of the dorsal columns: Preliminary clinical report. Annest Analg 46: 489–491
26. Trübestein G, von Bary S, Breddin K et al. (1989) Intravenous prostaglandin E1 versus pentoxifylline therapy in chronic arterial occlusive disease – a controlled randomised multicenter study. Vasa. Suppl 28: 44–49

Author's address:
L. G. Y. Claeys, MD
Academic Teaching Hospital Cologne-Porz
Dept. of General and Vascular Surgery
Urbacher Weg 19
D-51149 Cologne
FRG

Spinal Cord Stimulation for Angina Pectoris

Neurophysiological mechanisms of pain relief by spinal cord stimulation in angina pectoris

R. D. Foreman

Department of Physiology, University of Oklahoma Health Sciences Center, Oklahoma City, Oklahoma, USA

Introduction

A number of clinical reports, including chapters in this book, demonstrate the clinical efficacy of epidural spinal cord stimulation and transcutaneous electrical nerve stimulation to reduce or suppress cardiac pain in patients who experience severe angina pectoris (13, 14, 30–32, 35, 43). A strong consensus has grown to support the anti-anginal effects of stimulation measures (42), but the neurobiology of the mechanisms of action remains a major and yet unresolved clinical problem. Clinical reports identify several possibilities, including reduction in sympathetic discharge to the heart, activation of endogenous opioid systems, release of prostaglandins, and production of a placebo effect. These implications provide an urgent impetus to understand the mechanisms and to provide additional support so that this novel therapeutic approach can be recommended for safe and effective use.

The purpose of this chapter is to summarize what is known about basic neural mechanisms that underlie angina pectoris and the neural effects evoked during spinal cord stimulation. The focus of this review will be directed to the pain processing and its inhibition, but this information sets the stage to address autonomic mechanisms because parallels exist between these two systems. The first brief section will discuss the possible neural mechanisms underlying angina pectoris. The second section will provide evidence to show how spinal cord stimulation might reduce pain associated with severe myocardial ischemia. In the third section discussion will focus on the activity of neurons of the upper cervical segments that are excited by vagal afferent excitation. This section also will provide speculation about how neurons in the upper cervical segments and vagal afferents might participate in pain control related to spinal cord stimulation.

Neural mechanisms of angina pectoris

Pain of angina pectoris is often sensed over a wide area of the thorax, left or sometimes right shoulder and arm, and occasionally in the neck, jaw and teeth (18, 35, 41). Clinical descriptions of referred pain associated with angina pectoris can be categorized into three main characteristics to explain pain that originates from the heart, but is referred to somatic structures. Pain of angina pectoris: 1) is dependent on afferent information that originates from the heart and is conveyed to the same spinal segments as the overlying somatic areas; 2) is referred to proximal and axial body areas, but not to distal regions (9); and 3) is described generally as a deep, unbearable pain and not as a superficial or cutaneous pain (25).

A systematic study of the organization and response properties of the spinothalamic tract (STT) system supports the characteristics described in patients (Fig. 1) (20). Cardiopulmonary afferent input excite spinothalamic tract cells located in the C_3 to C_6 and T_1 to T_6 segments of the spinal cord, but has little input to the cells of the C_7 and C_8 segments. The STT cells of the C_3 to C_6 segments and the T_1 to T_6 segments receive convergent somatic input predominately from muscle of the proximal arm and chest. In contrast, the STT cells located in the C_7 and C_8 segments are activated predominately by cutaneous receptive fields located on the hand and lower arm regions. Thus, viscerosomatic convergence of cardiopulmonary afferent input and the predominately proximal muscle input arising from the somatic fields provides the neurophysiological basis to support the clinical descriptions of angina pectoris (Fig. 1).

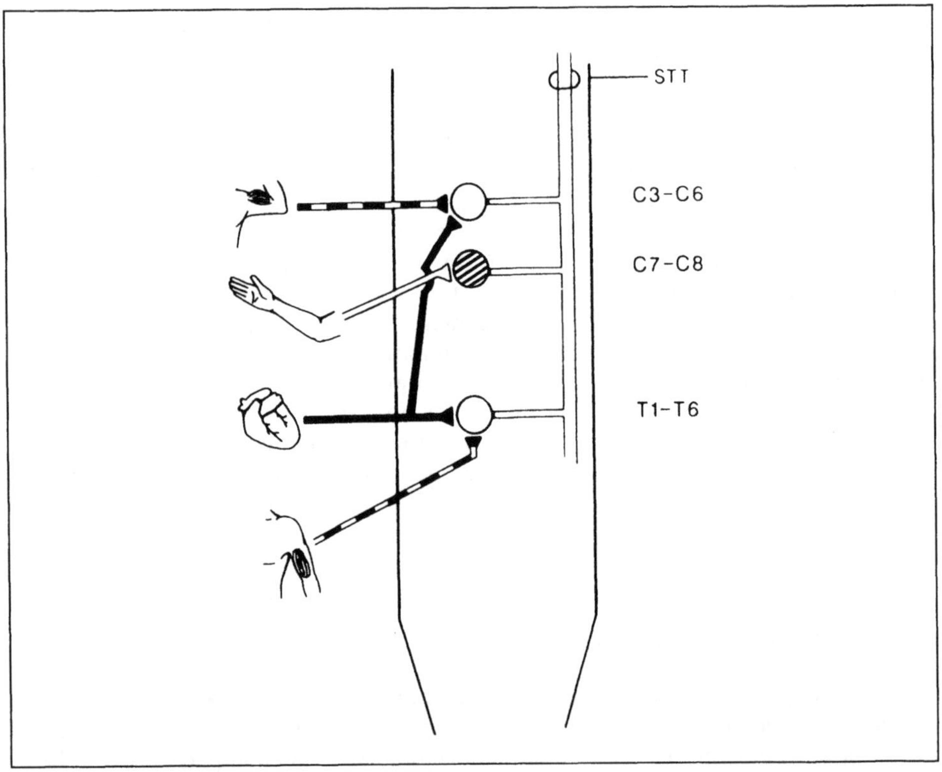

Fig. 1. Schematic diagram of spinal neural mechanisms that may explain the characteristics of angina pectoris. This figure illustrates the organization of the spinothalamic tract (STT) afferent fibers in the spinal cord to describe processing of information from the heart and somatic structures. Dashed lines are somatic afferent fibers and solid lines are sympathetic afferent fibers. Sympathetic afferent fibers from the heart converge on cells of the C3–C6 and T1–T6 STT cells that also receive primarily muscle input from the upper arm and chest. The hand and arm represent the predominately cutaneous (somatic) afferent input to the C7–C8 segments of the STT tract.

Effects of spinal cord stimulation on STT cell activity

Spinothalamic tract cells are selected for this type of study because they represent the classical pain pathway relevant to angina pectoris. These neurons have the potential to process noxious information from the heart and from the somatic structures that characteristically present the anginal pain (3, 4, 8, 20). Antidromic activation of these cells proved that they project to the ventroposterior lateral nucleus of the thalamus. This nucleus is critical for relaying noxious information to areas of the cortex that are important for contributing to pain sensation. In fact, locations for antidromic stimulation in our experiments are in or close to the thalamic area in a human patient where electrical stimulation produces the sensation of angina pectoris (24).

Extracellular action potentials of STT neurons located in the gray matter of the C_8–T_5 spinal cord segments were recorded to determine the effects of spinal cord stimulation. Somatic receptive fields for these cells are located in the left arm, axilla, and/or chest region. To demonstrate that spinal cord stimulation affects noxious information arising from the heart, the potentially algesic chemical bradykinin was used to activate cardiac receptors of sympathetic afferent fibers projecting to the T_1–T_5 segments of the spinal cord. Bradykinin is an algesic chemical that is found in the effluent of the coronary sinus during myocardial ischemia (19, 23). Approximately 2–4 μg/kg of bradykinin was injected into the left atrium to activate receptors. Our laboratory has shown that intracardiac injections via this route activates primarily cardiac receptors (7).

Spinal cord stimulation was administered while STT cells increased their activity as a result of the bradykinin injections. To simulate spinal cord stimulation performed in human studies (30) a monopolar ball electrode was placed on the left dorsal column in the lower cervical segments and the parameters also mimicked the human study. Current intensity varied between 1 and 350 μA and frequency varied between 50 and 200 Hz with the duration set at 250 μs. Activity of STT cells increased approximately 10 s after bradykinin was injected into the left atrium. The delayed activation of the cell is a common characteristic of receptor activation (4, 7, 29). During peak evoked activity of the STT cells, ipsilateral dorsal columns were stimulated by using a ball electrode and making direct contact with the surface. An example of the stimulation effects is shown in Fig. 2 and a summary of the responses is illustrated in Fig. 3. Spinal cord stimulation also reduced spontaneous activity and noxious evoked activity that resulted from pinching the somatic receptive fields (11). Stimulation of the dorsal column below but not above a spinal transection activated STT cells to the same extent as the intact spinal cord (11).

Paresthesia associated with spinal cord stimulation for angina pectoris might be explained using somatic characteristics of the STT cells (3, 6, 20). The paresthesia is crucial for proper placement of the stimulating electrodes in patients (5, 15, 30). In general, STT cells can be separated into four categories: 1) high threshold or nociceptive specific cells responding only to noxious somatic stimulation; 2) high threshold inhibitory are cells that are excited by noxious stimuli, but inhibited during innocuous stimulation such as hair movement or light touch; 3) wide dynamic range neurons are excited slightly by innocuous stimuli but the frequency of discharge is much greater at noxious intensities; 4) low threshold cells are excited only with innocuous stimuli, but the discharge rate does not increase at higher intensities. Spinal cord stimulation more likely inhibited activity of high threshold and high threshold inhibitory cells than activity of the wide-dynamic range and low threshold cells (11). These results are

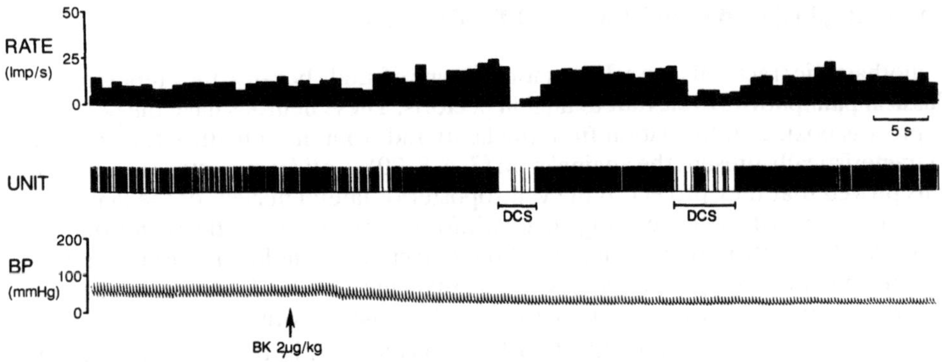

Fig. 2. Effects of dorsal column stimulation (DCS) on the activity of a STT cell after injecting the algesic chemical bradykinin into the heart (11). The dorsal column was stimulated (80 μA, 80 Hz, 250 μs) after a bradykinin injection (2 $\mu g \cdot kg^{-1}$) was made into the heart and the STT activity increased. The top tracing is the discharge rate of the cell in impulses/second (Imp/s), the middle tracing is unit activity where each vertical deflection represents the output of a window discriminator which is triggered by an extracellular action potential. The rate meter trace lags the unit trace by 1 s. The bottom tracing is blood pressure (BP) in mmHg. The arrow indicates the time bradykinin is injected into the heart and the horizontal lines above DCS represent the stimulation period.

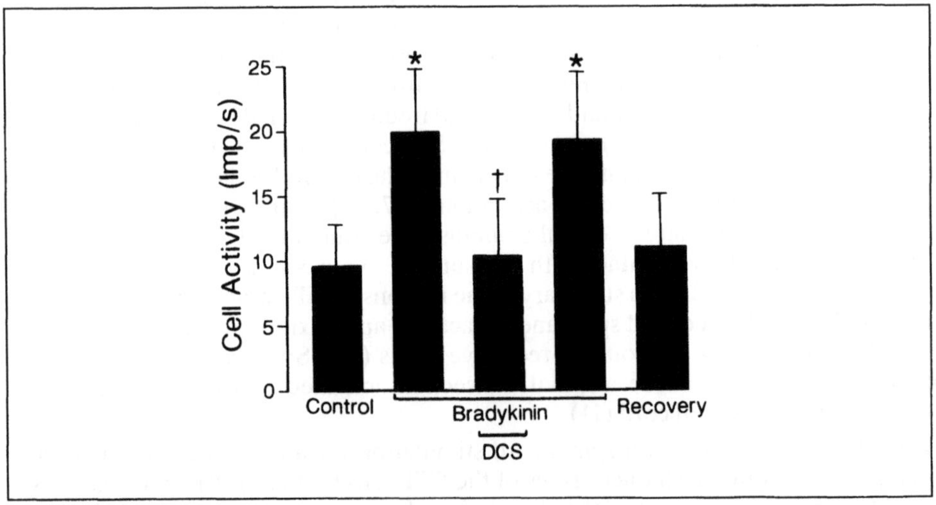

Fig. 3. Summary of the inhibitory effects of dorsal column stimulation (DCS) on the activityof STT evoked after intracardiac injections of bradykinin (n = 7) (11). Control = spontaneous activity; Bradykinin = activity evoked by intracardiac bradykinin; DCS = dorsal column stimulation applied during the bradykinin-evoked activity; Recovery = spontaneous activity following the bradykinin response. The long horizontal bar above Bradykinin indicates that the responses to bradykinin and DCS were measured at different times during single bradykinin injections. Cell activity of the first bar was measured near the peak of the bradykinin response, the results of the second bar was measured a short time later, but was still near the peak of the response, and the third bar was measured after DCS was terminated, but bradykinin effects were still present. ANOVA for repeated measures, $p < 0.001$ (n = 7); post-hoc Tukey's test, *compared to control, †compared to bradykinin-evoked activity.

consistent with the concept that spinal cord stimulation reduces the amount of information projecting to the thalamus and higher cortical regions because it decreases the discharge rate of STT cells that is generated as the result of activating small caliber spinal afferents. Paresthesia may be present during spinal cord stimulation as a result of activating the large diameter fibers of the wide dynamic range cells (11). Thus, these wide dynamic range neurons may be necessary for patients to sense the paresthesia in the somatic region related to the referral of their anginal pain (14, 30, 35).

A common feature of spinal cord stimulation is its long lasting effects after the stimulus is turned off (30, 31). The STT cell responses were stimulus locked, i.e., their activity was reduced at the onset of the stimulus and returned to control levels of discharge after the stimulus was terminated. The time course of inhibition for STT cells does not account for the prolonged relief of anginal symptoms. Two important differences between this study and the clinical effects are that electrical stimulation procedures are applied for much longer periods than the short length of time used in this study and the procedures are performed in anesthetized preparations.

In summary, the study provides physiological mechanisms to explain the efficacy of using spinal cord stimulation to reduce angina pectoris. The explanation is that impulses originating from the heart and transmitted in a major pain pathway of the spinothalamic tract are blocked during spinal cord stimulation of the dorsal column (Fig. 4).

Vagal stimulation

The most common placement of spinal cord stimulation for relieving angina pectoris is in the high thoracic regions, as described by Mannheimer and DeJongste in other chapters of this book. In one clinical report, however, the spinal cord stimulating electrode was placed on the left dorsal side of the dura mater at the superior edge of the C_2 laminae (17). Electrical stimulation of segments beneath this electrode elicits paresthesia on the left side and affects the lateral aspect of the neck, shoulder, upper thoracic region and hand, and eventually extended over the entire arm. Electrical stimulation significantly reduces the number of anginal attacks per week and significantly increases the double product (heart rate x systolic blood pressure). This section of the chapter provides evidence that may, in part, explain the neural mechanisms producing these clinical results.

Anatomical studies and clinical reports raise the possibility that vagal afferent fibers from the heart terminate in the C_1–C_3 spinal segments. A small population of vagal afferent fibers terminates directly in the upper cervical spinal cord after bypassing the nucleus tractus solitarius (22, 34). Clinical reports provide indirect evidence that the information carried from the heart to the brainstem in the vagal afferent fibers produce pain referred to the neck and trigeminal somatic distribution after sympathectomy (26, 44, 45). In carefully selected patients, sympathectomies were successful in approximately 80 % of the cases. In some of the patients, sympathectomy alleviated anginal pain referred to the upper chest and arm, but in its place pain was expressed in the neck and jaw. The observations support the possibility that vagal afferents excite neurons in the upper cervical cord. Our laboratory has shown that upper cervical spinal neurons (16) and STT cells (11) are excited during electrical stimulation of vagal afferent fibers. Somatic receptive fields for the STT cells were located on the ipsilateral jaw, the left side of the face and ear, and extended to the neck and shoulder region, and occasionally extended down the left arm and chest.

In summary, vagal afferent input excites cells in the C_1 to C_3 segments of the spinal cord. These neurons most likely are the necessary ones to produce angina pectoris that is referred especially to the neck, jaw, and upper shoulder. Spinal cord stimula-

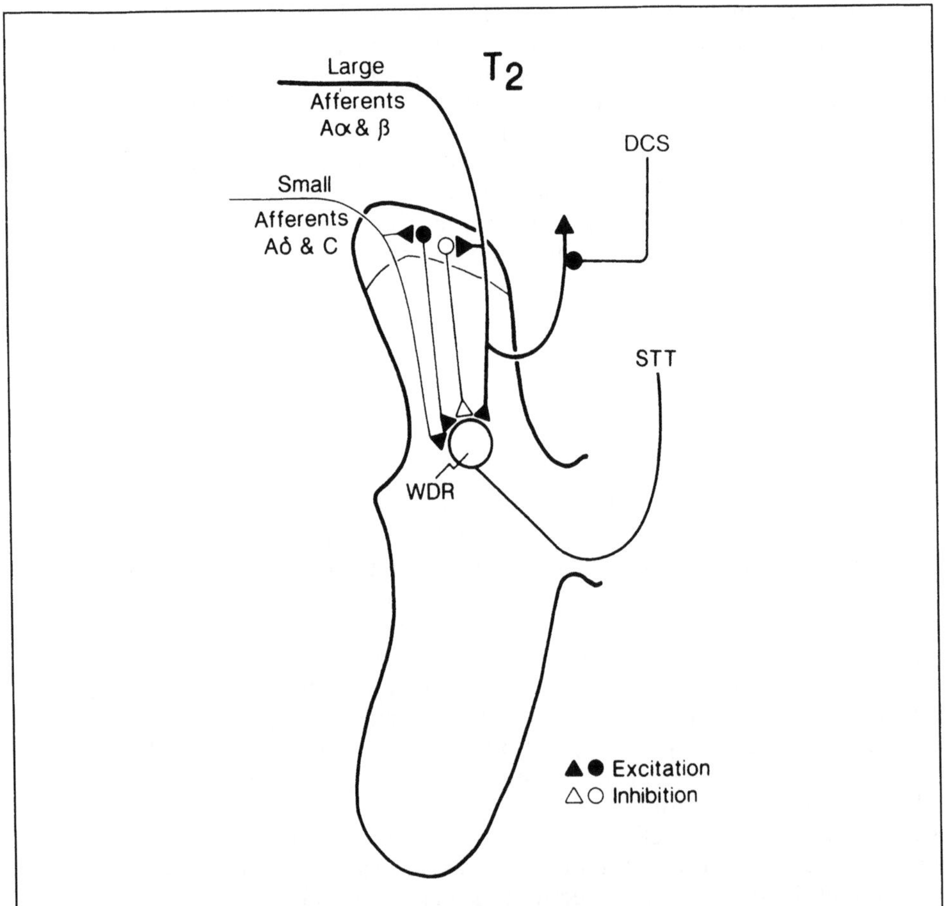

Fig. 4. Schematic diagram to explain the effects of dorsal column stimulation (DCS) on wide dynamic range (WDR) STT cells. This diagram is based on the gate control theory of Melzak and Wall (1988) to explain how activation of large afferent fibers may reduce activity of STT cells that are activated by a noxious stimulus, in this case from the heart. Dorsal column stimulation may antidromically excite large afferent fibers (Aα and β). Initially these afferent fibers could slightly excite the STT cell and produce parasthesia. These afferent fibers also could excite an inhibitory neuron in the substantia gelatinosa (lamina II). Noxious stimuli resulting from ischemia in the heart activate small afferent fibers (Aδ and C) that directly and possibly indirectly excite STT cells strongly. Activation of large afferent fibers applied during the ischemic episode might suppress the noxious input because DCS activates inhibitory neurons that synapse on the STT cell.

tion of electrodes placed in these C_1–C_3 segments also may block the impulses of the neurons in these segments and thus reduce the number of anginal attacks and improve the rate-pressure product (17). Based on the pain characteristics described in patients who experienced sympathectomies, just the elimination of the responses of these neurons might not reduce the most intense forms of referred pain that involve thoracic segments of the spinal cord.

One complication concerning the effects of vagal afferent stimulation is that in contrast to its strong excitatory effects on the activity of the cells in the upper cervical segments specifically the C_1 to C_3 segments, a large population of STT cells in the remaining segments of the spinal cord are inhibited (1, 2, 12, 20, 40). Recent studies provide evidence that the vagal system participates in an antinociceptive role (28, 29, 37, 38, 39).

The heart is of particular interest because its vagal afferent fibers may be the major source for producing antinociception or reduction in pain (Fig. 5). Experimental evidence provides support to focus on the heart. One part of the experimental evidence is based on the observation that electrical stimulation of the cardiac branch of the vagus decreases activity to the same extent as the inhibition resulting from stimulating the thoracic vagus (1). Additional support for vagal afferents from the heart

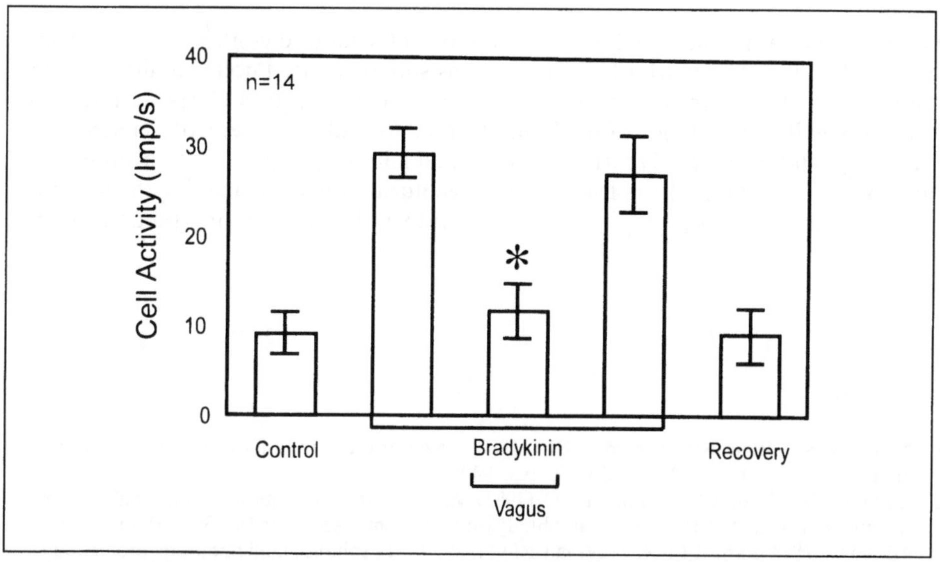

Fig. 5. Averaged STT responses to intracardiac injections of bradykinin and the effects of stimulating left thoracic vagus nerve on those responses. Control = spontaneous activity; Bradykinin = activity evoked by intracardiac bradykinin; Vagus = electrical stimulation of the vagus during the bradykinin-evoked activity; Recovery = spontaneous activity following the bradykinin response. The long horizontal bar above Bradykinin indicates that responses to bradykinin and DCS were measured at different times during single bradykinin injections for each of the 14 cells studied. Cell activity of the first bar was measured at the peak of the bradykinin response, the results of the second bar was measured a short time later while the vagus nerve was stimulated, but was still near the peak of the bradykinin response, and the third bar was measured after vagal stimulation was terminated. *$p < 0.001$ for effects of vagal stimulation compared to the first bar of the bradykinin response.

comes from the evidence that electrical stimulation of the vagal afferent fibers above the heart, but not below the heart, strongly suppresses spontaneous and noxiously-evoked activity of STT cells (1, 2, 21). Although both these pieces of evidence are indirect, vagal afferents arising from the heart appear to be important contributors for antinociception.

Is it possible that spinal cord stimulation of the cervical spinal cord activates the pathway or pathways producing antinociception? In a preliminary report, we have shown that electrical stimulation of the thoracic vagal afferent fibers excites a group of cells in the C_1–C_3 segments whose axons project down to at least the thoracic spinal cord (10). These cells were shown to be propriospinal neurons because they were antidromically activated by stimulating their axons in the thoracic, and in some cases in the lumbar segments of the spinal cord. We can only speculate at this point that these descending-projecting cells may be part of the inhibitory relay pathway of the upper cervical segments. Further work is designed to clarify this interesting pathway, but it does help to expand possibilities that the vagus may participate with spinal cord stimulation in cervical segments to produce pain relief. For example, stimulation parameters from the spinal cord stimulation may activate vagal afferents or other input to these cells and, in turn, they may initiate the inhibitory effects in cells of the thoracic segments.

Acknowledgements

The author gratefully acknowledges the important scientific contributions of Margaret J. Chandler. The work of the author was supported by Public Health Service Grant HL22732, and grants and contracts from the Medtronics Corporation, Presbyterian Health Foundation, Oklahoma Center for Advancement of Science and Technology, and American Heart Association, Oklahoma Affiliate. Special appreciation is expressed to D. Holston for providing technical assistance, making the illustrations and taking the photographs, and to C. Smith and C. Hulka for typing the manuscript.

References

1. Ammons WS, Blair RW, Foreman RD (1983) Vagal afferent inhibition of primate thoracic spinothalamic neurons. J Neurophys 50: 926–940
2. Ammons WS, Blair RW, Foreman RD (1983) Vagal afferent inhibition of spinothalamic cell responses to sympathetic afferents and bradykinin in the monkey. Circ Res 53: 603–612
3. Ammons WS, Girardot M-N, Foreman RD (1985) T_2–T_5 spinothalamic neurons projecting to medial thalamus with viscerosomatic input. J Neurophysiol 54: 73–89
4. Ammons WS, Girardot M-N, Foreman RD (1985) Effects of intracardiac bradykinin on T_2–T_5 medial spinothalamic cells. Am J Physiol 249: R147–R152
5. Barolat G (1993) Experience with 509 plate electrodes implanted epidurally from C_1 to L_1. Stereotactic & Functional Neurosurgery 61: 60–79
6. Blair RW, Weber RN, Foreman RD (1981) Characteristics of primate spinothalamic tract neurons receiving viscerosomatic convergent inputs in T_3–T_5 segments. J Neurophysiol 46: 797–811
7. Blair RW, Weber RN, Foreman RD (1982) Responses of thoracic spinothalamic neurons to intracardiac injection of bradykinin in the monkey. Circ Res 51: 83–94

8. Blair RW, Weber RN, Foreman RD (1984) Responses of spinoreticular and spinothalamic cells to intracardiac bradykinin. Am J Physiol 246: H500–H507
9. Bonica JJ (1990) Management of Pain. Lea & Febiger, London pp 133–179
10. Chandler MJ, Zhang J, Foreman RD (1994) Vagal and sympathetic afferent inputs excite upper cervical (C_1–C_3) descending propriospinal neurons in monkeys. Soc Neurosci Vol 20, p 550, # 233.4
11. Chandler MJ, Brennan TJ, Garrison DW, Kim KS, Schwartz PJ, Foreman RD (1993) A mechanism of cardiac pain suppression by spinal cord stimulation: implications for patients with angina pectoris. Eur Heart J 14: 96–105
12. Chandler MJ, Hobbs ST, Bolser DC, Foreman RD (1991) Effects of vagal stimulation on cervical spinothalamic tract neurons in monkeys. Pain 44: 81–87
13. Chauhan A, Mullins PA, Thuraisinghma SI, Taylor G, Petch MC, Schofield PM (1994) Effect of transcutaneous electrical nerve stimulation on coronary blood flow. Circulation 89: 694–702
14. DeJongste MJL, Hautvast RWM, Hillege HL, Lie KI (1994) Efficacy of spinal cord stimulation as adjuvant therapy for intractable angina pectoris: A prospective, randomized clinical study. J Am Coll Cardiol 23: 1592–1597
15. DeJongste MJL, Nagelkerke D, Hooyschuur CAM, Journee LH, Meyler WJ, Staal MJ, de Jonge P, Lie KI (1995) Stimulation characteristics, complications, and efficacy of spinal cord stimulation systems in patients with refractory angina. A prospective feasibility study. PACE (in press)
16. Fu Q-G, Chandler MJ, McNeill DL, Foreman RD (1992) Vagal afferent fibers excite upper cervical neurons and inhibit activity of lumbar spinal cord neurons in the rat. Pain 51: 91–100
17. Gonzàlez-Darder JM, Canela P, Gonzàlez-Martinez V (1991) High cervical spinal cord stimulation for unstable angina pectoris. Stereotact Funct Neurosurg 56: 20–27
18. Harrison TR, Reeves TJ (1968) Patterns and causes of chest pain. In: Principles and Problems of Ischemic Heart Disease. Year Book Medical Publishers, Chicago, pp 197–204
19. Hashimoto K, Hirose M, Furukawa S, Haykawa H, Kimura E (1977) Changes in hemodynamics and bradykinin concentration in coronary sinus blood in experimental coronary artery occlusion. Jpn Heart J 18: 679–689
20. Hobbs SF, Chandler MJ, Bolser DC, Foreman RD (1992) Segmental organization of visceral and somatic input onto C_3–T_6 spinothalamic tract cells of the monkey. J Neurophys 68: 1575–1588
21. Hobbs SF, Oh UT, Chandler MJ, Foreman RD (1989) Cardiac and abdominal vagal afferent inhibition of primate T_9–S_1 spinothalamic cells. Am J Physiol 257: R889–R895
22. Kalia M, Sullivan JM (1982) Brainstem projections of sensory and motor components of the vagus nerve in the rat. J Comp Neurol 211: 248–264
23. Kimura E, Hashimoto K, Furukawa S, Hayakawa H (1973) Changes in bradykinin level in coronary sinus blood after the experimental occlusion of coronary artery. Am Heart J 85: 635–647
24. Lenz FA, Gracely RH, Hope EJ, Baker FH, Rowland LH, Dougherty PM, Richardson RT (1994) The sensation of angina can be evoked by stimulation of the human thalamus. Pain 59: 119–125
25. Lewis T (1942) Pain. Macmillan, New York
26. Lindgren I, Olivecrona H (1947) Surgical treatment of angina pectoris. J Neurosurg 4: 19–39
27. Maixner W, Touw KB, Brody MJ, Gebhart GF, Long JP (1982) Factors influencing the altered pain perception in the spontaneously hypertensive rat. Brain Res 237: 137–145
28. Maixner W, Randich A (1984) Role of the right vagal nerve trunk in antinociception. Brain Res 298: 374–377
29. Malliani A (1982) Cardiovascular and sympathetic afferent fibers. Rev Physiol Biochem Pharmacol 94: 11–74
30. Mannheimer C, Augustinsson L-E, Carlsson C-A, Manhem K, Wilhelmsson C (1988) Epidural spinal electrical stimulation in severe angina pectoris. Br Heart J 59: 56–61
31. Mannheimer C, Carlsson C-A, Emanuelsson H, Vedin A, Waagstein F, Wilhelmsson C (1985) The effects of transcutaneous electrical nerve stimulation in patients with severe angina pectoris. Circulation 71: 308–316
32. Mannheimer C, Eliasson T, Andersson B et al. (1993) Effects of spinal cord stimulation in angina pectoris induced by pacing and possible mechanisms of action. Br Med J 307: 477–480
33. Melzak R, Wall PD (1982) The Challenge of Pain. Basic Books Inc, New York, pp 222–261

34. McNeill DL, Chandler MJ, Fu Q-G, Foreman RD (1991) Projection of nodose ganglion cells to the upper cervical spinal cord in the rat. Brain Res Bull 27: 151–155
35. Murphy DF, Giles KE (1987) Dorsal column stimulation for pain relief from intractable angina pectoris. Pain 28: 365–368
36. Procacci P, Zoppi M (1989) Heart pain. In: Textbook of Pain. Churchill Livingstone, Edinburgh, pp 410–419
37. Randich A, Aicher S (1988) Medullary substrates mediating antinociception produced by electrical stimulation of the vagus. Brain Res 445: 68–76
38. Randich A, Maixner W (1984) Interactions between cardiovascular and pain regulatory systems. Neurosci Biobehav Rev 8: 343–367
39. Ren K, Randich A, Gebhart GF (1988) Vagal afferent modulation of a nociceptive reflex in rats: involvement of spinal opioid and monamine receptors. Brain Res 446: 285–294
40. Ren K, Randich A, Gebhart GF (1991) Effects of electrical stimulation of vagal afferents on spinothalamic tract cells in the rat. Pain 44: 311–319
41. Sampson JJ, Cheitlin MD (1971) Pathophysiology and differential diagnosis of cardiac pain. Prog Cardiovasc Dis 23: 507–531
42. Sanderson JE (1990) Electrical neurostimulators for pain relief in angina. Br Heart J 63: 141–143
43. Sanderson JE, Brooksby P, Waterhouse D, Palmer RBG, Neubauer K (1993) Epidural spinal electrical stimulation for severe angina: a study of its effects on symptoms, exercise tolerance and degree of ischemia. Eur Heart J 13: 628–633
44. White JD and Bland EF (1948) The surgical relief of severe angina pectoris. Methods employed and end results in 83 patients. Medicine 27: 1–42
45. White JD and Sweet WH (1968) Pain and the neurosurgeon. CC Thomas, Springfield IL. pp 525–559

Author's address:
Robert D. Foreman, PhD
Professor and Chair
George Lynn Cross Research Professor
Department of Physiology
The University of Oklahoma Health Sciences Center
P.O. Box 26901, BMSB 653
Oklahoma City, OK 73190
USA

Spinal cord stimulation in severe angina pectoris – presentation of current studies, indications and practical experience

C. Mannheimer, T. Eliasson

Multidisciplinary Pain Center, Department of Medicine, Östra University Hospital, Göteborg

Introduction

Spinal cord stimulation has been used in clinical practice for several years in the treatment of chronic pain, mainly of neurogenic origin (31). Since 1976 several reports have been published on the favorable effects of spinal cord stimulation in advanced peripheral arterial vascular disease in the lower extremities. The treatment appears to produce increased local peripheral perfusion which leads in turn to improved healing of arterial leg ulcers (1, 5, 17).

Despite the development of pharmacotherapeutic and surgical treatment alternatives in coronary disorders a group of patients with severe angina remains resistant to therapy. Pain alleviation is a fundamental measure in the treatment of severe angina pectoris, not only to relieve symptoms but also because the pain itself aggravates the myocardial ischemia by generally and segmentally increased sympathetic activity. Breaking this vicious circle is therefore a matter of the greatest concern.

Against this background, transcutaneous electrical nerve stimulation (TENS) was introduced for patients with severe angina pectoris, despite optimal pharmacotherapy, in whom further coronary surgery was not possible. Several studies have been published and the results of these have been presented previously (24). In summary, TENS appeared to be a safe method, even for patients with myocardial ischemia, without any side-effects in the form of arrhythmias (22). The treatment also appeared to have a beneficial effect on the patients' angina and seemed to be associated with a reduction in myocardial ischemia. At Östra University Hospital in Göteborg, Sweden, TENS is routinely used today in patients with severe angina who do not respond to conventional treatment methods. The method is also used at several centers in Europa and Australia. However, about 10 – 15 % of patients develop skin irritation as a reaction to the electrodes, which makes the use of this therapy more difficult. This applies, above all, to patients who require continuous stimulation. TENS is also an impractical method for long-term treatment. Against this background, spinal cord stimulation was introduced for this patient category.

This survey presents mainly the results from current studies investigating the mechanisms behind the pain-relieving effect of spinal cord stimulation, but practical experiences relating to indications, patient selection and long-term results are also discussed.

Implantation and stimulation techniques

After local anesthetic an incision is made at the T6–T8 level, and a quadripolar electrode is introduced in the epidural space via a guidewire. The tip of the electrode is guided through the epidural space under x-ray monitoring, usually to the level of the T1–T2 vertebrae. During the peroperative stimulation, the patient experiences paresthesiae in the chest. It is important to adjust the position of the electrodes so that the paresthesiae in the chest cover the area to which the patient subjectively localizes the anginal pain, even if it is atypically localized. This is the only way for the implanting surgeon to ensure that the area innervating the heart is really stimulated. A common cause of inadequate effect is inappropriate localization of the electrode. If the electrode is correctly placed, complete regression of the anginal pain is obtained after 20 – 120 s of high-intensity stimulation, provided that the pain is caused by myocardial ischemia.

As soon as adequate paresthesiae are obtained, an electric cable is tunneled subcutaneously to below the left costal arch, where it is connected to a subcutaneous pulse generator of about the same size as a pacemaker. The system is thus completely closed, and the patient can move about freely and experiences no practical restrictions in his daily life. The stimulator is switched on and off by a magnet passed over the pulse generator, which is set by an external programmer. The patient can also use the magnet to switch between the preset stimulation strengths: one stronger, used in the case of an established or expected attack, and a weaker setting, used as "maintenance therapy" (stimulation for at least 2 h four times daily).

Presentation of current studies

Safety aspects

The most common objection to this treatment method is the fear that treatment with a spinal cord stimulator would block only the pain signal without affecting the myocardial ischemia and would therefore constitute a risk to the patients. In a study on monkeys Chandler et al. have shown that electrical stimulation of the spinal cord inhibits the transmission of nociceptive signals in the spinothalamic tract from the heart (3).

A study of the safety aspects was performed to investigate whether spinal cord stimulation causes increased myocardial ischemia or malignant arrhythmias on ECG during 24-h ambulatory ECG recording (10). Nineteen patients with advanced coronary heart disease and severe angina with a spinal cord stimulator implanted were investigated. There were no signs of increased myocardial ischemia or arrhythmias during stimulation compared with control recordings. Similar results were obtained in a study with 24-h ECG recordings performed in the Netherlands (6, 7).

Mechanisms of action

The acute effects of spinal cord stimulation were investigated in a study on ten patients (24). The patients performed a number of exercise tests during ECG recording. Depression of the ST-segment on the ECG is considered to be a quantitative measure of myocardial ischemia. Spinal cord stimulation resulted in reduction of the angina, increased exercise capacity, and a reduced degree of ST segment depression during comparable work load, indicating that the effects are related to a reduced degree of myocardial ischemia. However, at maximum work load during stimulation, the same degree of ST-segment depression and angina as during the control situation was observed, indicating that myocardial ischemia during stimulation gives rise to angina, and that the treatment does not block the pain signal selectively.

Similar results were obtained in studies in which pharmacological provocation, among other things, was used (15 patients) and in another study in which regional myocardial ischemia was studied noninvasively by means of positron emission tomography (8 patients) (8, 20, 30).

Atrial pacing is a common experimental method to induce myocardial ischemia (13, 32). The heart is paced by a gradually increased frequency until ischemia occurs as a result of the increase in frequency (shortening of diastole). This method offers good possibilities to study metabolic myocardial events when venous blood from the coronary sinus in the heart is studied at the same time as arterial blood with respect to oxygen saturation, lactate concentration, catecholamines, etc.

A recent report presented an account of the effects of spinal cord stimulation on myocardial metabolism and coronary hemodynamics in pacing-induced angina in 20 patients with advanced coronary disease (27). The purpose of the trial was to study how the treatment influences coronary flow and the oxygen consumption of the myocardium. The results are presented in Table 1. In summary, the results show that spinal cord stimulation has favorable effects in the form of increased tolerance to pacing, improved lactate metabolism (lactate production during control pacing changed to lactate extraction during stimulation), and a reduced degree of ST-segment depression on ECG at a comparable pacing frequency. There was a parallel decrease in oxygen consumption and coronary blood flow. At maximum pacing frequency during stimulation all the patients again experienced angina. Lactate metabolism, the

Table 1. Effect of spinal cord stimulation during pacing, with regard to tolerance to pacing, ST segment level, lactate metabolism, coronary sinus blood flow, and myocardial oxygen consumption.

		Spinal cord stimulation	
	Control (C)	P_1	P_2
Heart rate (bpm)	128 ± 13	128 ± 14	149 ± 15 ($P < 0.001$ P_2 vs. C, $P < 0.001$ vs. P_1)
Lactate extraction ratio (%)	−8 ± 33	8 ± 21 ($P = 0.003$ vs. C)	−3 ± 21 ($P = 0.001$ vs. P_1)
ST segment depression (mm)	−1.8 ± 0.9	−1.0 ± 0.6 ($P = 0.001$ vs. C)	−1.8 ± 1.0 ($P = 0.004$ vs. P_1)
Coronary sinus blood flow (ml/min)	136 ± 65	124 ± 63 ($P = 0.01$ vs. C)	145 ± 55 ($P = 0.003$ vs. P_1)
Myocardial oxygen consumption (ml/min)	19 ± 11	16 ± 9 ($P = 0.02$ vs. C)	19 ± 9 ($P = 0.002$ vs. P_1)

Table 2. Investigation program for patients with therapy-resistant angina pectoris.

- Myocardial scintigraphy during exercise testing and simultaneous ECG examination
- Echocardiography at rest and during stress, i.e., provocation with intravenously infused dobutamine or adenosine
- Long-term ECG (24 – 48 h Holter) recording and/or vector cardiography
- Psychometric testing
- Evaluation by psychiatrist with special interest in the problem of pain

degree of ST-segment depression, coronary flow, and oxygen consumption returned to the same order of magnitude as in the control situation.

A study on 12 patients with so-called syndrome X (angina pectoris, objective demonstrable myocardial ischemia, normal coronary angiography) showed increased exercise capacity, reduced severity of chest pain and less severe myocardial ischemia (9).

Discussion

The symptom of angina is caused by a nociceptive stimulus, secondary to threatening tissue injury due to oxygen deficiency in the myocadium – myocardial ischemia – and is thus a warning signal to the patient. Chandler et al. expressed concern that spinal cord stimulation would only block the pain signal and thereby constitute a risk in clinical use (3). However, long-term ECG studies provide no support for the hypothesis that the stimulation has negative effects in the form of increased myocardial ischemia or induction of arrhythmias (6, 9). Furthermore, studies on the effects of TENS and spinal cord stimulation in angina show that the antianginal effect is associated with reduced myocardial ischemia and that myocardial ischemia during stimulation gives rise to angina (6, 10, 19, 22, 24, 25, 29). There is thus no indication that the treatment constitutes a risk to these patients.

Theoretically the anti-ischemic effect of spinal cord stimulation may be due to three mechanisms; increased coronary flow, decreased cardiac oxygen consumption, or direct pain relief which produces a secondary reduction of the myocardial ischemia.

The coronary flow was reduced in connection with spinal cord stimulation at a comparable pacing frequency in the invasive study referred to above (27). Previous studies have provided no support for the hypothesis that the anti-ischemic effect of TENS and spinal cord stimulation during increased cardiac work is secondary to a general increase in coronary flow (8, 11, 23, 26). A microvascular redistribution of the flow to ischemic areas is, however, possible and has been thought to be the cause of the favorable effects of spinal cord stimulation in peripheral arterial circulation insufficiency (16). However, there are data indicating that the mechanism responsible for the anti-ischemic effects of spinal cord stimulation, produced both by TENS and spinal cord stimulation during rest, is secondary to increased coronary flow (4, 8, 9).

Chauhan et al., for instance, have recently shown that TENS increases coronary flow in patients with coronary insufficiency and normal coronary vessels, determined by intracoronary flow measurement using Doppler technique (4). No increase in coronary flow was obtained in heart-transplanted patients in whom the heart is denervated. It appears that intact innervation to the heart is required to obtain an increase in coronary flow by means of TENS. Previous studies have also shown that TENS and spinal cord stimulation in other conditions give rise to increased flow (15, 21). Hosobuchi, for instance, obtained an increase in the ipsilateral cerebral flow through cervical spinal cord stimulation in man (15). In another study on humans TENS was found to increase the blood flow in ischemic skin flaps, which led to healing (21).

The other alternative means that the anti-ischemic effect of spinal cord stimulation is secondary to reduced myocardial oxygen demand. The oxygen consumption of the myocardium has been shown in a large number of studies to clearly be the most important factor regulating the coronary flow (12, 18, 28, 29). The relationship is a linear one; if, for instance, the consumption is reduced, the flow is correspondingly reduced, and vice versa. If spinal cord stimulation reduces the oxygen consumption of the myocardium, this effect gives rise to a reduction in the coronary flow, as seen in the invasive study referred to above (27).

As regards the third alternative, spinal cord stimulation probably reduces the pain signal at the spinal level (4). Previous investigations indicate that treatments which primarily reduce anginal pain also reduce the sympathetic activity to the heart and thereby reduces the oxygen consumption of the myocardium (2, 19). Pain inhibition per se could thus give rise to a reduction in myocardial ischemia.

In summary, TENS and spinal cord stimulation increased coronary flow at rest. However, if the heart is subjected to increased load, the stimulation appears instead to reduce the myocardial oxygen consumption, which explains the anti-ischemic effect in connection with physical stress.

Practical experiences, indications and patient selection

The majority of implanted patients have severe angina secondary to coronary disease despite optimal pharmacotherapy and surgical treatment. Another important group are patients with therapy-resistant angina with objectively demonstrable myocardial ischemia despite angiographically normal coronary vessels, the so-called syndrome X.

So far 230 patients with severe angina have been implanted. Retrospective long-term follow-up shows that about 80 % of patients enjoy a lasting, good effect of the treatment, in the form of reduced frequency of attacks and consumption of short-acting nitroglycerin, as well as increased physical activity and improved quality of life. This result compares favorably with the long-term results of spinal cord stimulation in chronic neurogenic pain (about 50 %) or in severe peripheral arterial circulation insufficiency (60 – 70 %) (16). In patients who respond inadequately to the treatment psychological factors are often a major contributor to the development of the chest pain, or the chest pain cannot be correlated to on-going myocardial ischemia. Furthermore, patients who are physically active and have good left ventricular function seem to adapt more easily to a higher stress level after implantation. The result is offen initial improvement, followed by a preimplantation attack frequency, although at a higher level of activity.

Placebo effects most probably contribute considerably to the positive effects. However, these decrease with time and are considered to be negligible after 2 – 3 months (33). Reduced myocardial ischemia during stimulation, as well as the fact that the clinical effects last for several years, indicate that other mechanisms in addition to placebo are involved. This is also supported by the fact that patients with battery dysfunction deteriorate, so that the angina recurs or the number of attacks increases. However, further controlled, randomized studies are needed to confirm the positive clinical effects of the treatment. A prospective randomized study is therefore being carried out at present comparing the effects of coronary surgery with those of spinal cord stimulation on groups of patients in whom surgery would not improve the prognosis.

Complications and side effects are rare compared with medical or surgical treatment. The actual implantation is a relatively minor operation. Superficial postoperative wound infections have been reported in three patients, and there have been no cases of epidural or intrathecal infection. Electrode revision, occasioned by inadequate paresthesiae, has been performed on five patients. One patient was reoperated on due to electrode breakage.

The stimulator is relatively easy to handle for the patients, who can usually be released from hospital 1 – 2 days after the implantation and after having been given oral and written instructions. Use of the stimulator requires basic compliance, and implantation in patients with impaired short-term memory or poor intellectual capacity should therefore be avoided. It is also important to ensure that the patient's chest pain is indeed secondary to on-going myocardial ischemia, on which spinal cord stimulation has a good and rapidly obtained effect, while the effect on chest pain of other origin is fairly moderate. If no current myocardial ischemia can be demonstrated, implantation should be used with restriction, regardless of whether the patient has a known coronary disease or not, above all, if functional factors are thought to play a prominent role.

One group of patients that constitutes a major clinical problem are those with severe coronary insufficiency and very severe pain problems who do not respond to pharmacotherapy or surgical treatment. An investigation program has been developed by the Östra University Hospital Pain Center to clarify the connection between on-going pain and reversible myocardial ischemia, quantify the degree of ischemia, and determine which and the extent to which other components control the patient's perception of pain (Table 2). Several of these patients have undergone coronary bypass surgery twice and, in some cases, three times. This kind of surgical intervention requires the use of a heart-lung machine, entailing a considerable risk of anoxic brain damage with secondary cerebrolesional syndrome that may lead to altered pain perception. Signs of diffuse anoxic brain damage are often seen in these patients which may contribute to the poor response to traditional antianginal therapy. Also patients in whom no apparent clinical signs of brain damage can be seen sometimes show signs of clear ischemic brain damage when tested psychometrically.

After the implantation the patients are closely followed up by physicians and other personnel with special experience of and interest in electrostimulation. Intially they are seen frequently, and reprogramming of the stimulator is almost always necessary to optimize the treatment. It is important to ensure that the patient uses the stimulator correctly. It is a great advantage if the treating physician (cardiologist or internist) is also able to check the patient's stimulator.

To summarize, spinal cord stimulation is a therapeutic alternative for patients with severe angina when conventional treatment strategies have been exhausted. As coronary disorders are one of the major causes of disease and disability, this is a rapidly growing group of patients. Many patients with syndrome X are difficult to treat. Spinal cord stimulation would thus add to the range of possible treatments. It is essential that the patient is able to observe basic compliance, and that the chest pain really is related to on-going myocardial ischemia.

References

1. Augustinsson L-E, Carlsson C-A et al. (1985) Epidural electrical stimulation in severe limb ischemia. Ann Surg 202: 104–10
2. Blomberg S, Curelaru I et al. (1989) Thoracic epidural anesthesia in patients with unstable angina pectoris. Eur Heart J 10: 437–44
3. Chandler M, Brennan T et al. (1993) A mechanism of cardiac pain suppression by spinal cord stimulation: implications for patients with angina pectoris. Eur Heart J 14: 96–105
4. Chauhan A, Mullins P et al. (1994) Effect of transcutaneous electrical nerve stimulation on coronary blood flow. Circulation 89: 694–702
5. Cook A, Aygar A et al. (1976) Vascular disease of the extremities. Electrical stimulation of spinal cord and posterior roots. NY State J Med 76: 366–68
6. De Jongste M, Haaksma J et al. (1993) Effects of spinal cord stimulation on daily life myocardial ischemia in patients with severe coronary artery disease. Br Heart J 71: 413–418
7. De Jongste M, Hautvast R, Hillege HL et al. (1994) Efficacy of special cord stimulation as an adjuvant therapy for intractable angina pectoris: A prospective randomized clinical study. JACC 7: 1592–1597
8. De Landsherre C, Mannheimer C et al. (1992) Effect of spinal cord stimulation on regional myocardial perfusion assessed by positron emission tomography. Am J Cardiol 69: 143–49
9. Eliasson T, Albertsson P et al. (1993) Spinal cord stimulation in angina pectoris with normal coronary arteriograms. Coronary Artery Disease 4: 819–27
10. Eliasson T, Jern S et al. (1994) Safety aspects of spinal cord stimulation in severe angina pectoris. Coronary Artery Disease (submitted)
11. Emanuelsson H, Mannheimer C et al. (1987) Catecholamine metabolism during pacing-induced angina pectoris and the effect of transcutaneous electrical nerve stimulation. Am Heart J 114: 1360–66
12. Feigl EO (1983) Coronary physiology. Physiol Rev 63: 1–205
13. Forrester J, Helfant R et al. (1971) Atrial pacing in coronary heart disease. Am J Cardiol 27: 237
14. Gybels J, Kupers R (1987) Central and peripheral electrical stimulation of the nervous system in the treatment of chronic pain. Acta Neurochir 38 (suppl): 64–75
15. Hosobuchi A (1985) Electrical stimulation of the cervical spinal cord increases cerebral blood flow in humans. Appl Neurophysiol 48: 372–76
16. Illis L (1992) Spinal cord dysfunction, vol III. Functional stimulation. Oxford. Oxford University Press
17. Jacobs MS, Jörning P et al. (1990) Foot salvage and improvement of microvascular blood flow as a result of epidural spinal cord electrical stimulation. J Vasc Surg 12: 354–60
18. Knabb R, Ely S et al. (1983) Consistent parallel relationships among myocardial oxygen consumption, coronary blood flow and pericardial infusate adenosine concentration with various interventions and betablockade in the dog. Circ Res 53: 33–41
19. Kröger K, Schipke J et al. (1989) Poststenotic ischaemic myocardial dysfunction induced by peripheral nociceptive stimulation. Eur Heart J 10: 179–82
20. Kujacic V, Eliasson T et al. (1993) Assessment of the influence of spinal cord stimulation (SCS) on left ventricular function in patients with severe angina pectoris: an echocardiographic study. Eur Heart J 14: 1238–44

21. Lundberg T, Kjartansson J et al. (1988) Effect of electrical nerve stimulation on healing of ischaemic skin flaps. Lancet 24: 712–14
22. Mannheimer C (1984) Transcutaneous electrical nerve stimulation (TENS) in angina pectoris. Thesis. University of Göteborg, Sweden
23. Mannheimer C, Carlsson C-A et al. (1985) The effects of transcutaneous electrical nerve stimulation in patients with severe angina pectoris. Circulation 71: 308–16
24. Mannheimer C, Carlsson C-A et al. (1986) Transcutaneous electrical nerve stimulation (TENS) in angina pectoris. Pain 26: 291–300
25. Mannheimer C, Augustinsson L-E et al. (1988) Epidural spinal electrical stimulation in severe angina pectoris. Br Heart J 59: 56–61
26. Mannheimer C, Emanuelsson H et al. (1989) Influence of naloxone on the effects of high frequency transcutaneous electrical nerve stimulation in angina pectoris induced by atrial pacing. Br Heart J 62: 36–42
27. Mannheimer C, Eliasson T et al. (1993) Effects of spinal cord stimulation in angina pectoris induced by pacing and possible mechanisms of action. BMJ 307: 477–80
28. Miller W, Belardinelli L et al. (1979) Canine myocardial adenosine and lactate production, oxygen consumption, and coronary blood flow during stellate ganglia stimulation. Circ Res 45: 708–18
29. Mosher P, Ross J et al. (1964) Control of coronary blood flow by an autoregulatory mechanism. Circ Res 14: 250–9
30. Sanderson JE, Brooksby P et al. (1992) Epidural spinal electrical stimulation for severe angina: a study of its effects on symptoms, exercise tolerance and degree of ischaemia. Eur Heart J 13: 628–33
31. Siegfried J, Lazorthes Y (1982) Long-term follow-up of dorsal column stimulation for chronic pain syndrom after multiple lumbar operations. Appl Neurophysiol 45: 201–4
32. Sowton G, Balcon R et al. (1967) Measurement of the angina threshold during atrial pacing. Cardiovasc Res 1: 301
33. White L, Tursky B et al. (1985) Placebo. Guilford press, New York

Author's address:
Clas Mannheimer
Multidisciplinary Pain Center
Department of Medicine
Östra University Hospital
S-41685 Göteborg
Sweden

Spinal cord stimulation for intractable angina

J. E. Sanderson

Department of Medicine, Chinese University of Hong Kong,
Prince of Wales Hospital, Shatin, Hong Kong

Introduction

Spinal Cord Stimulation has been used in chronic intractable pain syndromes with mixed results. However, in patients with severe peripheral vascular disease it has been shown to lessen pain, hasten the healing of trophic ulcers, and this is associated with an increase in capillary blood flow and transcutaneous oxygen tension (10, 11). It also considerably improves the quality of life (7). It is logical therefore for this technique to be tried in patients with intractable angina which has not responded to the usual treatments of medical therapy, coronary bypass grafting, or balloon angioplasty. In 1987, Murphy and Giles (15) from Australia described 10 patients in which there were significant symptomatic improvement. In 1988, Mannheimer reported on the results in 10 patients again confirming symptomatic improvement and also increased exercise capacity (13). It appeared therefore that this technique was of some potential value in patients with angina, but there have been four major concerns; Firstly, does this therapy merely inhibit the sensation of pain due to ischemia; secondly, could ischemia be increased due to loss of warning; thirdly, will the pain of myocardial infarction be masked; fourthly, could mortality be increased? We have conducted a number of studies in 23 patients with SCS units to try to answer these questions (4, 16, 17, 18, 19, 20).

Indications for spinal cord stimulation in patients with angina

It is very important to select the patients carefully. We have taken great care to make sure that the pain is of cardiac origin by either reproducing the pain on treadmill exercise testing or confirming that the pain is associated with ST-segment depression on 24-h ECG Holter monitoring. The pain has to be disabling psychologically or physically or both. The patient should have had standard surgical or medical therapy if it is possible. In some of our patients because of age or general condition surgery was not feasible and therefore they were referred for Spinal Cord Stimulation. In most of our patients we also carried out a trial of Transcutaneous Electrical Nerve Stimulation (TENS) Therapy. It cannot be stressed enough that the correct selection of patients is paramount. Spinal Cord Stimulation is not very effective for non-cardiac or musculo skeletal pains. One of the problems in conducting trials in this area is that a double blind method is impossible with this technique because the patient experiences paraesthesiae and the stimulation artifacts are apparent on ECG recordings. This also means that SCS units need to be briefly switched off to measure ST-segment depression during exercise testing and that special filters have to be employed on Holter monitors.

We have implanted SCS units in 23 patients (18 males) mean age 59.3 (range 46–81 years). In these patients the duration of angina symptoms was for a mean (SD) of 9.1 (5.0) years and in 18 of these patients angiography performed preimplantation showed; three-vessel disease in 12, two-vessel disease in four, and two patients had single vessel disease. Five patients did not have angiography because of age or other contraindications to surgery. Coronary artery surgery had been carried out in 17 patients; nine patients had two operations and one patient had three procedures. Five patients were not surgical candidates. Angioplasty was also performed in six patients (and twice in one patient).

Implantation technique

This has been well described elsewhere (13, 18). We used a standard technique with the pulse generator placed in the axilla. The stimulation units were Itrel I, Itrel II and Cordis. The patients were instructed to use the units regularly for 1 h three times a day, for relief of an attack of angina or prophylactically before exercise.

The effect of SCS on symptoms (Table 1)

For the whole group, mean (SD) NYHA grade decreased significantly ($p < 0.1$) from 3.1 (0.8) preoperatively to 2 (0.9) immediately after operation, and was 2.1 (1.07) at the latest follow-up. Three patients improved by three grades, five patients by two grades, nine patients by one grade, and in six patients there was no significant change (five of these six patients were graded two preoperatively desite their complaints of severe symptoms). This illustrates the point that those who objectively have mild symptoms (despite their severe complaints) do less well with SCS. In general, those who were in the higher grades (three or four) preoperatively showed the best

Table 1. Overall changes in angina symptoms classified by NYHA class (% patients in each grade) assesed before implantation, immediately after operation and at the latest follow-up

Grade	Baseline	Immediately after operation	Latest follow-up
I	0	23	35
II	26	55	35
III	39	18	15
IV	35	4	15
Mean (SD)	3·1 (0·8)*	2·0 (0·9)*	2·1 (1·1)

*$p < 0.01$.

improvement (Fig. 1). There was a slight regression in symptomatic improvement at the latest follow-up with fewer patients in class 2 and slightly more in class 4 (Table 1). However, a few patients continued to improve, moving from class 2 to class 1 during the period from immediately after operation to the latest follow-up (Table 1). GTN consumption fell from an average of 9.0 tablets per day (4–20) to 1.5 and was 0 in 11 patients.

A symptom questionnaire was used to assess the degree of angina and dyspnea. Patients were asked to score the pain from 0 to 5 (5 = severe pain) at rest, walking on the flat, uphills and stairs. Any breathlessness was similarly scored. The results confirmed general improvement of angina at rest and or exercise. The mean (SD) score for the severity of angina while walking on the flat was 3.3 (1.5) before the operation and 1.8 (1.6) after the operation ($p = < 0.05$), and for the severity of angina while walking uphill from 4.8 (0.4) before the operation to 2.9 (1.4) after the operation ($p = < 0.01$) the symptom of breathlessness was also improved during exercise, but not at rest.

Effect on exercise capacity

Our results confirm those of Mannheimer (13, 14). Exercise testing was done using the modified Bruce protocol. Test were performed with the neural stimulator off, on and off again with at least 30 min between each test. The sum of ST-segment depression was measured in all leads as an index of ischemia and the rate-pressure product (heart rate x systolic blood pressure x 10^{-3}) as an indirect assessment of myocardial oxygen consumption.

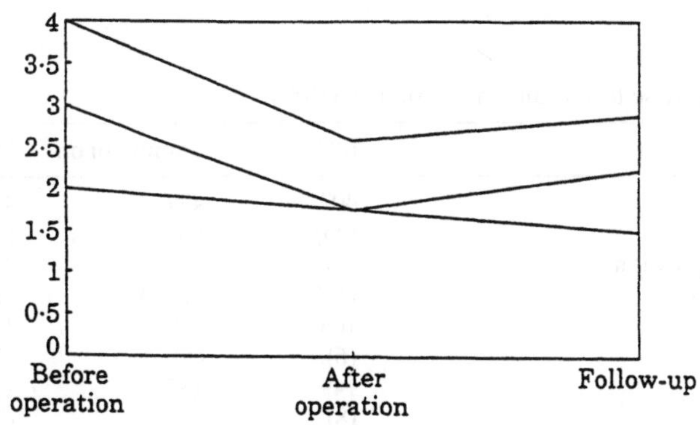

Fig. 1. Changes in angina symptoms (NYHA class) related to initial NYHA class. Those with the worst symptoms (highest class) had the best improvement. (From Sanderson et al., 1994)

Sixteen patients were able to adequately perform three exercise tests. Results are shown in Table 2. The duration of exercise was significantly increased ($p < 0.01$) from a mean (SEM) of 407 (45) s with the stimulator off, to 499 (46) s with the stimulator on. There was a slight "hang-over" effect in that the third exercise period was also slightly improved compared to the first (mean 434) s ($p = < 0.05$). Total ST-segment depression was slightly lower at peak exercise with the stimulator on, but this was not significant. Rate-pressure product was also marginally but not significantly increased at peak exercise with the stimulator on.

Effect of SCS on myocardial ischemia

In a previous study, we assessed the effect of SCS on pacing-induced ischemia (19). Pacing with continuous ECG monitoring was started at a rate of 100 beats per minute and increased in increments of 10 beats per minute at 2-min intervals; blood pressure was taken every 2 min during pacing and after 10 min following termination. Pacing was stopped at the request of the patient because of symptoms (angina or dyspnea) or when a rate of 160 beats per minute was reached. Pacing was done with the neural stimulator off, on and off with a 30-min interval. Total ST-segment depression and rate-pressure product at each pacing rate and at peak heart rate were calculated. The results showed that the total ST-segment depression was less at all heart rates, reaching significance at rates of 120 and 130 beats per minute (Fig. 2). Rate-pressure product was not significantly different at peak heart rates despite the higher rates because of a fall in systolic blood pressure when the neural stimulator was on.

In a small group of subjects (seven patients), we carried out 48-h ST-segment monitoring. Surprisingly, in two patients there were no significant ST-segment changes suggestive of ischemia during the recording period; in one patient the quality of the recordings was inadequate. In four remaining patients the mean (SD) number of ischemic episodes was 19 (16) with the stimulators on, and 28 (15) with the

Table 2. Treadmill exercise test results (n = 16); mean (SEM)

Stimulator	off[1]	Stimulator on	Stimulator off[2]
Time to maximum exercise (s)	407 (45)	499* (46)	434† (43)
Total ST-segment depression at max. exercise (mm)	4·9 (1·4)	4·4 (1·25)	3·9 (1·25)
Max. heart rate (beats. min^{-1})	106 (6)	109 (5)	106 (5)
Systolic BP at max. exercise (mmHg)	149 (8)	155 (7)	139 (7)
Rate-pressure product at max. exercise (beats. min^{-1} mmHg $\times 10^{-3}$)	16·2 (1·7)	17·2 (1·6)	14·9 (1·3)

* $p < 0.01$ (on compared to off[1]); $p < 0.04$ (off[2] compared to on).

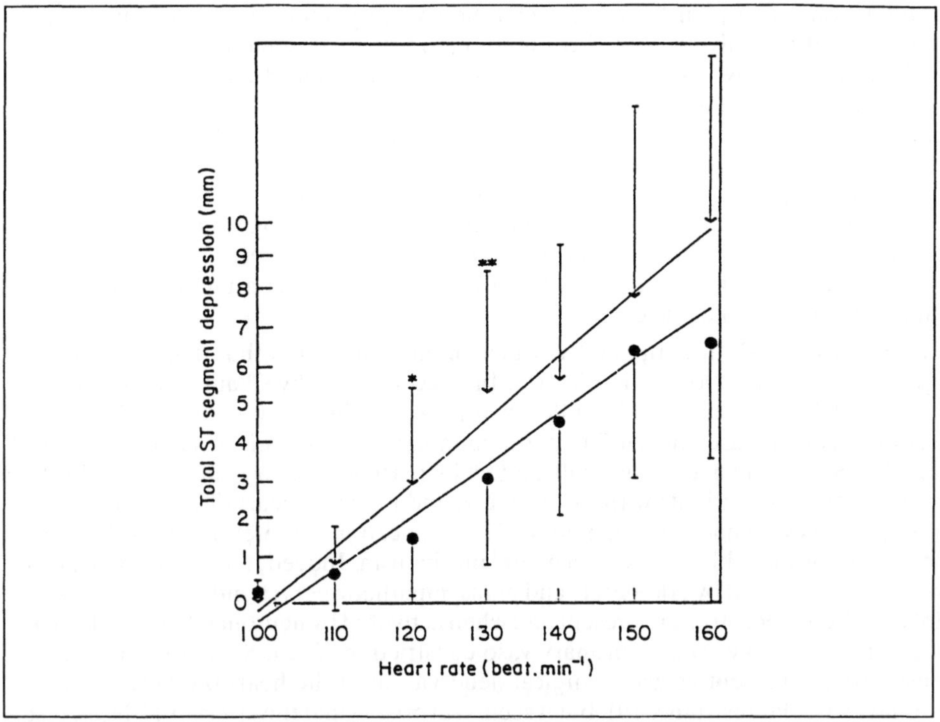

Fig. 2. Total ST-segment depression (mean ± CI) at different heart rates during RA pacing (v = mean with neurostimulator off; • = mean value with neurostimulator on). (From Sanderson et al., 1992)

stimulator off. The total duration of ischemic episodes was reduced in all four patients from a mean of 365 (331) s (with the stimulator off) to 221 (232) s (with the stimulator on). This was marked in one patient in whom the total duration of ischemic episodes was reduced from 627 to 310 s with SCS. These results have now been confirmed in a larger group of patients as part of a collaborative study (4).

The clinical results in these various studies therefore confirm that SCS can improve the symptoms of chronic intractable angina, increase exercise capacity and in some cases, reduce myocardial ischemia. Furthermore, recent work suggest's that SCS does not mask the pain of myocardial infarction (1). In our series two patients had myocardial infarctions which presented in the usual way and which were clinically obvious.

Mechanism of action for spinal cord stimulation for angina

There are at least four possibilities to be considered to explain the action of SCS in angina. Firstly, direct inhibition of pain fibers within the spinal cord (i.e., a purely analgesic effect); secondly, a reduction of reflex sympathetic activity consequent on the reduction in pain; thirdly, a direct inhibition of sympathetic activity within the spinal cord; and fourthly, increased coronary blood flow via some unspecified neural mechanism. There would appear to be little doubt that reduction of pain alone will reduce reflex sympathetic nerve stimulation to the heart and thereby will tend to reduce myocardial oxygen consumption by lowering heart rate and inotropic action. However, it does appear that SCS has a more direct antiischemic effect and it is interesting to speculate why this could be so. Mannheimer's group believe that the mechanism is secondary to a decrease in myocardial oxygen consumption (14). They found in their study with SCS that there were no significant effects of stimulation on coronary sinus blood flow, and a fall in myocardial oxygen consumption, an effect comparable to beta blockade.

In contrast, work in peripheral vascular disease suggested that there may be an increase in capillary blood flow (10, 11). In a recent study by Chauhan et al. (3) the effect of TENS on coronary blood flow was measured in patients with Syndrome X, ischemic heart disease and cardiac transplantation. This study is of some interest as TENS appeared to have a remarkable effect increasing coronary blood flow velocity by nearly 50 % in patients with Syndrome X and ischemic heart disease, but not in those patients who had transplantation. The implication is therefore that TENS was increasing coronary blood flow by a neural mechanism. Indeed, the coronary arteries are richly innervated by adrenergic and parasympathetic nerves and both alpha 1 and alpha 2 adreno receptors are present and when activated by neuronally released or circulating epinephrine, cause coronary vaso constriction (2, 8). Some tonic coronary constriction is present as acute surgical denervation of the heart produces a fall in coronary vascular resistance (9), but it seems surprising that the effect of TENS at rest should be so large. We have tried to reproduce these results in patients with Syndrome X (17). However, preliminary data from 11 patients with Syndrome X failed to confirm the result of Chauhan et al. In our study the mean coronary blood flow velocity was unchanged or fell during TENS therapy. There was little significant change of coronary artery diameter measured by quantitative coronary angiography. There was however a significant effect on the rate-pressure product which fell during TENS therapy and this was associated with a small fall in mean coronary blood flow velocity and a compensatory rise in coronary vascular resistance. This was very similar to that of nitroglycerine which in our studies also produced a fall in rate-pressure product and coronary blood flow velocity with a compensatory small rise in coronary vascular resistance.

As any mechanism of TENS is likely to be neurally mediated, we studied the effect of the cold pressor test which is known to cause vaso constriction in patients with ischemic heart disease and mild vaso dilatation in patients with normal coronary arteries consequent upon the rise in arterial pressure. In our patients with Syndrome X the cold pressor test increased coronary vascular resistance, which is an abnormal response indicating that there are abnormalities within the coronary circulation in these patients. However, TENS therapy had no effect on the response to the cold pressor test. These results in Syndrome X patients are in keeping with previous work from Mannheimer's group (5, 12 13, 14) that the primary effect of TENS and SCS is to reduce myocardial oxygen consumption and rate-pressure product i.e.: a largely peripheral effect without any direct or immediate action on coronary blood flow. This does not however rule out the possibility that TENS and SCS have a direct action on stenotic coronary arteries. In the areas of stenosis it may be that coronary tone is more influenced by neural regulation. Constriction of stenotic lesions has been seen during coronary angiography which has been demonstrated to be mediated by the nervous system and alpha adreno-receptors (6, 8). We are currently undertaking a study to assess the effect of TENS on coronary artery stenosis using a Doppler-flow wire which allows measurement of the gradient across a stenosis.

Because it appears that TENS may have an action on the sympathetic nervous system, we have assessed the effect of high-frequency TENS on a variety of standard tests of the autonomic nervous system in 10 normal subjects (17). Tests were done on 4 consecutive days at the same time and TENS therapy was randomly allocated on 2 days each. The results showed that TENS appeared to have a mild anti-sympathetic effect, shown by a significant reduction in the rise of diastolic blood pressure during isometric exercise (hand grip test). There was no significant effect on the parasynthetic nervous system tested by the valsalva ratio and the heart rate ratio (Tilt test). These results will confirm that TENS appeared to have a mild action on the sympathetic nervous system which is more apparent when the stimulation is greater, such as during isometric exercise. These results are also in keeping with the previous findings which have shown reduced levels of circulating adrenaline and noradrenaline.

Conclusion

Several clinical studies have now confirmed that SCS has a beneficial effect on symptoms, exercise tolerance, and some indices of myocardial ischemia. Our follow-up data also confirms that SCS appears to be safe. There is no evidence for increased ischemia or masking of serious symptoms such as myocardial infarction. To date, no long-term mortality study has been carried out and although there is no evidence from our study that mortality is increased, a larger long-term study needs to be done. The mechanism of action of SCS is likely to be multifactorial. The techniques are very crude and will produce major changes within the spinal cord and thus affect various pathways and physiological responses. It appears likely that the predominant action is a combination of inhibition of pain pathways, which by itself reduces reflex autonomic activity, and a more direct inhibitory effect on the autonomic nervous system especially sympathetic activity. It is also possible that there is an effect on locally released neuropeptides that moderate the relation between ischemia and pain and which also may be involved in tissue regulation of blood flow.

References

1. Andersen C, Hole P, Oxhøj H (1994) Does pain relief with spinal cord stimulation for angina conceal myocardial infarction? Br Heart J 71: 419–21
2. Braunwald E, Sobel BE (1992) Coronary blood flow and myocardial ischemia. In: Braunwald E (ed.) Heart Disease, 4th edn. Philadelphia: WB Saunders, 1161–99
3. Chauhan A, Mullins PA, Thuraisingham SI, Taylor G, Petch MC, Schofield PM (1994) Effect of transcutaneous electrical nerve stimulation on coronary blood flow. Circulation 89: 694–702
4. de Jongste MJL, Haaksma J, Hautvast RWM, Hillege HL, Meyler PWJ, Staal MJ, Sanderson JE, Lie KI (1994) Effects of spinal cord stimulation on myocardial ischemia during daily life in patients with severe coronary artery disease; a prospective ambulatory electrocardiographic study. Br Heart J 71: 413–418

5. Emanuelsson H, Mannheimer C, Waagstein F, Wilhelmsson C (1987) Catecholamine metabolism during pacing-induced angina pectoris and the effect of transcutaneous electrical nerve stimulation. Am Heart J 114: 1360–6
6. Feigl EO (1987) The paradox of adrenergic coronary vasoconstriction. Circulation 76: 737–45
7. Hersch S, Claeys L (1994) Epidural spinal cord stimulation in the treatment of severe peripheral arterial occlusive disease. Ann Vasc Surg 8: 468–474
8. Heusch G (1990) Alpha-adrenergic mechanisms in myocardial ischemia. Circulation 81: 1–13
9. Holtz J, Mayer E, Bassenge E (1977) Demonstration of alpha adrenergic coronary control in different layers of canine myocardium by regional sympathectomy. Pflugers Arch 372: 187–94
10. Jacobs MHJM, Jorning PJG, Soures RJ et al. (1988) Epidural Spinal Cord Electrical stimulation improves microvascular blood flow in severe limb ischemia. Ann Surg 207: 179–183
11. Jacobs MJHM, Jorning PJG et al. (1990) Foot salvage and improvements of microvascular blood flow as a result of epidural spinal cord electrical stimulation. J Vasc Surg 12: 354–60
12. Mannheimer C, Carlsson C-A, Emanuelsson H, Vedin A, Waagstein F, Wilhelmsson C (1985) The effects of transcutaneous electrical nerve stimulation in patients with severe angina pectoris. Circulation 71: 308–316
13. Mannheimer C, Augustinsson L-E, Carlsson C-A, Manhem K, Wilhelmsson C (1988) Epidural spinal electrical stimulation in severe angina pectoris. Br Heart J 59: 56–61
14. Mannheimer C, Eliasson T, Andersson B et al. (1993) Effects of spinal cord stimulation in angina pectoris induced by pacing and possible mechanisms of action. Br Med J 307: 477–80
15. Murphy DF, Giles KE (1987) Dorsal Column stimulation for pain relief from intractable angina pectoris. Pain 28: 365–8
16. Sanderson JE, Tomlinson B, Lau MJW, So KWH, Cheung AHK, Critchley JAJH, Woo KS (1995) The effects of transcutaneous nerve stimulation (TENS) on the autonomic nervous system. (Clin. Autonomic Res.)
17. Sanderson JE, Woo KS, Chung HK, Chan WM, Tse KK, White HD: TENS: The Effect of Transcutaneous Electrical nerve stimulation on coronary and systemic hemodynamics in Syndrome X. (Submitted)
18. Sanderson JE (1990) Electrical neurostimulators for pain relief in angina. Br Heart J 63: 141–3
19. Sanderson JE, Brooksby P, Waterhouse D, Palmer RBG, Neubauer K (1992) Epidural spinal electrical stimulation for severe angina: a study of its effects on symptoms, exercise tolerance and degree of ischemia. Eur Heart J 13: 628–33
20. Sanderson JE, Ibrahim B, Waterhouse D, Palmer RBG (1994) Spinal electrical stimulation for intractable angina; long term clinical outcome and safety. Eur Heart J 15: 810–814

Author's address:
J. E. Sanderson, MD, FRCP
Department of Medicine
Chinese University of Hong Kong
Prince of Wales Hospital
Shatin, N.T.
Hong Kong

Pain modulation by spinal cord stimulation in patients with symptomatic coronary artery disease not accessible to surgical reconstruction

T. Eliasson[2], C. Mannheimer[2], L-E. Augustinsson[1]

Institute of [1]Clinical Neuroscience, Department of Neurosurgery, Sahlgrenska University Hospital, and [2]Multidisciplinary Pain Center, Östra University Hospital, Göteborg, Sweden

Introduction

Spinal cord stimulation (SCS) has been used for neuropathic pain since more than 25 years. More than 100000 implants have been performed, with a very low rate of severe complications (1). The long term follow up results in most independent series show a success rate of approximately 50 % in chronic pain conditions (2).

Chest pain is a common problem and one of diverse etiology. In this context it is of importance to distinguish between pain of neuropathic origin (e.g., after sternothomy) and true angina pectoris which is caused by reversible myocardial ischemia. The clinical presentation of these principally different pain conditions of the chest can be identical. In true angina the typical central chest pain is often accompanied by referred pain.

Chest pain due to neuropathy has been treated with spinal cord stimulation (SCS) since this technique was routinely introduced in the beginning of the 1970s, and with varying success. It is thus of major importance to discriminate between the two etiologies because clinically the symptoms may be very similar and also respond to SCS. SCS has been used to treat severe angina pectoris since 1985. In our total material of 250 patients we have consequently avoided including neuropathic pain patients.

This paper focuses particularly on the effects of SCS on pain, surgical technique, intraoperative physiology, complications, and side effects.

Background

All the patients treated with SCS were referred to us by specialists in cardiology. The clinical cardiological status of the patients was assessed as class III or IV (New York Heart Association classification). About 80 of the patients had undergone one or two coronary by pass operations and suffered from recurrent angina, and the others were not operable for technical reasons. Thirty patients suffered from vasospastic coronary disease, the so-called syndrome X (angina pectoris, normal coronary angiograms, and objective criteria of myocardial ischemia).

Surgical technique

All 250 patients except two were operated on with percutaneous implantation of a quadripolar wire lead. In two patients it was necessary to perform a small laminectomy in order to implant the electrode because of advanced degenerative changes of the osseous structures of the spine. However, all were operated on under local anaesthesia. The prone position was used, and the lead was generally placed at about C7–T1. A subcutaneous pouch was made in the left fossa ilicca for the pulse generator, and the extension wire was tunneled to the midline incision in the back. The entire system was connected and implanted. A prophylactic antibiotic was given postoperatively (Cefuroxime 1.5 g x 3).

Intraoperative physiology

When using any kind of electrical stimulation technique for the treatment of pain it is imperative to cover the painful area with stimulation-induced paresthesiae. Whether the paresthesiae are effective on their own in the pain alleviation achieved or merely a paraphenomenon is not known; however, clinical experience shows that results are poor in the absence of adequate paresthesia . The most common sites for anginal pain are precordial, retrosternal, segmental, and interscapular with referred pain to the left arm, both arms, jaws, back, shoulder, and axillae. The corresponding spinal levels for lead placements are C7 (arms), T1, T2 (upper chest and arms), and T3, T4 (lower chest, back). The stimulator parameters generally used 50 – 80 Hz, pulse width 210 μs amplitude 3 – 6 V.

Complications and side effects

No severe complications, such as epidural hematoma or abscess, occurred. Mild complications included two lead fractures, one pulse generator pouch infection, and seven lead tip migrations. The overall complication rate was 10:250 x 100 = 4 %. Since 1985 some patients have undergone reoperation with replacement of the pulse generator because of battery depletion. In all patients the Medtronic quadripole lead and fully implantable pulse generator were used (Medtronic, Minneapolis: QUAD plus and ITREL II).

Clinical effect on pain and quality of life

For SCS in various neuropathic pain conditions the long-term success rate is about 50 % (up to 60 % in some series), although the results are better in certain subgroups such as peripheral posttraumatic pain (3). In peripheral vascular disease the long term pain relief/success rate is about 80 %, which has been demonstrated independently by different authors. In a prospective randomized study by Jivegård et al. the pain relief with SCS was significant (P = 0.05) compared to controls (4). In our series with SCS in angina pectoris almost all patients responded. This is reflected by a minimum intake of analgesics including nitrates when stimulation is used. The onset of pain relief after stimulation is rapid (seconds). After 1 year or more 90 % of the patients still use their stimulators on a regular basis and experience an enhanced quality of life.

Conclusion

The painrelieving effects of SCS in cardiac ischemic pain (angina pectoris) are good, even during long-term follow-up. This is accompanied by an improvement in the patients' quality of life. Medical treatment, coronary by pass surgery and percutaneous transluminal coronary angioplasty are the first choice treatment methods in angina pectoris and coronary artery disease. However, many patients are unsuitable for surgery, and the rate of recurrence of symptoms after open heart surgery is a clinical reality, making SCS an attractive and promising form of treatment in severe angina pectoris. Syndrome X is another indication for SCS. By definition syndrome X can not be treated surgically. The anti-anginal and anti-ischemic properties of SCS in ischemic heart disease have been amply demonstrated in a number of scientific publications (5–16). A prospective randomized study comparing open coronary bypass surgery with SCS in surgical high-risk patients suffering from coronary artery disease has recently been completed (100 patients), and the last patients' 6 month follow-up will be finished in June 1995, after which the study will be analyzed and published.

References

1. Manman D, Larsson S, Sances A (1985) Spinal cord stimulation for pain. In: Mycklebust J (ed) Neural stimulation. Boca Raton: CRC Press: 148–154
2. Illis L, Krainick J (1992) Spinal cord stimulation for pain. In: Illis L (ed) Spinal cord dysfunction. Oxford: Oxford University Press 3: 264–269
3. Illis L (1992) Spinal cord dysfunction vol III-Functional stimulation. Oxford: Oxford University Press
4. Jivegård L, Augustinsson L-E (1987) Long-term results of epidural spinal electrical stimulation (ESES) in patients with inoperable severe ischemia. Eur J Vasc Surg 1: 345–349
5. De Jongste M, Haaksma J, Hautvast R et al. (1993) Effects of spinal cord stimulation on myocardial ischemia during daily life in patients with severe coronary artery disease. Br Heart J 71: 413–418
6. De Landsherre C, Mannheimer C, Habets A et al. (1992) Effect of spinal cord stimulation on regional myocardial perfusion assessed by positron emision tomography. Am J Cardiol 69: 1143–1149
7. Eliasson T, Jern S, Augustinsson L-E, Mannheimer C (1994) Safety aspects of spinal cord stimulation in severe angina pectoris. Coronary Artery Dis 5: 845– 850
8. Eliasson T, Mannheimer C (1995) Spinal cord stimulation in severe angina pectoris-presentation of current studies, indications and practical experience. Pain (submitted)
9. Mannheimer C, Augustinsson L-E, Carlsson C-A, Manhem K, Wilhelmsson C (1988) Epiural spinal electrical stimulation in severe angina pectoris. Br Heart J 59: 56–61
10. Mannheimer C, Emanuelsson H, Waagstein F, Wilhelmsson C (1989) Influence of naloxone on the effects of high frequency transutaneous electrical nerve stimulation in angina pectoris induced by atrial pacing. Br Heart J 62: 36–42
11. Mannheimer C, Emanuelsson H, Larsson G et al. (1991) Myocardial release of endogenous opioids in the human heart and the effects of epidural spinal electrical stimulation in pacing-induced angina pectoris. J Am Coll cardiol 17: 107
12. Mannheimer C, Eliasson T, Andersson B et al. (1993) Effects of spinal cord stimulation in angina pectoris induced by pacing and possible mechanisms of action. BMJ 307: 477–480
13. Sanderson JE (1990) Epidural neurostimulators for pain relief in angina. Br Heart J 63: 141–143
14. Sanderson JE, Brooksby P, Waterhouse D, Palmer RBG, Neubauer K (1992) Epidural spinal electrical stimulation for severe angina: a study of its effects on symptoms, exercise tolerance and degree of ischaemia. Eur Heart J 13: 628–633

15. Sanderson J, Ibrahim B, Waterhouse D, Palmer R (1994) Spinal cord stimulation for intractable angina-long-term clinical outcome and safety. Eur Heart J 15: 810–814
16. Mannheimer C, Waagstein F, Eliasson T et al. (1994) Myocardial metabolism of endogenous opioids and calcitonin gene-related petide in the human heart and the effects of spinal cord stimulation on pacing-induced angina pectoris. Circulation 90: 1–160

Authors' adress
T. Eliasson, MD PhD
Östra Hospital
Multidisciplinary Pain Center
S-41685 Göteborg
Sweden

Neurostimulation for angina pectoris irresponsive to standard therapies

G. A. J. Jessurun, R. W. M. Hautvast, M. J. L. de Jongste

Dept. of Cardiology, University Hospital Groningen, Groningen, Netherlands

In the majority of patients, coronary artery disease induces angina pectoris, a discomfort in the chest, usually occurring during exercise. In the majority of patients, angina pectoris can be accurately treated with medication (1) or revascularization procedures. However, in an increasing number of these patients, a revascularization procedure is not a feasible option anymore due to, for instance, a diffuse affliction of the coronary arteries (18). The seriously disabled patients suffer from "intractable angina pectoris". In these patients any therapy that improves the quality of life without aggravating their desease would be of great importance. Neurostimulation may be one of these therapies.

Neurostimulation was reinvented after 1965 when Melzack and Wall published the "Gate Control" theory (12). This theory comprehends a model in which the nociceptive, unmyelated C-fibers' afferents are inhibited by stimulation of non-nociceptive myelinated A-fibers' afferents. Although the model of the "gate control" theory does not appear tenable in all its aspects (17), the basic ideas of noxious evoked activity by myelinated non-nociceptive afferent A-fibers remain unchanged.

Defining the problem of intractable angina

In respect to incidence, morbidity, and mortality, little is known about patients with angina pectoris which is therapeutically intractable. However, it can be expected that despite pharmacological, cardiological, and surgical improvements, the number of patients will increase. The patients with intractable angina perform limited activities. Moreover, the psychological stress caused by the awareness of the increased risk on a myocardial infarction often forms an additional burden on the patient and his family.

Any therapy that would alleviate the chronic symptoms of patients with intractable angina and would improve the qulity of life of these patients without worsening the prognosis, would be of great importance. However, it should be emphasized that such a therapy does not necessarily include a better life expectancy. It has been shown that neurostimulation improves exercise capacity with a concomitant reduction in ischemia in patients with intractable angina (13, 14). A major question is whether the improvement in quality of life is based on a reduction in pain perception of these patients, or on a reduction in myocardial ischemia. A reduction in pain perception resulting in an increase in exercise capacity would increase myocardial ischemia. As a consequence, the life expectancy of the patients would decrease. On the other hand, if neurostimulation results in a decrease in myocardial ischemia, this would imply that the improvement in quality of life of the patient is not related to a worsening in prognosis.

Considering the relative low incidence of patients suffering from intractable angina pectoris and the potential complication rate of the technique a limited number of implantation centers is preferable.

Neurostimulation for angina

From observational studies it is concluded that spinal cord stimulation (SCS) in patients with severe angina resulting from coronary artery disease produces: 1) a decrease in the number of anginal attacks, 2) a decrease in the intake of short-acting nitrates, 3) an increase in exercise capacity, and 4) a concomitant decrease in ST-segment depression during exercise (19, 20). However, these results may be biased by the study design. A cross-over protocol or a blinding of therapy is not feasible since SCS provokes paresthesias and stimulation artifacts on the ECG. Moreover, the duration of the eventual effects of SCS is unknown. This implies that in patients in the Treatment group, who are crossed from the Treatment group to the Control group, the effects of SCS may be maintained after witholding therapy during the Control period (carry-over effect). Nevertheless, a randomized study on SCS in patients with intractable angina is still feasible.

Own experiences

The different aspects of neurostimulation were studied in a multidisciplinary "Working Group on Neurocardioloy" in which a neurosurgeon, a cardiologist, a physiotherapist, and a neurologist participated. Later, other basic scientists became involved, in order to solve some of the elementary problems mentioned above.

Patient selection

Patients with intractable angina are included in the study, if they meet the following criteria: 1) coronary angiographically documented significant coronary artery disease without options for a revascularization procedure and 2) compared to the ECG at rest, at least 0.1 mV ST depression at maximum exercise, during an exercise test. Exclusion criteria mainly refer to the inability to perform an exercise test, a short life expectancy, conduction disturbances, and insurmountable problems concerning the implantation of the electrode.

Since 1987, patients referred by various Dutch hospitals, including the University Hospital of Groningen, were seen at our outpatient clinic for assessing their suitability to receive SCS according to our protocol (4). Patients unsuitable for surgery and ineligible for treatment with SCS received transcutaneous electrical nerve stimulation (TENS), a method proven to be effective in angina (15), provided they had angina pectoris NYHA class III–IV and the antianginal therapy was optimized. The pulse intensity was variable and was individually tailored to the patients' requirements. As preventive treatment, the patients were stimulated three times per day for 1 h continuously, and additionally at the onset of an anginal attack.

Baseline characteristics of all referred patients with intractable angina

Within a period of almost 8 years we have examined 164 patients. Their age ranged from 31 to 81 years with a mean of 65.3 ± 9.0 years for the 62 women and a mean of 61.5 ± 8.1 years for the 102 men. All 164 patients had documented significant coronary artery disease. Coronary angiography revealed one-vessel disease in 37 patients, two-vessel disease in 48 patients, and three-vessel disease in 79 patients. A positive exercise test was found in 48 patients and signs of ischemia on myocardial thallium-201 scintigraphy were demonstrated in another 10 patients. Of those 164 patients, 47 patients all with myocardial ischemia were eventually treated with spinal cord stimulation, 97 with TENS, two patients appeared to be eligible for revascularization and in 18 patients conventional treatment was continued for various reasons. The patients treated with SCS were relatively young (63 ± 3.8 years), they had suffered from coronary artery disease for an average duration of 10 years, and they had a relative moderately hampered left ventricular ejection fraction of about 48 ± 10 %, on average.

In a randomized pilot study we evaluated the effects of spinal cord stimulation in five patients (5). Though activities of daily living incresed, and both angina attacks and the consumption of short-acting nitrates decreased, no increase in exercise capacity was observed. To make our randomized study results comparable with other (non-randomized) studies, we modified our protocol in concert with Mannheimer et al. (14) by exercising the patients during active stimulation. In the protocol one alteration was made to exclude the influence of a learning curve of the patients, and one other to prevent an operation bias (4).

Protocol for the evaluation of spinal cord stimulation (4)

During neurostimulation the patients were aware of the paresthesias and the physician saw the artifacts on the ECG, which made it impossible to undertake a double-blind or cross-over study. However, a randomization into a Treatment and a Control group was still possible. Originally, in the Treatment group, the spinal cord stimulator was implanted at the beginning of the study period, and in the Control group after the study period. The patients equipped with a spinal cord stimulator needed 6 weeks to learn the procedure of activating the SCS device. Consequently, the study protocol was extended from 2 to 3 months. In addition, to prevent an operation bias, we implanted the device in the Control group at the beginning of the study, without having the device activated in the Control group during this 3-month study period. After the 3-month study period, the device was switched to active stimulation mode in the

Control group. The patients were no longer randomized and served as their own controls during the follow-up period.

Efficacy of spinal cord stimulation

In a prospective randomized study with a 2-month follow-up, the efficacy of SCS was evaluated through exercise capacity and quality of life in patients with intractable angina. Exercise capacity was assessed by treadmill exercise tests, and quality of life by registering the short acting nitrate intake and the number of anginal attacks in a diary, and scoring of activities of daily living (ADL). The unmistakable conclusion was that SCS improved both exercise capacity and quality of life. The increase in exercise capacity and rate pressure product, in conjunction with the reduction in ST-segment despression, suggested that SCS improved the oxygen supply to the heart. It is uncertain whether SCS employed its electro-analgesic effect as a result of its anti-ischemic action on the heart, or vice versa. The effects of SCS on ST segment depression was further studied in detail (6).

Anti-ischemic effect of spinal cord stimulation

To study a potential anti-ischemic effect of SCS, the patients performed treadmill exercise tests and 48-h ECG monitoring. Exercise capacity was assessed by a standardized treadmill protocol in patients randomly assigned into a Treatment group and a Control group. To evaluate a potential operation bias wie implanted the spinal cord stimulator in half of the Control group patients before the 3-month study period and in the other half of the Controls after the study period. The exercise capacity of patients treated with SCS increased with a concomitant reduction in ST-segment depression (4). Moreover, we could not explain the significant improvement in the Treatment group only by an operation bias. The study using 48-h ECG recording was not randomized, since only 10 of the 47 patients had significant ST-segment changes. However, in this group of 10 patients, a significant reduction in ST-segment depression on 48-h ambulatory monitoring was demonstrated, after implantation of the spinal cord stimulation device (7).

Follow-up and contra-indications

The implantation of a spinal cord stimulator can be considered as a standardized surgical procedure similar to the implantation of a pacemaker. Complications of the neurosurgical procedure are rare and include a.o. infections and leakage of cerebrospinal fluid (8). During 1-year follow-up the stimulation threshold did not change significantly. This implies that no adaptation in the provoked paresthesias occurred. Neurostimulation by an implanted device in combination with an implanted cardiac pacemaker, carries the risk of interference with the function of the cardiac pacemaker. However, this risk can be minimized by taking into account some precautions (8).

Indications of transcutaneous electrical nerve stimulation

In the majority of our patients with severe angina, resulting from coronary artery disease, documented by coronary angiography, ischemia could not be demonstrated by treadmill exercise or ambulatory ECG recordings. The absence of ischemia in these patients, despite severe complaints, was probably related to the beta-blocker, which reduced the heart rate to a level at which ischemia does not occur. Moreover, in patients with severe three-vessel disease, cancellation of ST-segment may occur in the same way as sometimes seen during a myocardial infarction. These patients were not included in the study on SCS; they were treated with transcutaneous electrical nerve stimulation (TENS) (16).

Studies on mechanisms of neurostimulation

To date, it is not yet known which higher structures in the central nervous system are involved in SCS. The periaqueductal gray (PAG) might be one of the structures involved. In animal experiments we have demonstrated that stimulation in specific parts of the PAG produces an increase in femoral, carotid and coronary blood flow. This effect was even more expressed when, intermittently, a coronary artery was occluded (9).

The mechanism of action of SCS on the heart might be the result of a direct beneficial effect on myocardial ischemia. Recently, an increase in coronary flow has been showed using TENS in patients with myocardial ischemia (3). SCS may act by improving both myocardial perfusion and metabolism. On the other hand, this hypothesis could not be established in a positron emission tomography (PET) study using SCS for intractable angina (11). Although the symptoms of angina and the electrocardiographic signs of ischemia decreased, the investigators did not find a significant change in regional myocardial perfusion. The absence of an increase in myocardial perfusion might be related to patient selection, protocol, or even PET camera or PET tracer. In our PET study on patients treated with SCS for intractable angina, SCS induced a more homogenious distribution in myocardial blood flow. This finding suggests an anti-ischemic effect of SCS. However, total coronary blood flow during dipyridamole stress decreased with SCS. The reduction in dipyridamole induced total coronary blood flow during SCS may be related to the adenosine metabolism. Therefore, we speculate that neurostimulation might inhibit the effect of adenosine.

The physiologic level of adenosine, which is believed to play an important role in the pathogenesis of angina pectoris, is increased under hypoxic conditions (2). Dipyridamole blocks cellular re-uptake of interstitial adenosine. In addition to adenosine another important compound with algesic properties is bradykinine. To evaluate the influence of both compounds on angina, we performed the Cardiac Adenosine Myocardial Bradykinine and Angina study (CAMBRIA). In this study, angina pectoris, which was scored by a questionnaire, was compared to the mRNA density of bradykinine and adenosine (in situ hybridization). Tissue to determine the mRNA was obtained during coronary artery bypass surgery. The preliminary results indicate a significant relation between adenosine and the quality of pain. Moreover, adenosine was inversely correlated with age, but not with the severity of anginal pain.

To study the involvement of the autonomic nervous system when SCS is applied, we performed an animal study. In rats electrodes were introduced into the epidural space and fixated at the T1 level. By stimulation of the spinal cord we could study the expression of the proto-oncogene c-fos and the Heat Shock Protein (HSP 72) in the brain. We found c-fos labeling in specific parts of the autnomic nervous system (such as the periaqueductal gray matter, DMNX, nucleus (retro)ambiguus, etc.) after SCS. No neuronal HSP 72 staining was found. Therefore, brain damage is not induced by SCS (10).

Safety and efficacy of the therapy. Is a placebo effect involved?

In some patients the safety and efficacy of neurostimulation in refractory angina pectoris has been documented for more than 5 years (21). A placebo response is unlikely since the effects lasted for 1 year, and up to 3.5 years (19). In our patient group, the survival during the 1-year follow-up did not appear to be adversely influenced by SCS.

Future developments and implantation rates

In Europe, more than 700 patients (±150/year) are treated for angina with SCS devices for angina. There is no evidence yet that afferent nerve fiber stimulation will produce any deleterious effect in conditions such as angina pectoris which is refractory to standard therapies (22). Nevertheless, in addition to the elucidation of the mechanism of action, the safety of spinal cord stimulation has to be established, preferably by a mortality study. Therefore, studies on both cost-benefit (utility, efficacy) and on the psychological effect of neurostimulation are required. From clinical experience we had the impression that in some patients neurostimulation resulted in "addictive-like" behavior. It is not known whether this supposed behavior is based on metabolic alteration (increase in endogenous opiates), psychological dependency, or other mechanisms.

Conclusions

Any therapy for patients with coronary artery disease, who are chronically badly disabled by their intractable angina pectoris, is a very important addition to the presently available therapies. Spinal cord stimulation may be such a treatment for patients with severe angina pectoris. Although the mechanism by whih neurostimulation acts is not yet clarified, a mortality study is mandatory to exclude potentially harmful effects of neurostimulation. However, the available data suggest that neurostimulation is an effective longterm therapy for angina pectoris. In addition, an increase in exercise capacity with a concomitant reduction in ischemia was found. An important factor is also that the surgical procedure, necessary to achieve SCS, is simple and can be performed without major complications.

References

1. Corne RA (1987) Risk stratification in stable angina pectoris. Am J Cardiol 59: 695
2. Crea F, Pupita G, Galassi AR et al. (1990) Role of adenosine in pathogenesis of anginal pain. Circulation 81: 164–172
3. Chauhan A, Mullins PA, Thuraisingham SI et al. (1994) Effect of transcutaneous electrical nerve stimulation on coronary blood flow. Circulation 89: 694–702
4. De Jonste MJL, Hautvast RWM, Hillege JL et al. (1994) Efficacy of spinal cord stimulation as an adjuvant therapy for intractable angina pectoris – a prospective randomized clinical study. J Am Coll Cardiol 23: 1592–7
5. De Jongste MJL, Lie KI, Linde ven der MR et al. (1989) A longterm randomized study on the efficacy of spinal cord stimulation as an adjuvant therapy for severe angina pectoris. Proceedings of the 1st ICESS congress Groningen, The Netherlands (abstract)
6. De Jongste MJL, Staal MJ (1993) Preliminary results of a randomized study on the clinical efficacy of spinal cord stimulation for refractory severe angina pectoris. On behalf of the Groninger Working Group on Neurocardiology. Acta Neurochir 58: 161–4
7. De Jongste MJL, Haaksma J, Hautvast RWH et al. (1994) Effects of spinal cord stimulation on myocardial ischemia during normal activity in patients with severe coronary artery disease. A prospective ambulatory ECG study. Br Heart J 71: 413–8
8. De Jongste MJL, Nagelkerke D, Hooyschuur CM et al. (1994) Stimulation characteristics, complications and efficacy of spinal cord stimulation systems in patients with refractory angina. A prospective feasibility study. Pace 17 (11): 1751–1760
9. De Jongste MJL, Cowie RJ, Holstege G (1993) Neural regulation of coronary bloodflow and its impact on angina pectoris and myocardial ischemia. In: Neurohumoral regulation of coronary flow. Role in endothelium. van Gilst WH, Lie KI (eds.) Kluwer Academic Publishers, Dordrecht
10. Hautvast RWM, Homminga SA, De Jongste MJL et al. (1994) C-Fos expression in the central nervous system of the rat after myocardial infarction and neurostimulation. Eur Heart J 15: 810–814
11. Landsheere CH de, Mannheimer C, Habets A et al. (1992) Effect of spinal cord stimulation on regional myocardial perfusion assessed by positron emission tomography. Am J Cardiol 69: 1143–1149
12. Melzack R, Wall PD (1965) Pain mechanisms: a new theory. Science 150: 971–979
13. Murphy DF, Gilles KE (1987) Dorsal column stimulation for pain relief from intractable angina pectoris. Pain 28: 365–368
14. Mannheimer C, Augustinsson LE, Carlsson CA et al (1988) Epidural spinal electrical stimulation in severe angina pectoris. Br Heart J 59: 56–61
15. Mannheimer C, Carlsson CA, Emmanuelsson H et al. (1985) The effects of transcutaneous electrical nerve stimulation in patients with severe angina pectoris. Circulation 71: 308–316
16. Meyler WJ, De Jongste MJL, Rolf CAM (1994) Clinical evaluation of pain treatment with electrostimulation. A study on TENS as a routine therapy in patients with different pain syndromes. Clin J Pain 10: 22–7
17. Nathan PW (1976) The gate-control theory of pain, a critical review. Brain 99: 123–58

18. Silverman KJ, Grossman W (1984) Angina pectoris – natural history and strategies for evaluation and management. New Eng J Med 310/26: 1712–1717
19. Sanderson JE, Ibrahim B, Waterhouse D et al. (1993) Eidural spinal electrical stimulation for severe angina: a study of its effects on symptoms, exercise tolerance and degree of ischemia. Eur Heart J 13: 628–633
20. Sanderson JE, Ibrahim B, Waterhouse D et al. (1994) Long term clinical results and safety of epidural spinal cord stimulation (ESES) for angina. J Am Coll Cardiol special issue (abstract) 389A
21. Sanderson JE, Ibrahim B, Waterhouse D et al. (1994) Spinal electrical stimulation for intractable angina – Long-term clinical outcome and safety. Eur Heart J 15: 810–814
22. Santiesteban J (1985) Applications of transcutaneous electrical nerve stimulation for postoperative, cardiopulmonary and obstetric patients. In: *Textbook of Pain*, chapter 8: 179–197

Authors' address:
Gillian A. J. Jessurun, MD
University Hospital Groningen
Department of Cardiology
Oostersingel 59, PO Box 30001
9700 RB Groningen
Netherlands

Spinal cord stimulation for coronary vascular pathology: our experience

S. Greco, M. Santini

Department of Heart Diseases, San Filippo Neri Hospital, Rome, Italy

In cooperation with two other hospitals in Rome, in 1992, we began a randomized study (Table 1) regarding the clinical improvement and survival of patients treated with a permanent pacemaker for spinal cord stimulation (SCS).

All patients were suffering from intractable angina and most of them had already undergone coronary bypass surgery (Table 2, 3). A second operation would have been very difficult technically, for a too high risk and low benefit, because of either the anatomy of distal vessels or a poor ejection fraction. Fifteen coronary patients were implanted with a pacemaker in the neurosurgical department of our hospital.

Table 1. Patients population

- ► From March 1992 to May 1994 we randomized 21 pts affected by intractable angina pectoris
- ► 15 pts received a pacemaker for spinal cord stimulation
- ► 6 pts were included in a control group
- ► Scheduled follow-up: 12 months

Table 2. Clinical characteristics

	age	sex (m/f)	prev. m.i. (ant/inf)	prev. bypass (y/n)
L. S.	62	m	inf	y
T. S.	49	m	inf	y
P. G.	70	m	/	n
D. M.	64	f	ant	n
S. M.	79	f	ant	n
P. M.	82	f	/	y
D. O.	82	m	inf	n
D. C.	63	m	ant	y
B. G.	70	m	/	y
T. N.	62	f	ant	n
D. M.	69	f	ant + inf	y
C. R.	77	m	inf	y
P. G.	76	f	inf	n
S. G.	43	m	inf	y
M. G	80	m	ant	n

Table 3. Clinical characteristics

age (yrs)	68.5 ± 11.7 (43–82)
sex (m/f)	9 m
	6 f
Previous M. I. (ant/inf)	5 ant
	6 inf
	1 ant + inf
Previous Bypass	8 pts

The scheduled follow-up should have been 12 months for each patient, but 1 year ago, considering the favourable published experiences, we decided to abolish the control group. Since then, we recommend the SCS to all otherwise intractable patients and now we are evaluating the possibility to implant a pacemaker also to surviving control group patients. The number of our cases is too small to allow any statistical result.

Currently we are considering to stimulate all the candidates, and in the next week two admitted patients will receive a pacemaker. We hope that future funding from our hospital will be enough to support this technique. All the implantations have been performed by the same neurosurgeon and up to now we have not observed any severe complication. Only one patient suffered from a little dislocation of the spinal electrocatheter one year after the operation.

Out of 15 implanted patients, 12 have a high quality of life but 3 patients died: the first from intestinal cancer, the second after vascular surgery, and the last one from myocardial infarction (Table 4).

Initially we used to keep the generator on continuosly; now we are evaluating turning it on only three times a day: 1 h on and 7 h off. The mild paresthesia felt in the left side of the thorax is generally well tolerated. We tried to increase the voltage in one of our patients suffering from four crises of angina per day; after 2 days we observed a reduction of anginal crises, anyway the paresthesia was unbearable and we had to return to the previous values.

Before and after the implantation of pacemakers, five patients performed an exercise thallium 201 myocardial scintigraphy and we did not observe any significant difference in coronary blood flow.

Last June, we presented a paper to the Annual Congress of Hospital Cardiologists in Florence on "Heart rate variability in spinal cord stimulated patients". The aim of our study was to evaluate possible changes in sympathovagal autonomic balance. We

Table 4. Clinical follow-up

3 pts died of
- intestinal cancer
- peripheral vascular surgery
- myocardial infarction

1 pt dropped out because of coronary bypass

studied the HRV in the frequency domain and observed a reduction of low frequencies when the pacemaker was on. That is to say that SCS patients showed a change in autonomic drive towards a decreased sympathetic activity.

In conclusion, the results of our observations on SCS have shown an impressive reduction of anginal weekly crises, particularly in the first 3 months after the pacemaker implantation. Later, we have observed a trend to a stable higher number of anginal crises which occured, in any case, less frequently than before the treatment.

References

1. De Jongste M, Raymond W, Hautvast M et al. (1994) Efficacy of spinal cord stimulation as adjuvant therapy for intractable angina pectoris: a prospective, randomized clinical study. Jaac 23: 1592–1597
2. De Landsheere C, Mannheimer C, Habets A et al. (1992) Effect of spinal cord stimulation on regional myocardial perfusion assessed by positron emission tomography. Am J Cardiol 69: 1143–1149
3. Emanuelsson H, Mannheimer C, Waagstein F (1991) Changes in arterial levels and myocardial metabolism of catecholamines during pacing induced angina pectoris. Clin Cardiol 14: 567–572
4. Greco S, Cardinale M, Antonini L et al. (1994) Variabilita del ciclo cardiaco nei portatori di pacemaker per neurostimolazione. Giorn It Cardiol, Atti del Congresso ANMCO 24 (suppl. 1) 619, abstract
5. Kujacic V, Eliasson T, Mannheimer C et al. (1993) Assessment of the influence of spinal cord stimulation on left ventricular function in patients with severe angina pectoris; an echocardiographic study. Eur Heart J 14: 1238–1244
6. Mannheimer C, Augustiansson LE, Carlsson CA et al. (1988) Epidural spinal electrical stimulation in severe angina pectoris. Br Heart J 59: 56–61
7. Mannheimer C, Eliasson T, Andersson B et al. (1993) Effect of spinal cord stimulation in angina pectoris induced by pacing and possible mechanism of action. BMJ 307: 477–480
8. Melzack R, Wall PD (1965) Pain mechanism: A new theory. Science 150: 971–979
9. Naver H, Augustiansson LE, Elam M (1992) The vasodilating effect of spinal column stimulation is mediated by sympathetic nerves. Clin Auton Res 2: 41–45
10. Wall PD, Sweet WH (1967) Temporary abolition of pain in man. Science 155: 108–109

Authors' address
Dr. Salvatore Greco
Via Flaminia Nuova 219
I-00191 Roma
Italy

Buerger's Disease – Miscellaneous

Buerger's Disease: an Overview

S. Shionoya

Emeritus Professor of Nagoya University, Sanjay Gandhi Post-Graduate Institute of Medical Sciences, Lucknow-226001, India

Introduction

After many changes, Buerger's disease has become an independent clinical entity; the condition is no longer a disease of misconceptions. Specificity of the disease is characterized by peripheral ischemia of an inflammatory nature and with a self-limiting course. The clinical name of the disease, "Buerger's disease", is preferred to its pathological name, "Thromboangitis obliterans", which tends to be associated with imprecise histopathological criteria (11).

The incidence of the disease is low in Europe and the USA, but its management remains a major problem for vascular surgeons in Asia where its incidence is higher.

Clinical diagnostic criteria

Our clinical criteria for the diagnosis of Buerger's disease are: a history of cigarette smoking; onset before the age of 50 years; infrapopliteal arterial occlusive lesions; either phlebitis migrans or upper-limp involvement; and absence of atherosclerotic risk factors other than smoking (10). Confident clinical diagnosis of the disease may be made when all five requirements have been fulfilled.

From 1977 to 1988, 255 patients with Buerger's disease were treated at Nagoya University Hospital; 249 (98 %) were men and six (2 %) women. The mean (s.d.) age of onset was 35.8 ($\pm$ 7.7) (range 19–49) years. From symptom onset to the end of the 12-year follow-up, gangrene or ulceration occured in 184 patients (72 %), phlebitis migrans in 109 (43 %), and involvement of the upper-limb in 230 (90 %). Both upper-limb involvement and thrombophlebitis migrans occured in 84 (33 %) of the main patient group. However, no significant difference was found in ischemic symptoms and clinical course between patients presenting with two symptoms and those with only one. Hence, upper-limb involvement and thrombophlebitis migrans are important features, either of which supports the clinical diagnosis of Buerger's disease (10).

Foot claudication, severe ischemia of the plantar muscles, is almost pathognomonic of Buerger's disease, especially when associated with upper-limb involvement or phlebitis migrans.

Should Buerger's disease affect older men (> 50 years), their response may differ from that of younger men who develop the condition. Such differences may reflect degenerative changes in the arterial wall in older patients. Identification of atherosclerotic risk factors in patients with Buerger's disease late in life should not hinder diagnosis of the condition. Whether this is a coincidence or whether atherosclerosis becomes superimposed on Buerger's disease through a predisposition of the arterial tree to the disease is unknown.

Smoking

Aetiology of Buerger's disease remains unknown, but there is a clear relationship between tobaco abuse and its occurence or recurrence; complete cessation of smoking renders the disease benign. Essentially all patients with Buerger's disease are smokers. Some investigators insist that the condition occurs only in smokers, while others cite evidence of cases in non-smokers. This discrepancy may result from a lack of objective evidence that these patients are "true" non-smokers.

Carbon monoxide hemoglobin (COHb) in blood is not specific to nicotine intake; COHb levels are influenced by the concentration of carbon monoxide in the environment. Cotinine, the major metabolite of nicotine, may be used to assess either active of passive smoking (Fig. 1). It has a relatively long plasma half-life (20 h) and urinary cotinine levels can indicate nicotine intake (4). Based on the measurement of urinary cotinine excretion in smokers and non-smokers with or without passive smoking (Figs. 2, 3), patients with urinary cotinine levels of > 50 ng/mg of creatinine (Cr) were considered active smokers, those with levels of 10 – 50 ng/mgCr passive smokers, and those with levels of < 10 ng/mgCr non-smokers not subjected to significant passive smoking; urinary cotinine excretion is expressed as ng per mg of creatinine to avoid the influence of urinary volume (6).

Although it remains unknown whether non-smokers will develop Buerger's disease, a cooperative epidemiological and clinical study to assess long-term effects of involuntery smoking on health may indicate whether passive smoking can cause the disease or not (2).

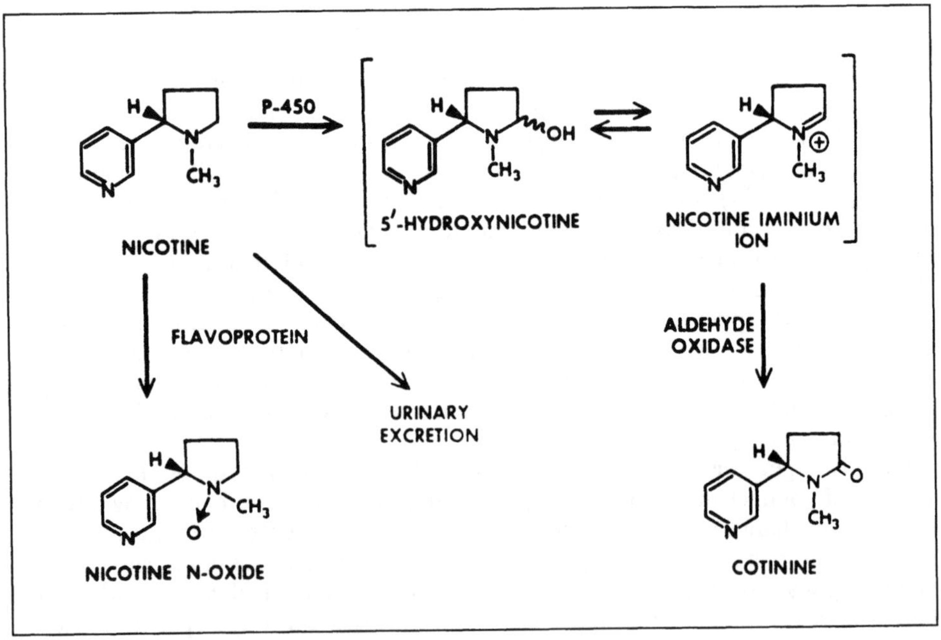

Fig. 1. Metabolic pathway of nicotine to cotinine.

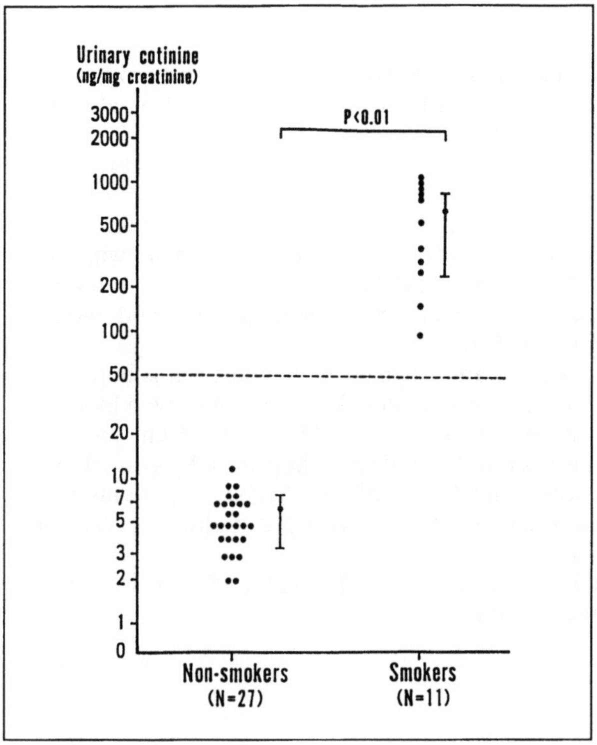

Fig. 2. Urinary cotinine excretion in non-smokers and smokers.

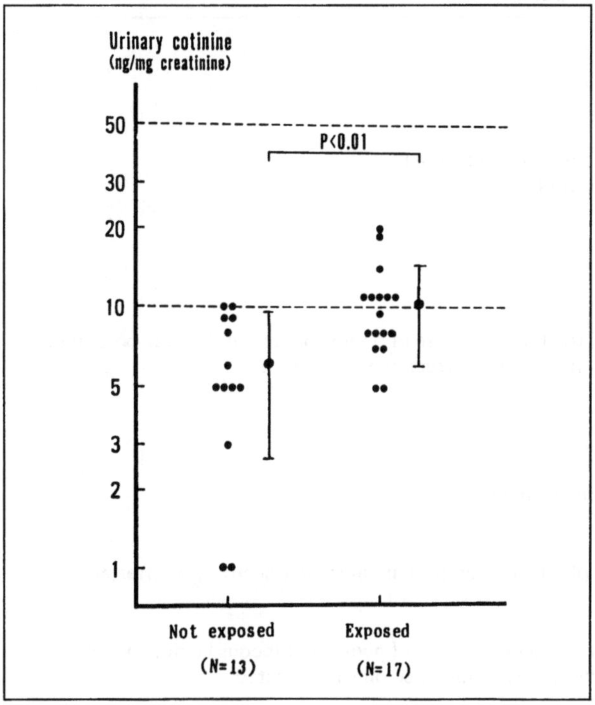

Fig. 3. Effect of passive smoking on urinary cotinine excretion in non-smokers.

Treatment

Total abstinence from smoking remains the sole means of halting disease progression and must accompany any therapeutic procedure if the latter is to succeed; a reduction in the number of cigarettes smoked is useless.

The general approach to management of Buerger's disease is shown in Table 1. Initial management of all patients with Buerger's disease should be conservative since several arteries may be unaffected. The goal of conservative management is to encourage blood flow through intact vessels and compensatory collateral network. At present, there are two means of increasing the blood flow through the collateral network; physical method, including exercise (8); and pharmacological method, including intra-arterial infusion of vasodilators (9).

Vasospastic symptoms such as coldness and Raynaud's phenomenon is improved by protection from exposure to cold. Intermittent claudication is improved by walking training and exercise. Sympathectomy is not indicated for intermittent claudication, because circulation in the muscles is not significantly improved by sympathetic denervation. Arterial reconstruction is not frequently applicable to patients with Buerger's disease, because of widespread arterial occlusions at multiple levels with prevalence in the distal extremities.

A matter of primary concern in the treatment of Buerger's disease is how to manage intractable pain and necrotic lesion.

Table 1. Management plan for therapy of Buerger's disease

A	Acute stage	
		Bridging treatment.
B	Chronic stage	
	I	Upper extremities
		Raynauds phenomenon, coldness and paresthesia:
		Protection from exposure to cold.
		Arm claudication:
		Physical exercise.
		Rest pain:
		Drug treatment.
		Gangrene or ulceration:
		Pharmacotherapy and local treatment. In case of poor spontaneous healing potential, thoracic sympathectomy or arterial reconstruction is indicated.
	II	Lower extremities
		Coldness and paresthesia:
		Protection from exposure to cold.
		Intermittent claudication:
		Walking training and physical exercise.
		Rest pain:
		Drug treatment.
		In case of poor response to pharmacotherapy, lumbar sympathectomy or arterial, reconstruction is indicated.
		Gangrene or ulceration:
		Pharmacotherapy and local treatment. In case of poor spontaneous healing potential, arterial reconstruction and/or lumbar sympathectomy is indicated.

Analgesia

Patients must be helped through the difficult period between onset of severe ischemia and eventual clinical improvement; typically, severe intractable pain must be controlled. "Bridging treatment" is the term we use for appropriate application of epidural anesthesia, prostaglandin infusion, antithrombotic agents, and hyperbaric oxygen to help the patient through an acute exacerbation (3). Reducing the dependent edema facilitates healing of ischemic tissue. In most cases pain is alleviated and the patient's mental state also improved. This approach allows a therapeutic plan to be formulated that is based on the degree of ischemia and its response to such symptomatic treatment (11). Application of spinal cord stimulation has opened a new field in the treatment of intractable ischemic pain (5). Out of five patients with Buerger's disease suffering from severe pain in our series, the pain was improved in four cases and ulceration was healed in one by means of this technique. Although there is need for a randomized controlled trial, spinal cord stimulation may be indicated for ischemic rest pain and superficial tissue loss.

Pharmacotherapy

In managing trophic lesions of the extremity, it is an indispensable step to evaluate spontaneous healing potential of the lesions. Spontaneous healing potential of the ischemic lesion may be objectively evaluated with thallium-201 scintigraphy.

Ischemic ulcers in the foot are classified into four types according to the presence and degree of the inherent inflammatory response of the lesion in both the initial and delayed distributions after simultaneously intravenous injection of 2mCi of thallium-201, with releasing of the cuff pressure, 50 mmHg above the brachial systolic pressure, applied above the ankle (7).

Type I: a prominant localized increase of thallium accumulation (hot spot) in the postocclusive initial distribution, and a decreased accumulation in the delayed (3 h later) one.

Type II: a hot spot in the initial distribution, and an increased accumulation in the redistribution.

Type III: no hot spot in the initial distribution, but one demonstrated in the delayed phase.

Type IV: no hot spot at all in either distribution.

Judging from the therapeutic results, lesions of type I and II have a good spontaneous healing potential and will be healed in response to conservative treatment; those of type III will be healed with conservative management owing to fair healing potential, but surgical procedure may be advised to prevent protracted hospitalization; and those of type IV require arterial reconstruction if there is a hope for success, because of no healing potential (7). With noninvasive diagnostic techniques, the minimum requirements for spontaneous healing potential of ischemic trophic lesions might be as follows:

Skin blood pressure	> 40 mmHg
Ankle blood pressure	> 50 mmHg
Toe blood pressure	> 30 mmHg
Transcutaneous PO2	> 30 mmHg
Foot blood velocity	> 1.0 cm/sec
Scintigram with T1-201	+ a hot spot

Ischemic lesions in patients with Buerger's disease have much better spontaneous healing potential than generally expected.
Prostaglandins provide a major therapeutic approach to the management of critical limb ischemia (1, 9). However, psotaglandins cannot be considered as a panacea for the treatment of arterial insufficiency, and it is important to determine which patient will respond to PG-therapy. Of 255 patients in our series, 40 limbs had intractable ischemic ulceration for which arterial reconstruction was not feasible. The patients underwent continuous intra-arterial infusion of PGE1 (0.03–0.5 (mean 0.17) ng/kg/min). Infusion continued for 13–84 (mean 44) days, after which ulcers were healed in 12 limbs (30 %), improved in 21 (52 %), and unchanged in 7 (18 %). Intravenous infusions of PGE1 have become popular since they possess practical advantages (9).

At present, measurement of blood flow, blood pressure, transcutaneous oxygen tension and skin temperature in the target area is not sensitive enough to detect hardly discernible hemodynamic change in microcirculation by pharmacotherapy. Being mindful of an adverse effect, the drug-induced clinical response must be carefully observed in each patient.

Arterial reconstruction

Sympathectomy has been indicated for superficial trophic lesions of the skin. However, in hindsight, it appears that the lesions healed after sympathectomy would have been improved conservatively without sympathetic denervation.

Postsympathectomy neuralgia and dry skin was problematic in some, and careless abuse of this technique must be avoided.

Bypass grafts were performed in 44 (17 %) of 255 patients with Buerger's disease in the present series. Indications for arterial reconstruction were gangrene or ulceration in 28 limbs (55 %), rest pain in 10 (20 %), claudication in 11 (22 %), and graft infection in 2 (4 %). Follow-up ranged from 1 to 12 years; the cummulative actuarial patency rate of the 12 suprainguinal grafts was 90 % at 1 year, 70 % at 2 years, and 70 % at 10 years; that of 34 infrainguinal grafts was 56, 48, and 32 %, respectively. As the majority of graft failures occured within 2 years after operation, it is a great problem to mediate a way out of the intermediate pass for the grafts surviving the perioperative period. Postoperative anticoagulant and antiplatelet treatment will not salvage poor vascular reconstruction (12).

Of the 255 patients, below-knee amputation was required in six and above knee amputation in one (overall major amputation rate 2.7 %). Six of the seven patients continued to smoke despite advice to the contrary. In spite of the high incidence of digital gangrene in patients with Buerger's disease, a functional foot was commonly preserved owing to good spontaneous healing potential of the lesion. In the present series, five patients died in the follow-up course of 12 years. Three died from mesenteric thrombosis; each had juxttarenal aortic occlusion, and age at death was 33, 47, and 60 years, respectively. Two patients died from myocardial infarction; age at death was 48 and 51 years, respectively. There was, however, no evidence of typical histopathological changes of thromboangiitis obliterans in the vessels examined at autopsy. Involvement of the visceral vessels is rare and this is supported by patients with Buerger's disease having similar life expectancy to normal subjects of the same age and sex (10).

Diagnosis of Buerger's disease is based on knowledge of the natural history of the disease, which aids prognosis and the decision to undertake surgical or conservative management. Treatment of Buerger's disease should avoid premature, possibly unnecessary, surgery. If the patient with Buerger's disease absolutely abandons smoking, his natural course is uneventful and favorable.

References

1. Carlson LA, Eriksson I (1973) Femoral artery infusion of prostaglandin E1 in severe peripheral vascular disease. Lancet i: 155–156
2. Davis JW, Shelton L, Watanabe IS et al. (1989) Passive smoking affects endothelium and platelets. Arch Intern Med 149: 386–389
3. Eastcott HHG (1984) Buerger's disease. In: Bergan JJ, Yao JST (eds) Evaluation and Treatment of Upper and Lower Extremity Circulation Disorders. Grune and Stratton, Orland, Florida, pp 483–497
4. Fiedling JE, Phenow KJ (1988) Health effects of involuntary smoking. N Engl J Med 319: 1452–1460
5. Horsch S, Claeys L (1994) Epidural spinal cord stimulation in the treatment of severe peripheral arterial occlusive disease. Ann Vasc Surg 8: 468–474
6. Matsushita M, Shionoya S, Matsumoto T (1991) Urinary cotinine measurement in patients with Buerger's disease – effects of active and passive smoking on the disease process. J Vasc Surg 14: 53–58
7. Ohta T (1985) Noninvasive technique using thallium-201 for predicting ischaemic ulcer healing of the foot. Br J Surg 72: 892–895
8. Ratschow M (1959) Kritisches zu Ätiologie und Grundlagen einer konservativen Therapie peripherer Durchblutungsstörungen. Langenbecks Arch Klin Chir 292: 188–197
9. Shionoya S (1984) Clinical experience with prostaglandin E1 in occlusive arterial disease. Int Angiol 3: 99–103
10. Shionoya S (1990) Buerger's Disease. Pathology, Diagnosis and Treatment. The University of Nagoya Press, Nagoya, pp 101–116, 170–184, 189–197
11. Shionoya S (1993) Buerger's disease: Diagnosis and management. Cardiovasc Surg 1: 207–214
12. Shionoya S, Sakurai T, Ueyama T et al. (1990) Effect of ticlopidine on graft patency following arterial reconstructive surgery in the lower extremity: a multicenter three-year prospective study. Vasc Surg 24: 541–547

Author's address:
Prof. S. Shionoya, MD PhD
Sanjay Gandhi Post-Graduate
Institute of Medical Sciences,
Raebareli Road,
Lucknow-226001
India

Spinal cord stimulation in the treatment of Buerger's disease

K. Ktenidis, L. Claeys, C. Bartels, S. Horsch

Dept. of General and Vascular Surgery, General Hospital Cologne-Porz,
Academic Teaching Hospital of the University of Cologne, Germany

Introduction

Buerger's disease is a segmental, inflammatory occlusive disease primarily involving small and medium-sized arteries and veins of the extremity, affecting males who are in the third or fourth decade of life and heavy smokers.

The etiology of this disease remains unclear. However, current opinion considers it to be not a variant of atherosclerosis. Medical supervision with elimination of the risk factors is the main treatment for Buerger's disease. Among the medical treatments proposed, only prostaglandins offer elements which favor their efficacy. Vascular reconstruction is rarely possible, sympathectomy is indicated less frequently and amputation is in many patients unavoidable.

Since two decades, spinal cord stimulation has been advocated as a method of pain relief for therapeutic refractory ischemic pain. Different authors reported also healing of trophic lesions under spinal cord stimulation (1, 2, 4, 6, 8, 9, 25), suggesting that spinal cord stimulation improves nutritional skin blood flow. This was confirmed in recent studies (12, 14).

In this paper we describe the long-term effects of spinal cord stimulation on ischemic pain in patients with non-reconstructible Buerger's disease.

Patients and methods

A pilot study was made in nine patients with non-reconstructible Buerger's disease receiving 21-day intravenous prostaglandin E1 therapy (PGE1: 2 x 40 μg) for non-healing ulcers or gangrene. In two patients both lower limbs were involved. All patients received adjunctive spinal cord stimulation as pain treatment. Entry criteria included presence of ulcers or gangrene, and arteriographic evidence of non-reconstructible distal vessels.

Diagnosis of Buerger's disease was made according to the clinical criteria proposed by Shionoya (Table 1) (27). All patients were men and heavy smokers. Mean age was 35 years (range 18 – 48 years).

Typical atherogenic risk factors were not noted and there was no clinical or laboratory evidence for connective tissue disease.

Arteriographies were obtained in all patients to rule out an eventual indication for angioplasty or bypass surgery.

Spinal cord stimulation was only considered in a non-reconstructible patient with disabling rest pain and was only performed after informed consent. Indeed, in order to adequately benefit from the stimulation therapy the patient must understand the

Table 1. Clinical criteria proposed by Shionoya (10)

1. Smoking habit
2. Onset of the symptoms before the age of 50 years
3. Infrapopliteal arterial occlusion
4. Phlebitis migrans or upper extremity involvement
5. Absence of atherogenic risk factors.

principles of this therapy. The stimulation will cause paresthesias and the patient must be willing to accept it.

A full vascular workup was done. Visual analogue scale was used to help quantify the pain. The ankle/brachial index (ABI) was used to assess the macrocirculation and transcutaneous oxygen measurements to assess the microcirculation. ABI was obtained by dividing the systolic pressure, measured over the posterior tibial or the anterior tibial artery, by the systolic brachial artery pressure. These measurements were performed with the patient in the supine position and at rest for 15 min using a bidirectional continuous wave Doppler.

The $TcPO_2$-electrodes (Clark-type oxygen-sensing electrodes) were attached to the skin, the heating element of the electrode was warmed to 45 °C. The measurements were performed with the patient resting in the supine position. One electrode was attached on the dorsum of the foot and one on the chest. The ratio between foot and chest $TcPO_2$ was referred to as the regional perfusion index (RPI) and can be interpreted similarly to the ABI (7, 10, 15, 22).

These investigations were performed at 3-month intervals during follow-up.

We considered three types of outcome: 1) success: defined as significant pain relief (> 75 %) and limb survival; 2) partial success: limb survival with pain relief between 50 and 70 %, and 3) failure: no or little pain relief under stimulation with limb loss.

Surgical technique

This involves placing a quadripolar lead into the epidural space by performing a percutaneous lumbar puncture (Pisces Quad 3487A, Medtronic). The lead is advanced under radioscopic control to the level of Th 11 – 12. Midline placement is preferable. Connecting a portable stimulator to the lead allows intraoperative test stimulation producing comfortable paresthesias in the painful foot or limb. During a trial period of 1 week the clinical effects are monitored. When the patient has experienced adequate pain relief an externally implantable pulse generator (IPG, Itrel II, Medtronic) is placed in a subcutaneous pocket of the abdomen. The usual initial settings are a pulse amplitude varying between 1.0 – 2.5 V, a frequency between 70 – 120 Hz, and a pulse of 180 – 450 microseconds. Stimulation can be given continuously or intermittently. During follow-up the parameters can be reset with the help of a portable computer.

Statistical analysis

The data are presented as mean values and standard deviations. Student's *t*-test was used and $p < 0.05$ was chosen as the level for statistical significance.

Results

Relief of ischemic pain

We achieved complete pain relief in three patients after 4 weeks of stimulation. Pain relief of more than 75 % was noted in eight patients. During follow-up, 78 % of the patients remained pain-free, two patients were classified as partial success. No patient complained of severe or unbearable pain during the follow-up period.

Amputations

The trophic lesions healed quickly in five patients. Two patients needed a minor amputation. Of the patients with bilateral disease, one had limb survival after bilateral minor amputation, the other patient had limb loss after 2 months of stimulation and ulcer healing after minor amputation at the other site. The minor amputations were performed during the first weeks of stimulation.

Effects on the vascular system

Ankle/brachial systolic pressure index (ABI) improved marginally from 0.62 to 0.81 ($p > 0.05$, NS) (1, 2).

The mean initial regional perfusion index was 0.33. The mean value at 1 year was 0.71. Final mean value was 0.81 ($p < 0.05$).

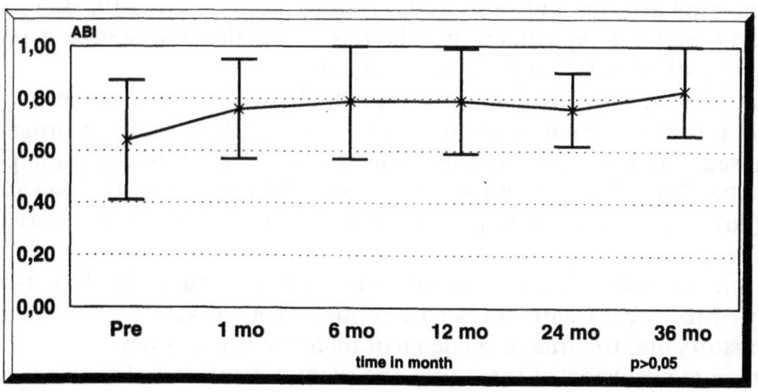

Fig. 1. No significant changes were noticed in the Ankle Brachial Index during the follow-up period.

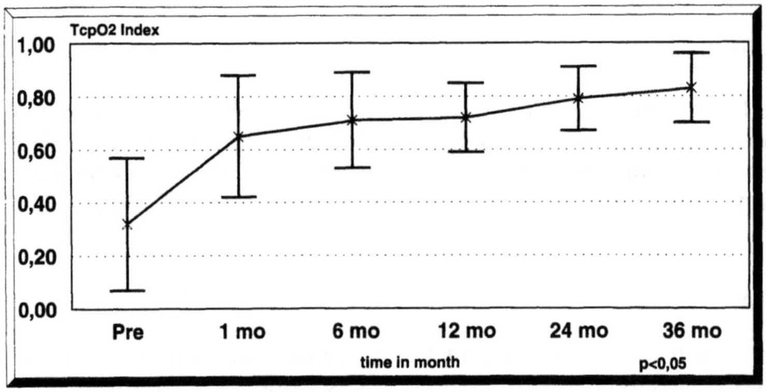

Fig. 2. $TcPO_2$ foot values and the Regional Perfusion Index increased significantly under longterm stimulation.

Complications

We observed one lead dislocation, after correction the system functioned properly again. Other complications like probe break, infection or liquor fistula were not noted.

Discussion

Buerger's disease is a segmental, inflammatory occlusive disease that involves small and medium-sized arteries and veins in the extremities. Patients with Buerger's disease have a normal life expectancy, but the risk of a major amputation is propably higher than that of atherosclerotic vascular disease.

The exact mechanisms involved in the pathophysiology have not been clearly established. Tobacco plays an essential part in the etiology and the prognosis of Buerger's disease and the incidence of acute attacks is linked to the resumption of tobacco intake. Therefore, stopping the tobacco intake is one of the essential prerequisites (26). Other factors discussed are vascular spasms and disturbances of the immune system.

The treatment consists of a local treatment and in the treatment of the ischemia. The quality of the local treatment is an essential element. Correct surgical wound care is mandatory and treatment of edema or infection is necessary.

The segmental occlusion of the crural and plantar arteries makes reconstructive vascular surgery impossible in most of the patients. However, a patient should only be declared as non-reconstructible when intraarterial arteriograms shows occluded crural and pedal arteries, not suitable for bypass surgery.

When vascular surgery is impossible, the following therapeutic options are available: 1) medical therapy (prostaglandins), 2) sympathectomy, and 3) spinal cord stimulation.

The therapeutic effects of prostaglandins are due to an increase in blood flow by relaxing the arterioles and precapillary sphincters and different rheological effects. Prostaglandins also improves the utilization of oxygen and glucose in ischemic tissue. A double-blind controlled and multicenter study evaluating the effects of prostaglandins on ischemic pain and ulcer healing in 152 patients with Buerger's disease, showed a significant difference in pain relief and ulcer healing in favor of the treatment with prostaglandins (11).

Sympathectomy, surgical or chemical, may lead to warming of the foot and some subjective improvement.

Spinal cord stimulation is a medically accepted therapeutic modality for the control of chronic pain (5, 13, 21, 23). It has been advocated as a method of pain relief for therapeutic refractory ischemic pain. Strikingly, in vascular patients not only pain relief could be achieved but also healing of ischemic ulcers. This suggests that spinal cord stimulation improves the nutritional skin blood flow. This was confirmed in recent studies.

The exact mechanisms underlying the effect of ESCS on ischemic pain and peripheral blood flow remain still uncertain. Presently the mechanisms proposed to be responsible for the modulation of ischemic pain are neurophysiological and neurohumoral in nature. The neurophysiology varies from simple blocking of impulse traffic in the spinothalamic tract, activation of supraspinal loops relayed via brainstem or thalamocortical system and activation of descending pain controlling pathways in the spinal cord. SCS might also induce the release of neurotransmitters involved in pain transmission (17, 18, 20, 24). The background for the therapeutic effects may als be an inhibition of sympathetically maintained peripheral vasoconstriction (19).

In the present study nine patients with Buerger's disease and non-reconstructible peripheral arterial occlusions were treated with PGE1 and spinal cord stimulation. Prostaglandin therapy was chosen as medical therapy and spinal cord stimulation as modality to treat the ischemic rest pain. The effects of this concept on ulcer healing and pain relief were studied. All patients received a standard wound care. The lesions healed quickly in five patients, three patients had limb survival after minor amputation. Only one major amputation was performed after 2 months of stimulation despite a good effect of the stimulation on the ischemic pain. The pain-relieving effect was stable and no patient complained of severe unbearable pain during the follow-up period.

SCS may have two inhibitory mechanisms to induce these improvements: 1) the inhibition of neuronal messages in the spinal cord, and 2) the inhibition of sympathetic vasoconstrictor neurons resulting in a relative vasodilation.

This study is not able to prove a limb-saving effect of spinal cord stimulation, since demonstration of such an effect requires a prospective randomized study.

It can be concluded that spinal cord stimulation is an effective method in the treatment of ischemic pain in patients with Buerger's disease. During follow-up, both ulcer healing and quality of life remained improved. Ulcer healing is most likely correlated to an increase in nutritional skin blood flow.

References

1. Augustinsson LE, Holm J, Carlsson CA et al. (1985) Epidural electrical stimulation in severe ischemia. Evidence of pain relief, increased blood flow and a possible limb saving effect. Ann Surg 202: 104–111
2. Broseta J, Barbera J, De Vera JA et al. (1986) Spinal cord stimulation in peripheral arterial disease. A cooperative study. J Neurosurg 64: 71–80
3. Cook AW, Oygar A, Baggenstos P et al. (1976) Vascular disease of the extremities: electrical stimulation of the spinal cord and the posterior roots. NY State J Med 76: 366–368
4. Dooley D, Kasprak M (1976) Modification of blood flow to the extremities by electrical stimulation of the nervous system. South Med J 69: 1309–11
5. Fiessinger J-N, Schäfer M (1990) Trial of Iloprost versus aspirin treatment for critical limb ischaemia of thromboangiitis obliterans. Lancet 335: 555–557
6. Fiume D (1983) Spinal cord stimulation in peripheral vascular pain. Appl Neurophysiol 46: 290–294
7. Franzeck UK, Talke P, Bernstein EF et al. (1982) Transcutaneous PO_2 measurements in health and peripheral arterial occlusive disease. Surgery 91: 156–163
8. Galley D, Elharrer C, Scheffer J et al. (1989) Neurostimulation et pathologie vasculaire: intéret thérapeutique a propos de 49 patients. Coeur 20: 35–44
9. Groth KE (1985) Spinal cord stimulation for the treatment of peripheral vascular disease. European multicenter study. In: Fields H (ed) Advances in Pain Research and Therapy. Raven Press, New York, pp 861–870
10. Hauser CL, Shoemaker WC (1983) Use of transcutaneous PO_2 regional perfusion index to quantify tissue perfusion in peripheral vascular disease. Ann Surg 197: 337–343
11. Hill GJ (1974) A rationale basis for the management of patients with Buerger's syndrome. r J Surg 61: 476–481
12. Horsch S, Claeys L (1994) Epidural spinal cord stimulation in the treatment of severe peripheral arterial occlusive disease. Annals of Vascular Surgery 8: 468–474
13. Hosobuchi Y (1990) Treatment of ischemic pain by neurostimulation. In: Lipton S, Tunks E, Zoppi M (eds) Advances in Pain Research and Therapy. Raven Press, New York, pp 223–226
14. Jacobs MJ, Jorning PJG, Beckers RCY et al. (1990) Foot salvage and improvement of microvascular blood flow as a result of epidural spinal cord stimulation. J Vasc Surg 212: 354–360
15. Jasczak P, Poulsen J (1983) Estimation of blood flow in transcutaneous PO_2 measurements. Acta Anaesthesiol Scand 27: 174
16. Linderoth B (1992) Dorsal column stimulation and pain: Experimental studies of putative neurochemical and neurophysiological mechanisms. Thesis, Stockholm, pp 11–19
17. Linderoth B, Stiller C-O, Gunasekera L et al. (1993) Release of neurotransmitters in the CNS by spinal cord stimulation: survey of present state of knowledge and recent experimental studies. Stereotactic Funct Neurosurg 61: 157–170
18. Linderoth B, Gazelius B, Franck J et al. (1992) Dorsal column stimulation induces release of serotonin and substance P in the cat dorsal horn. Neurosurgery 31: 289–297
19. Linderoth B, Herregodts P, Meyerson BA (1994) Sympathetic mediation of peripheral vasodilation induced by spinal cord stimulation: animal studies of the role of cholinergic and adrenergic receptor subtypes. Neurosurgery 35: 711–719
20. Linderoth B, Stiller C-O, Gunasekera L et al. (1994) Gamma-aminobutyric acid is released in the dorsal horn by electrical spinal cord stimulation: an in vivo microdialysis study in the rat. Neurosurgery 34: 484–489
21. Long DM, Erickson DE (1975) Stimulation of the posterior columns of the spinal cord for relief of intractable pain. Surg Neurol 4: 134–141
22. Matsen F, Wyss C, Pedegena L et al. (1980) Transcutaneous oxygen tension measurements in peripheral vascular disease. Surg Gynecol Obstet 150: 525–528
23. North RB (1993) The role of spinal cord stimulation in contemporary pain management. APS Journal 2: 91–99
24. Richardson DE, Dempesy CW (1984) Monoamine turnover in CSF of patients during dorsal column stimulation for pain control. Pain (Suppl 2): 224
25. Robaina FJ, Dominguez M, Diaz M et al. (1989) SCS for relief of chronic pain in vasospastic disorders of the upper limbs. Neurosurgery 24: 63–67

26. Shealy CN, Mortimer JT, Reswick JB (1978) Electrical inhibition of pain by stimulation of the dorsal columns: Preliminary clinical report. Anest Analg 46: 489–491
27. Shionoya S, Eastcott HHG (1992) Buerger's disease. In: Eastcott HHG (ed) Arterial Surgery. Churchill Livingstone, pp 153–173

Authors' address:
Prof. S. Horsch, MD PhD
Dept. of Vascular Surgery
Academic Teaching Hospital of the
University of Cologne
Urbacher Weg 19
D-51149 Köln
FRG

Spinal cord stimulation for upper extremity ischemic vascular disease

C. Bartels, L. Claeys, K. Ktenidis, S. Horsch

Department of Vascular Surgery, General Hospital Cologne-Porz,
Academic Teaching Hospital, University of Cologne, Cologne, Germany

Ischemic vascular disease of the upper extremity is less common than peripheral arterial vascular disease of the lower limbs. Peripheral vascular disease of the upper extremities as a result of severe generalized atherosclerotic disease or systemic vasospastic disorders presents a difficult therapeutic problem. In the presence of extensive distal atherosclerotic disease, arterial reconstruction is frequently impossible (14). Various vasospastic disorders may lead to severe ischemia of the upper extremity with distal necrosis and rest pain. Surgical treatment of these nonatherosclerotic lesions in the distal parts of the arterial tree is not feasible (15). Aggressive medical treatment has been the mainstay of treatment in these situations. However, medical treatment sometimes fails and tissue loss, dysfunctional limbs or major amputation may occur (15). The importance of the hand in daily living activities mandates aggressive therapeutic attempts.

Spinal cord stimulation (SCS) is an accepted therapeutic method for limb salvage, pain reduction, improvement of blood flow and healing of ulcers in severe peripheral arterial disease of the lower limbs (3, 5, 7, 8, 11, 12). Pain reduction and healing of otherwise therapy refractory ulcers has been observed in patients with different vasospastic diseases of the upper limbs treated by SCS (1, 10). The treatment of occlusive arterial disease of the upper extremity by SCS has never been evaluated. Therefore, the effect of SCS on limb salvage, pain reduction, transcutaneous oxygen tension ($TcpO_2$) and microcirculation in patients with severe vasospastic or peripheral occlusive arterial disease of the upper limbs was studied.

Methods

Patients

All patients required strong analgetics prior to implantation of the device; no vasoactive drugs were prescribed throughout the study period. Mean age of the patient cohort was 45 ± 17 years at time of implantation.

All patients with vasospastic disorders were female and refractory to conservative treatment, in all patients the right arm was more affected than the left one. Severe acrocyanosis was present in one young white female, primary Raynaud's syndrome was the underlying disease in another patient. Secondary Raynaud's syndrome occurred in two patients due to systemic lupus erythematosus, in one patient due to scleroderma, and in one patient due to mixed connective tissue disease. Irreversible necrosis of distal phalanges was present in two patients prior to treatment with SCS.

All but one patient suffered from rest pain. In two patients ischemia of the right arm was limb-threatening.

Peripheral arterial disease of the upper extremity was related to different underlying conditions; only male patients presented with arterial occlusive disease. In all patients the right upper extremity was the more afflicted site. One patient suffered from complete occlusion of all great arteries of the right arm due to a misdiagnosed thoracic outlet syndrome. This patient with a limb-threatening ischemia was referred to our institution for arterial reconstruction, however, reconstruction and concomitant thrombolytic therapy failed due to advanced irreversible distal arterial occlusion. In two other patients Winiwarter-Buerger's disease presents the underlying condition, both patients were still smoking more than 10 cigarettes per day. In one of these patients ischemia was limb-threatening; the other patient complained of severe rest pain. In another patient peripheral occlusive disease was due to a stab wound injury of the ulnar artery. Arterial reconstruction was not feasible in these cases.

Follow-up parameters

Parameters were assessed prior to implantation of the SCS device. After implantation the patient was controlled after the 1st week, the 1st month, the 3rd month, the 9th month, the 1st year and then at least every 12 months. All parameters were assessed after a rest period of at least 30 min in a supine position in a temperature-controlled room.

1) *Transcutaneous oxygen tension ($TcpO_2$)* was measured by the use of Clark's electrode (11). $TcpO_2$ measurements were performed at the dorsal site of both hands and at the chest wall to calculate $TcpO_2$ index (chest $TcpO_2$/hand $TcpO_2$).

2) *Pain intensity* was estimated from the patient's opinion of the degree of pain on a visual analogue scale (1 – 10; 1 = no pain) before implantation and during follow-up.

3) *Doppler wrist pressure index* was obtained (systemic systolic pressure/wrist pressure) by the use of a continous wave Doppler device (cw Doppler) and expressed in millimeters of mercury. Systemic systolic pressure was estimated from systolic pressure obtained by cw Doppler measurement of an unaffected extremity. The absence of arterial affliction of these unaffected extremities were validated by findings of cw-Doppler wave amplitude, B-scan and angiography.

4) *Microcirculation* was studied for nutritional capillary morphologic characteristics and capillary blood flow by means of intravital rest capillary microscopy at the distal phalanx of both hands. The technique of capillary microscopy has been described in detail elsewhere (6).

Dynamic capillaroscopy without dyes included the following parameters.

1) mean resting red blood cell velocity (rBCV, flying spot) (normal range: 0.55 – 0.7 mm/s) (13).

2) capillary density (normal range: 60 – 70/mm^2)

Classification of capillary morphology according to Fagrell was performed in patients with peripheral occlusive disease (4):

– Stage A: dot- or comma-shaped capillaries with good to decreased tonicity, occasional marked dilation or "micropools";
– Stage B: indistinct capillaries (e.g. edema, sclerosis) and/or capillary hemorrhages;
– Stage C: marked reduction of visible capillaries or no visible capillaries.

Results

The mean follow-up was 18.3 ±14 months. One patient with Winiwarter Buerger's disease died from lung cancer 12 months after implantation of SCS.

Pain reduction: Spinal cord stimulation induced excellent pain reduction immediately after implantation. During the follow-up period, pain intensity to a moderate degree reoccurred in two patients with secondary Raynaud's phenomenon due to intermittent aggravation of the underlying collagenosis. However, pain intensity was less severe than prior to SCS and after termination of these episodes complete pain reduction could be reachieved. In patients with arterial occlusive disease pain reduction was complete at rest and insignificant during exercise after treatment with SCS. Figure 1 depicts pain reduction of the study population.

Transcutaneous oxygen tension index: $TcpO_2$ index improved after SCS. The course of $TcpO_2$ index is shown in Fig. 2.

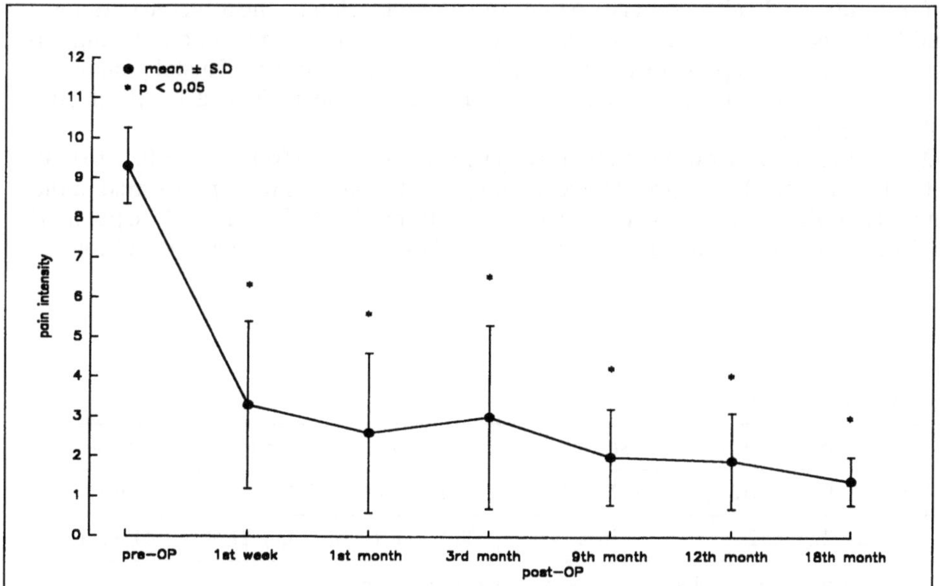

Fig. 1. Pain intensity

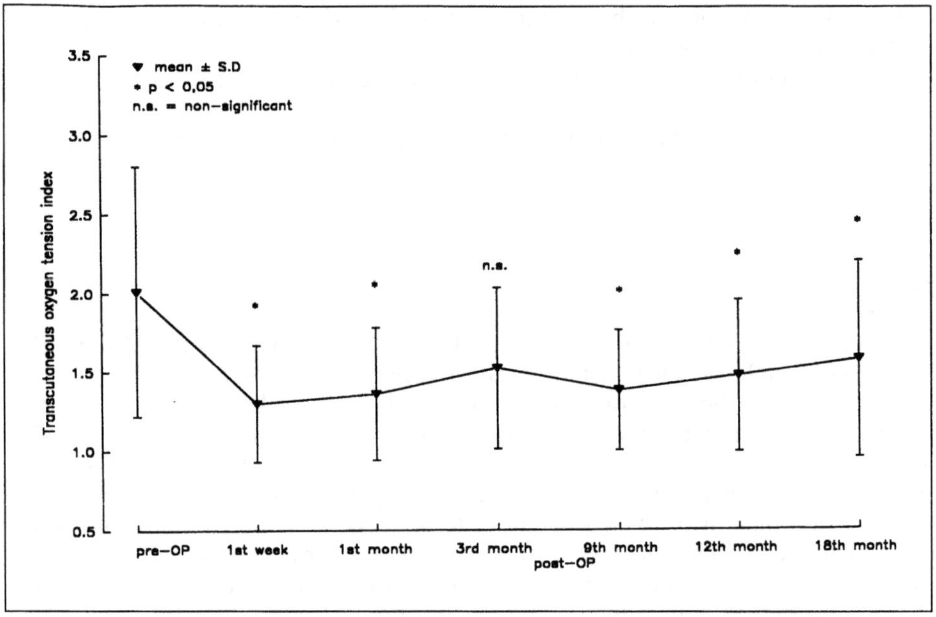

Fig. 2. Transcutaneous oxygen tension index

Doppler wrist pressure index remained unchanged throughout the follow-up period (0.8 – 1.0).

Limb-salvage: In all patients with limb-threatening ischemia the afflicted extremity could be preserved. Amputation was performed after clear demarcation of gangrenous areas on the two patients referred with preoperative necrosis of distal phalanges. Wound healing was primary in all cases. No further distal necrosis occurred during the follow-up period.

Microcirculation: Resting red blood cell velocity increased from 0.19 ± 0.12 to 0.46 ± 0.23 mm/s after 12 months. However, no provocation tests were performed in the studied population. Capillary density increased from 27.1 ± 12 to 41.3 ± 17.6 per mm^2 at 12-month follow-up. Results of dynamic capillaroscopy are summarized in Table 1.

Table 1: Dynamic capillaroscopy

	pre-operative	1st week	1st month	3rd month	1st year
rBCV	0.19 ± 0.12	0.26 ± 0.28	0.31 ± 0.14*	0.41 ± 0.21*	0.46 ± 0.23*
CD	27.1 ± 12	36 ± 14.6	38.5 ± 18.1	43 ± 21.5*	41.3 ± 17.6*

rBCV = mean resting red blood cell velocity (range 0.55 –0.7 mm/s);
CD = capillary density (range 60 – 70 per mm^2)
* = $p < 0.05$

In all patients with PAD capillary morphology was classified as Stage C according to Fagrell prior to stimulation (4). In one patient capillary morphology improved to such an extent that capillary morphology could be classified as Stage B after SCS. In the other cases amelioration was only minor and capillary morphology remained in Stage C throughout the follow-up.

Complications: Throughout the follow-up period spinal cord stimulation proved to be harmless, with no mortality and low morbidity. The latter centered around local infection of the lead in one patient and the break of the electrode in another patient. In the first patient the whole device was explanted and rest pain in the right hand reoccurred. In the other patient a new electrode was implanted without further complication.

Discussion

Severe ischemia of the upper extremity presents a therapeutic challenge to the vascular surgeon. If ischemia is related to more distal arterial occlusion or to vasospastic disease arterial reconstruction is frequently not feasible (14, 15). Our results demonstrate that even in cases with severe limb-threatening ischemia of the upper extremity treatment with spinal cord stimulation provides limb salvage and excellent pain reduction due to improved blood supply.

The use of SCS for treatment of vasospastic disease in a cohort of seven patients and in 37 patients with peripheral arterial disease of the lower limbs was studied by Augustinsson and co-workers (1). They found excellent pain relief in the patients with vasospastic disorders; the degree of pain relief in these patients was superior in comparison to patients with atherosclerotic vascular disorders of the lower limbs. However, the underlying immunologic disorder was not indicated and procedures examining the effect of thoracic SCS on blood supply were not performed. Robiana and co-workers studied the effect of SCS on pain relief, skin temperature, and peripheral blood flow in patients with primary Raynaud's disease and reflex sympathetic dystrophy (10). They experienced a good to excellent pain relief in 90 % of the patients. Increase of skin temperature and peripheral blood supply could be observed. The results of these two groups are in concordance with our findings, however, the degree of ischemia was minor in comparison to the present patient cohort, since no limb-threatening ischemia was studied by the other groups. In contrast to Augustinsson et al. pain reduction was more constant and more complete in patients with PAD of the arms in comparison to patients with vasospastic disease. However, the studied population was small and inhomogenous, and only patients with affection of the upper extremity were studied. Our results are the first to indicate that treatment with thoracic SCS can salvage upper limbs threatened by severe ischemia.

Currently no information concerning the treatment of peripheral arterial occlusive disease of the upper extremity by thoracic SCS is available. In most cases reconstructive surgery is feasible, however surgery may be impossible in some cases (14). More recently, arteriovenous reversal in six patients with arterial occlusive disease due to vasospastic and atherosclerotic disease of the upper limbs has been advocated with good results regarding limb salvage and pain relief (9). However, only two patients of this collective suffered from atherosclerotic disease, the remaining patients had an underlying vasospastic disease. In all patients with vasospastic disease a patent radial artery was present prior to arteriovenous reversal, this condition may explain the good surgical results. In the present study angiography of the patients with peripheral atherosclerotic disease revealed occluded major brachial arteries or major atherosclerotic changes. In two of these patients limb-threatening ischemia was present prior to SCS, in both cases the degree of ischemia deceased and rest pain disappeared. Our results demonstrate that even in cases with severe PAD of the upper limbs SCS provides a therapeutic method for limb salvage, pain reduction and increase of blood supply.

Tallis et al. demonstrated an increase of skin and muscle blood flow after SCS of the lower limbs by the use of radioactive tracers (12). Most clinical studies use the measurement of $TcpO_2$ for determination of skin blood flow, as $TcpO_2$ seems to be a reliable noninvasive index of tissue perfusion (5, 11). Since the skin $TcpO_2$ reflects systemic changes, e.g. pulmonary gas exchange, cardiac output a $TcpO_2$ index (chest $TcpO_2$/hand $TcpO_2$) was used (2). Fiume et al. and Sciacca et al. observed a significant increase of $TcpO_2$ in patients with PAD of the legs (5, 11). In concordance with these groups $TcpO_2$ increased significantly in the present investigation and paralleled the decrease in pain.

A reduction of capillary density has been observed in cases of secondary Raynaud's syndrome and acrocyanosis, however, capillary density is within normal limits in patients with primary Raynaud's phenomenon, though abnormal giant capillaries may be detected (6). In the same study decreased red blood cell velocity in patients with various vasospastic disorders has been described. Improvement of dynamic microcirculatory parameters after treatment with SCS has been observed by Jacobs et al. in patients with PAD of the lower limbs (7). In the present study rBCV and CD increased significantly, however these findings should be interpreted with caution. The first restricting factor is a small and inhomogeneous patient group: capillary morphology varies according to the underlying disease, vasospastic or arterial occlusive orign. Secondly no provocation tests were performed in these patients for ethical reasons and microcirculation at rest may be different from that at provocation status. As expected, no significant changes were observed in the patients with arterial occlusive disease concerning the classification of Fagrell, however, minor improvement was noted in two patients. Further studies with a larger and more homogeneous patient collective are warranted to study the effect of SCS on dynamic and qualitative capillary microscopic parameters.

The conclusions from this study are as follows:

1) SCS of the upper limbs is associated with low morbidity and no mortality.

2) Salvage of upper limbs can be achieved with the use of SCS.

3) SCS reduces the degree of pain by increasing the blood supply in patients with severe vasospastic or peripheral arterial disease.

4) SCS provides a successful way of treatment for refractory VD and PAD of the upper extremity.

References

1. Augustinsson LE, Holm J, Carlsson AC, Jivegard L (1985) Epidural electrical stimulation in severe limb ischemia. Evidence of pain relief, increased blood flow and a possible limb-saving effect. Ann Surg 202: 104–111
2. Blankensteijn JD, Abbott WM (1994) Evaluation of the skin microcirculation by photoplethysmography, laser Doppler velocimetry, and transcutaneous measurement of pO2. In: Horsch S, Claeys L (eds) Spinal Cord Stimulation. Steinkopff, Darmstadt, Berlin Heidelberg New York London Paris, pp 125–133
3. Claeys L, Ktenidis K, Horsch S (1994) Transcutaneous oxygen tension in patients with critical limb ischemia treated by spinal cord stimulation. In: Horsch S, Claeys L (eds) Spinal Cord Stimulation. Steinkopff, Darmstadt Berlin Heidelberg New York London Paris, pp 145–152
4. Fagrell B (1990) Techniques and normal findings. In: Bollinger A, Fagrell B (eds) Clinical Capillaroscopy. Hogrefe and Huber, Toronto New York, pp 1–9
5. Fiume D, Palombi M, Sciacca V, Tamorri M (1989) Spinal Cord Stimulation in peripheral ischemic pain. Pace 12: 698–704
6. Jacobs MJHM, Breslau PJ, Slaaf DW, Reneman RS, Lemmens HAJ (1987) Nomenclature of Raynaud's phenomenon. A capillary microscopic and hemorheologic study. Surgery 101: 136–145
7. Jacobs MJHM, Jörning PJG, Beckers RJG, Ubbink DT, van Kleef M, Slaaf DW, Reneman RS (1990) Foot salvage and improvement of microvascular blood flow as a result of epidural spinal cord electrical stimulation. J Vasc Surg 12: 354-360
8. Jacobs MJHM, Jörning PJG, Joshi SR, Kitslaar PJEHM, Slaaf DW, Reneman RS (1988) Epidural spinal cord electrical stimulation improves microvascular blood flow in severe limb ischemia. Ann Surg 207: 179–183
9. King TA, Marks J, Berrettoni BA, Seitz WH (1993) Arteriovenous reversal for limb salvage in unreconstructable upper extremity arterial occlusive disease. J Vasc Surg 17: 924–933
10. Robaina FJ, Dominguez M, Diaz M, Rodriguez JL, de Vera JA (1989) Spinal Cord Stimulation for relief of chronic pain in vasospastic disorders of the upper limbs. Neurosurgery 24: 63–67
11. Sciacca V, Mingoli A, Di Marzo L, Maggiore c, Fiume D, Cavallaro A (1989) Predictive value of transcutaneous oxygen tension measurement in the indication for Spinal Cord Stimulation in patients with peripheral vascular disease: preliminary results. Vasc Surg 23: 128–132
12. Tallis RC, Illis LS, Sedgwick EM, Hardwidge C, Garfield JS (1983) Spinal Cord Stimulation in peripheral vascular disease. J Neurol Neurosurg Psychiatry 46: 478–484
13. Tyml K, Ellis CG (1982) Evaluation of the flying spot technique as a television method for measuring red cell velocities in microvessels. Int J Micocirc Clin Exp 1: 145–155
14. Whitehouse WM (1984) Direct revascularisation for forearm and hand ischemia. In: Bergan JJ, Yao JST (eds) Evaluation and Treatment of Upper and Lower Extremity Circulatory Disorders. Grune and Stratton, New York
15. Yao JST, McDaniel MD, King TA (1984) Arterial surgery of the upper extremity. In: Bergan JJ (ed) Clinical Surgery International: Arterial Surgery. Churchill Livingstone, London, pp 201–224

Author's address:
C. Bartels, MD
General Hospital Cologne-Porz
Academic Teaching Hospital University of Cologne
Department of Vascular Surgery
Urbacher Weg 19
D-51149 Cologne
FRG

Mapping of sensory electrical responses to epidural spinal cord stimulation

G. Barolat

Thomas Jefferson University, Philadelphia, Pa, USA

Electrical stimulation of the spinal cord for therapeutic purpose has been performed since the early 1970s with variable success. More recently the application of spinal cord stimulation to treat ischemic peripheral vascular disease has been popularized in Europe. Exact electrode positioning in the spinal canal is a key factor in providing successful stimulation (4). Unfortunately, there are no published guidelines to intraspinal electrode(s) placement backed by a substantial number of observations in a large number of patients. This contrasts with the detailed observations obtained systematically, for instance, during stereotactic procedures in the deep brain structures. Our efforts have been directed in developing a database of responses to electrical stimulation of the neural intraspinal structures at various spine levels (2, 3, 5–8). All the testing and data collection was performed by professionals working full time in our neuroimplant program and with standardized electrical parameters. This minimized deviations from the protocol and assured a high degree of uniformity and reliability in the data.

For data collection the body surface was divided into 108 areas (Fig. 1). For data analysis some of the areas were merged to reduce the total to 20 areas. The latter correspond to the main parts of the body to which pain is usually referred to in the clinical setting.

Our data refer not to single electrode arrays, but to the individual contacts within the arrays. This results from the fact that with multi-contact electrodes the range of the contacts spans over more than one spinal level . The position of the electrode array does not therefore allow precise identification of the stimulated area. Only unipolar and bipolar combinations were analyzed, even though tri-, and quadri-polar combinations were also tested when indicated. In this report only the position of the contacts when they functioned as cathodes was studied; this is because the cathodal current is the prevalent factor in affecting the flow of the stimulation. As demonstrated in our previous work, anodal current has a much smaller, although not insignificant role (1).

A total of 3897 electrical combinations were collected and analyzed, 738 belonged to the cervical and 3159 to the thoracic / L1 area; 3000 combinations were bipolar and 159 were unipolar.

Our database contains data for electrodes implanted at all spine levels between C1–2 and L1. The data analysis reported in the work refers to 3549 combinations, of which 738 were from contacts located between C1 and C6 and 2811 between T6 and L1.

The level of the electrode contacts of each combination was derived from plain spine x-rays. The antero-posterior projection was found to be the most accurate for thoracic electrodes. For the cervical spine, instead, we relied on the lateral view. CT scan and plain x-ray analyses allowed to assess the position of the cathodes in the spinal canal in a medio-lateral direction. The distance from the radiological midline to the center of the contact was measured with the appropriate correction for magnification. The contacts were divided into two groups: the ones located within 3 mm from the radiological midline (classified as "midline"), and the ones located more than 3 mm from it (classified as "lateral").

To obtain a map that links the cathode positions on the spinal cord to the body surface areas where paresthesiae could be perceived, we devised a formula to measure

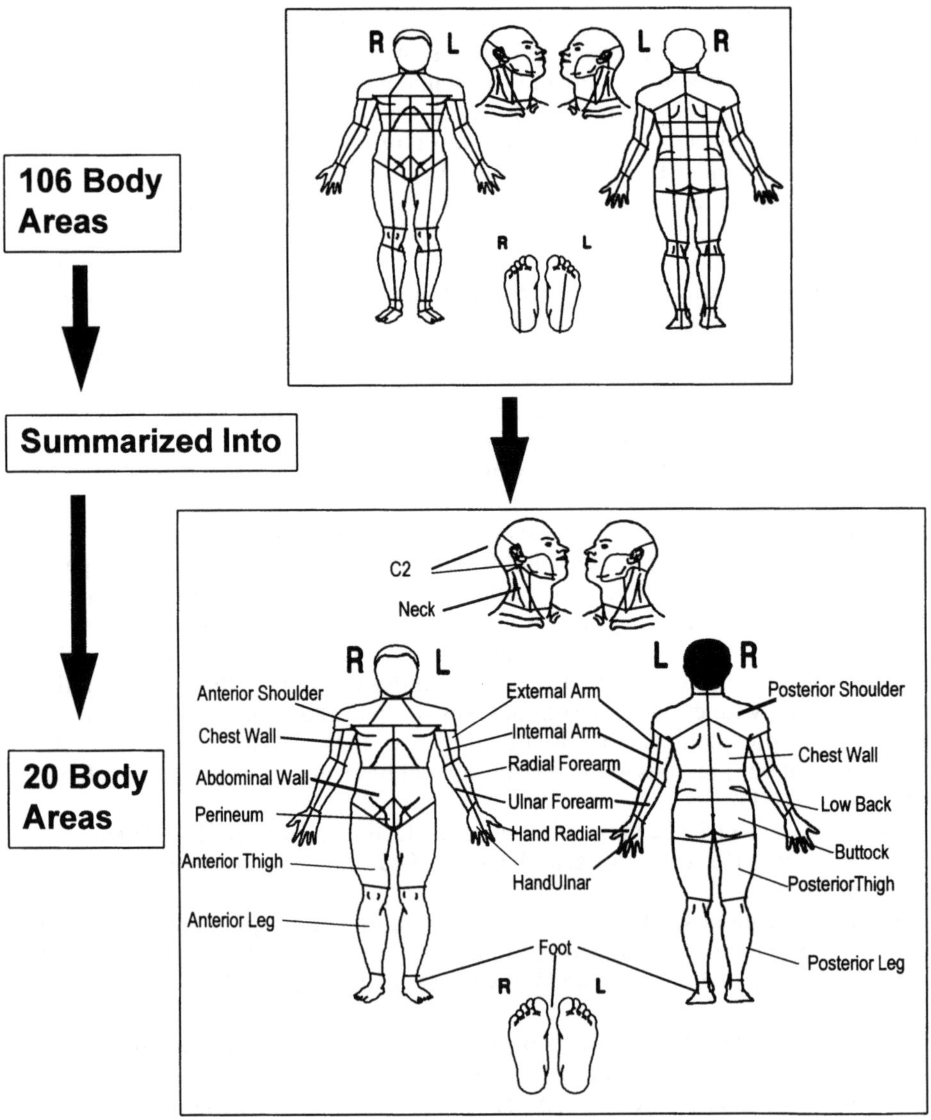

Fig. 1.

the effectiveness of eliciting sensation in various body parts by positioning the cathode on a specific spinal level. The formula was: { (number of combinations at the spine level eliciting paresthesiae in the designated body area X 100) / total number of combinations at the spine level.} The following example demonstrates how the formula works. Suppose there are 82 combinations tested with cathode position at C6. If 36 elicited stimulation in the lateral arm, then the effectiveness is 36 x 100 divided by 82 = 43.9 %. Each cathode stimulates multiple areas of the body. If 60 combinations also triggered paresthesiae in the hand, we can conclude that with cathode on C6 there is a 73.2 % effective rate of stimulation to hand and a 43.9 % effective rate of stimulation to lateral arm.

Data (Figs. 2 and 3)

Most of the data are shown in the illustrations. The discussion here will be limited to the most pertinent observations.

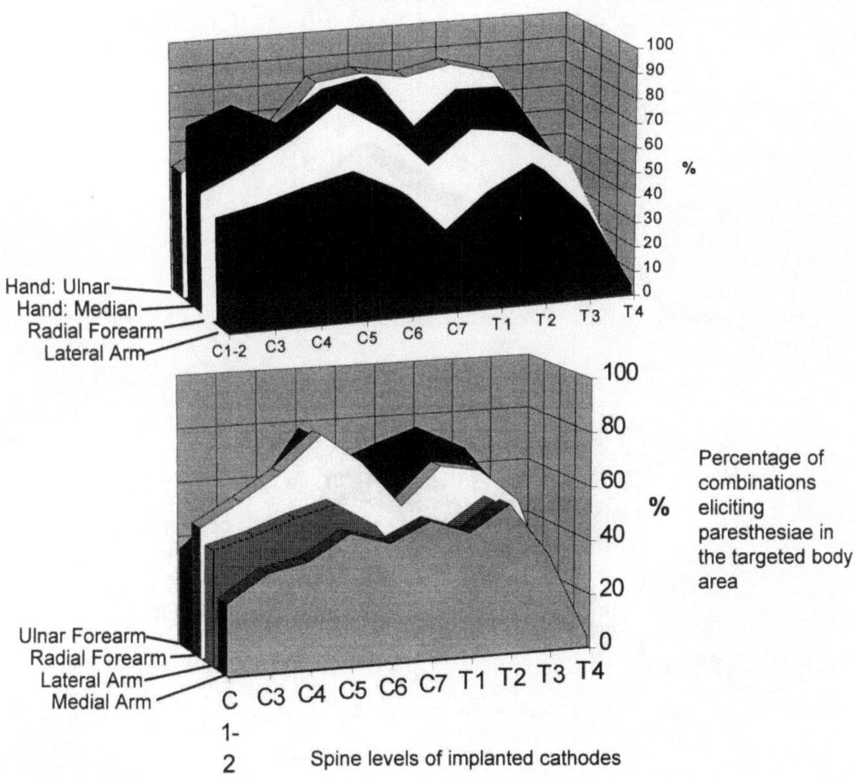

Fig. 2. Distribution of paresthesiae according to the various body areas

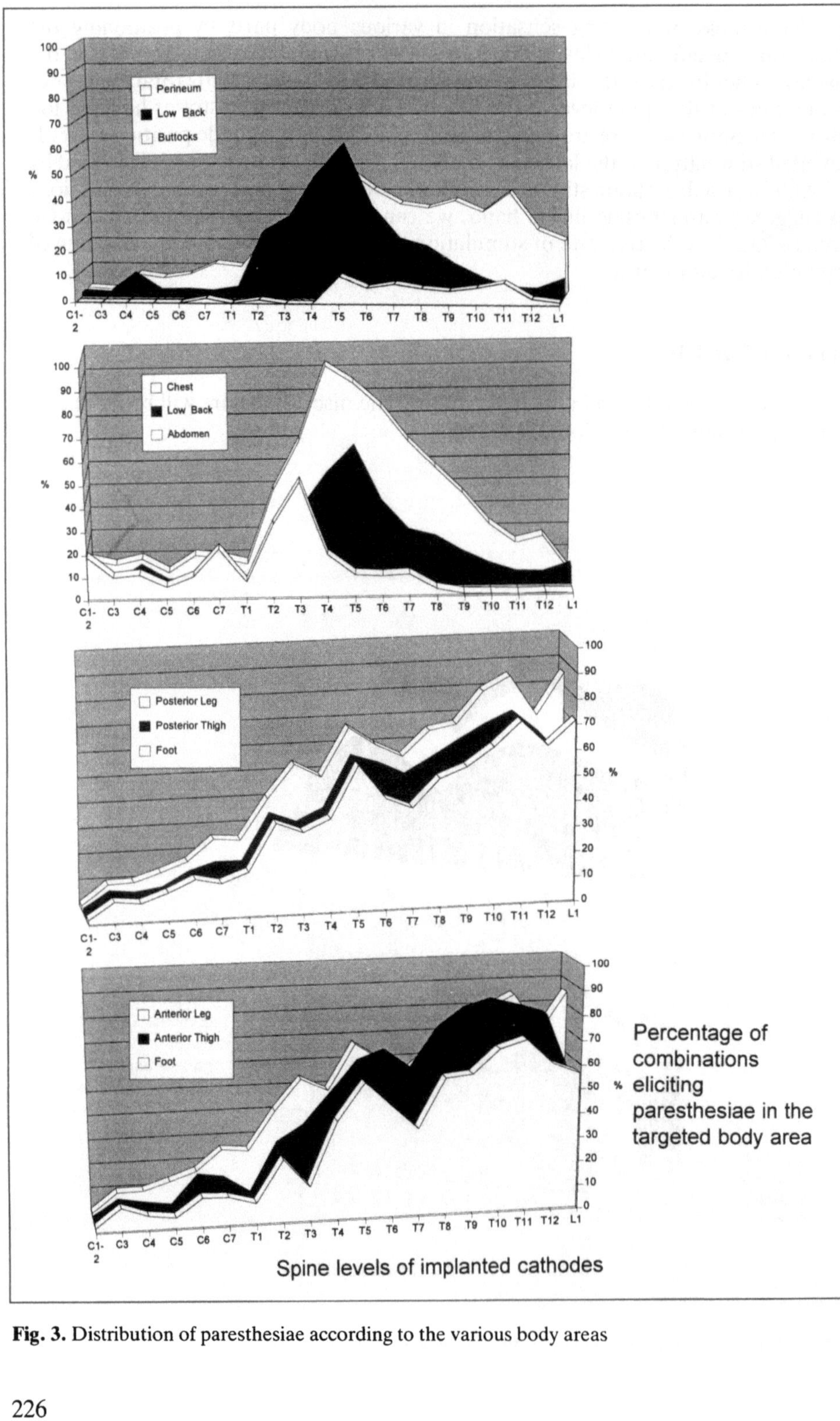

Fig. 3. Distribution of paresthesiae according to the various body areas

C2 area

The C2 distribution covers the ipsilateral posterior occipital area and the angle of the jaw. The C2 contribution to the angle of the jaw and the mandible is variable. In some individuals it covers only a small portion of the angle of the jaw; in others it covers a large portion of the mandible almost reaching midline. It never overlaps significantly with the V2 distribution. Paresthesiae in the C2 distribution are obtained with the electrode placed either under the arch of C1 or under the lamina of C2. The electrode has to be placed slightly off midline on the affected side. An excessively lateral placement stimulates the nerve root and generates undesirable motor contractions. In our experience the best arrangement to obtain paresthesiae in the C2 distribution is to have two electrodes side by side at C1–2, one in midline and one about 3 mm off midline. The preferred direction of current is between two adjacent contacts, with the cathode belonging to the laterally placed electrode. Other electrode arrangements might not yield as consistent a stimulation in the C2 distribution; this explains why in our database only a small percentage of combinations located at C1–2 stimulate the C2 area.

Neck

Neck stimulation is fairly difficult to obtain. The cathode must not be below C3. Optimal stimulation is usually obtained at the C1–2 spine levels. No major differences were found between midline or lateral contacts.

Shoulder

To stimulate the shoulder the cathode has to be at the C2–3–4 level. Below the C4 level shoulder stimulation is found erratically and the coverage is usually not satisfactory. Even with proper placement shoulder stimulation is not obtained as consistently as other areas such as the hand.

Hand

Stimulation of the median aspect of the hand is elicited from the large percentage of combinations with electrodes placed in the cervical area, irrespective of the level. We have observed combinations with cathodes at C1 giving rise to paresthesiae felt uniquely in the ipsilateral thumb. The ulnar side of the hand is not stimulated as consistently, and is often stimulated concurrently with the median side. To obtain complete coverage of the hand the electrode should be optimally placed at C5–6.

Chest / abdominal wall

Stimulation of the chest/abdominal wall is, in most instances, viewed as an undesirable side-effect of stimulation directed to other parts of the body, most frequently the low back. Chest wall stimulation is often perceived as an unpleasant constrictive band. Both sensory and motor activation are often obtained at the same threshold; this prevents the stimulation from obtaining any therapeutic effect. Stimulation of the chest/abdominal wall, unfortunately, is a prominent feature of stimulation through electrodes placed in the thoracic spine. Strict midline placement can minimize but not eliminate it. Even with a perfect midline electrode placement, in time chest/abdominal wall stimulation might become the most prominent feature, even if not so at the time of implantation. From our database, however, a larger percentage of contacts stimulating the chest/abdominal wall were located laterally.

Anterior thigh

Stimulation of this area is very frequently achieved with electrodes placed at the T11–12 spine level, especially if located slightly laterally. This type of stimulation could be attributed, in some instances, to direct stimulation of the dorsal L1–2–3 dorsal roots as they are laterally grouped in the spinal canal at that level. Anterior thigh stimulation due exclusively to activation of the dorsal column fibers can be obtained with electrodes placed at T7–8 or higher. In this case, however, other parts of the lower extremity are also simultaneously stimulated.

Posterior Thigh

Selective stimulation of the posterior thigh can be accomplished with electrodes placed at the T11–L1 level. In this instance stimulation is most likely due to activation of the S1 dorsal root fibers , which constitute a large, medially located bundle, or of the S1 dorsal root entry zone (DREZ), which is located at the L1 spine level in most individuals. A larger percentage of contacts eliciting these responses were located in midline. This parallels the trends for the buttock and the posterior leg and confirms the fact that the stimulation in this instance is most likely due to activation of the DREZ or dorsal root.

Foot

The foot is one of the areas that displays the highest likelihood of being covered by stimulation-induced paresthesiae. An electrode in the lower thoracic-upper lumbar area has over a 70 % chance of stimulating the foot fibers. This reaches almost 100 % when the cathode is at the L1 spine level. Foot fibers can also be stimulated from higher spine levels. We have seen several instances of perfectly midline placed cervical electrodes where the stimulation was initially felt in the bottom of the feet. Complete coverage of the foot, however, cannot always be obtained. Foot stimulation obtained from an L1 placed electrode might be more selectively perceived in the sole of the foot and not in the ankle. Further data are necessary to allow for a more accurate prediction of electrode placement.

Perineum

This area is very difficult to stimulate. Only a very small percentage of combinations elicit paresthesiae in the perineum/genitalia. Most of them come from electrodes located at T11–12–L1. To enhance the possibilities of stimulating this area, the electrodes have to be located in midline. Stimulation is also often simultaneously perceived in the anterior thigh area. Of the combinations that elicited paresthesiae in the perineum, a strikingly larger percentage was located in midline.

Low back

The low back area is very difficult to stimulate without intervening chest or abdominal wall stimulation. By overlapping the stimulation curves pertaining to the above structures, the following factors can be identified: a) the peak curve for low back stimulation coincides with the peak curve for the chest/abdominal wall; b) the chest

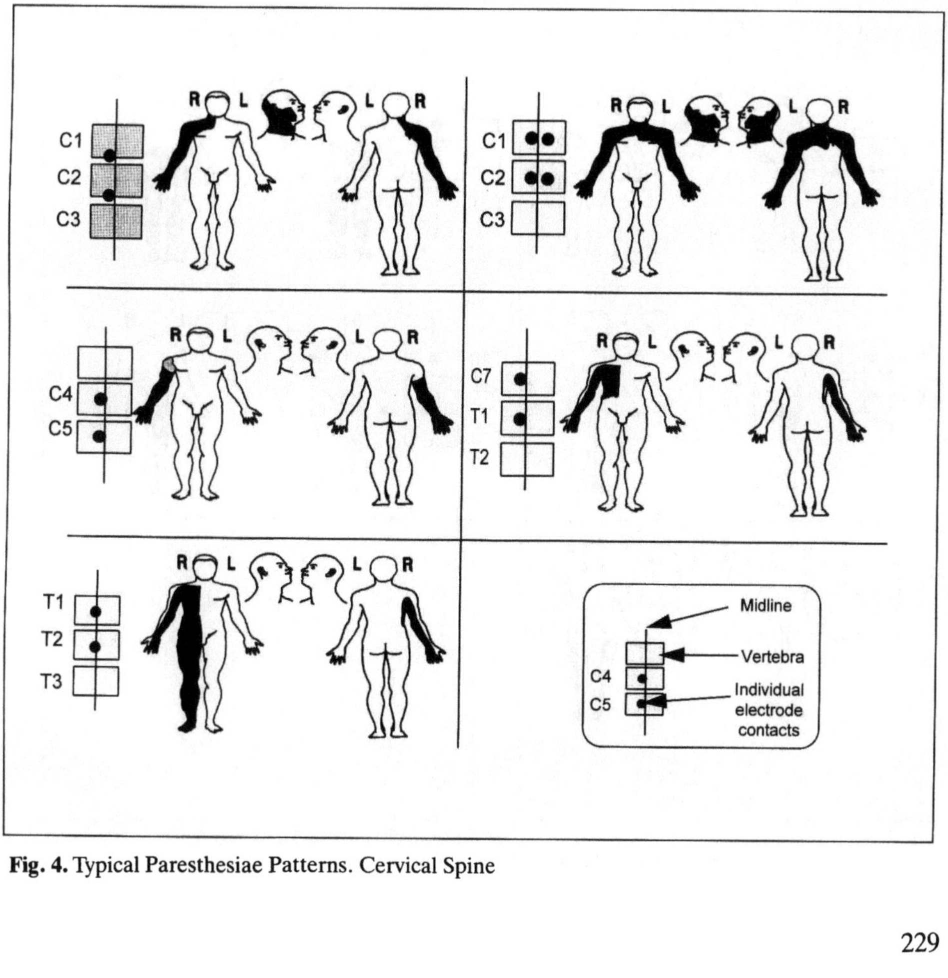

Fig. 4. Typical Paresthesiae Patterns. Cervical Spine

and abdominal wall have a higher possibility of being stimulated than the low back; c) the chest/abdominal wall has a lower stimulation threshold than the low back. All these factors contribute to the challenge of being able to direct stimulation selectively to the low back without interference from the body walls. In our experience the best location is at about T9–10 with an electrode placed strictly in midline. New electrode configurations are being developed which might allow a more exclusive activation the low back fibers.

Buttock

The buttock area can be activated more easily than the low back. This is most likely due to the fact that peak level for the buttock is located more caudally in the spine than the peak for the abdominal wall which therefore does not interfere with it. The buttock area still has a substantial representation at T11–T12–L1. The usual pattern

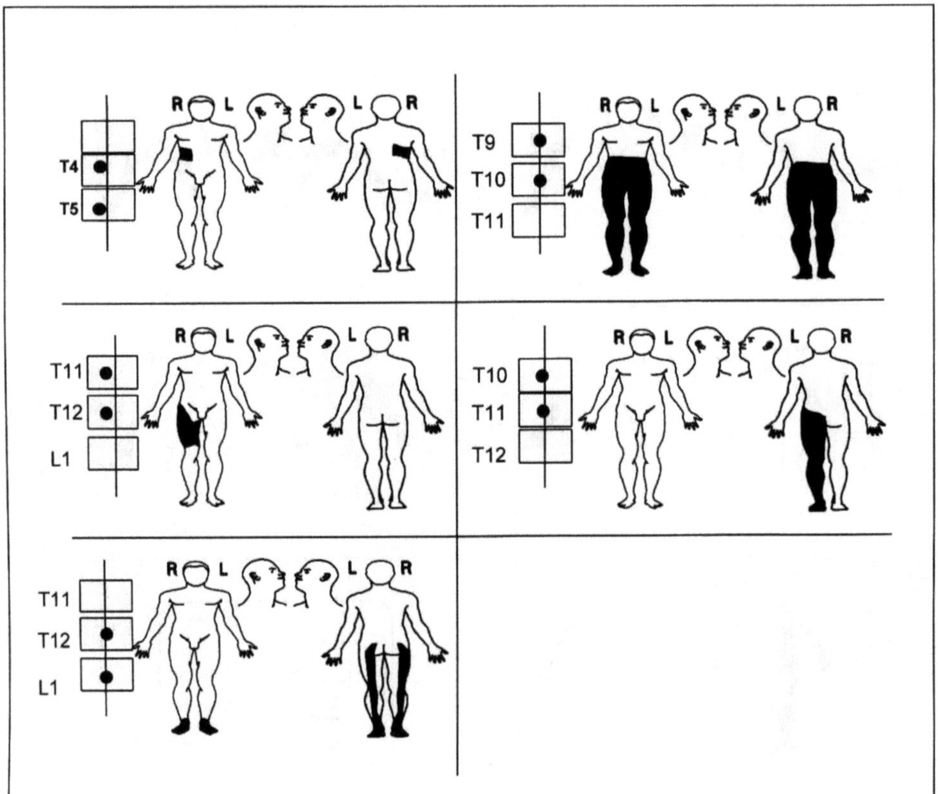

Fig. 5. Typical Paresthesiae Patterns. Thoraco-Upper Lumbar Spine

observed with an electrode at T11–T12 is that one activates first the posterior leg fibers, then the posterior thigh and last the buttock. We have never encountered isolated stimulation of the buttock area without prior involvement of the posterior aspect of the lower extremity. Following activation of the buttock area if the electrode is high enough in the spine, stimulation spreads to the low back.

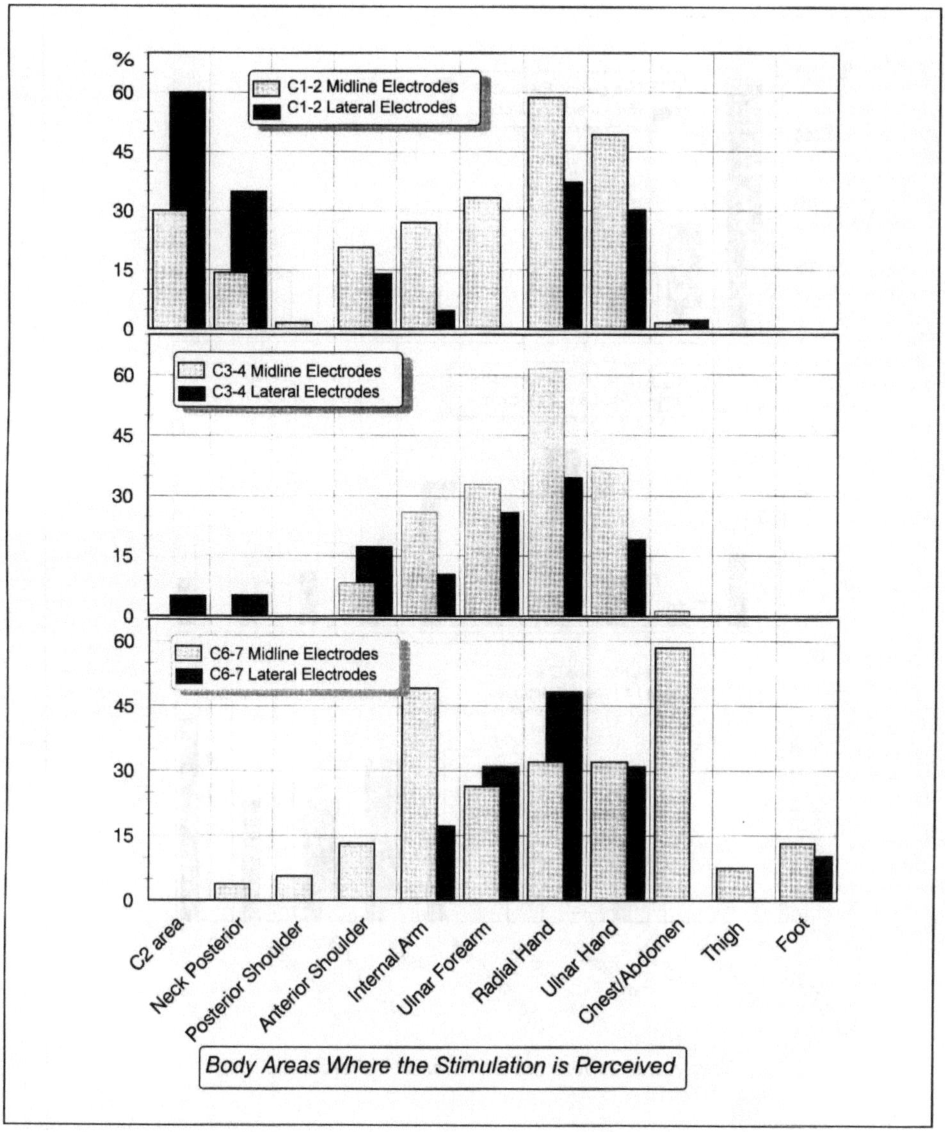

Fig. 6. Distribution of paresthesiae from spinal cord stimulation of perception threshold

The data can be analyzed in a different way, looking at the various spine levels where the electrodes are implanted and assessing which body parts receive sensory stimulation according to those levels. These data are presented in Figs. 4–7. The upper cervical area is the main target when the pain is in the C2 distribution, the neck and the upper extremity. The mid-cervical area is implanted when the pain is mostly in

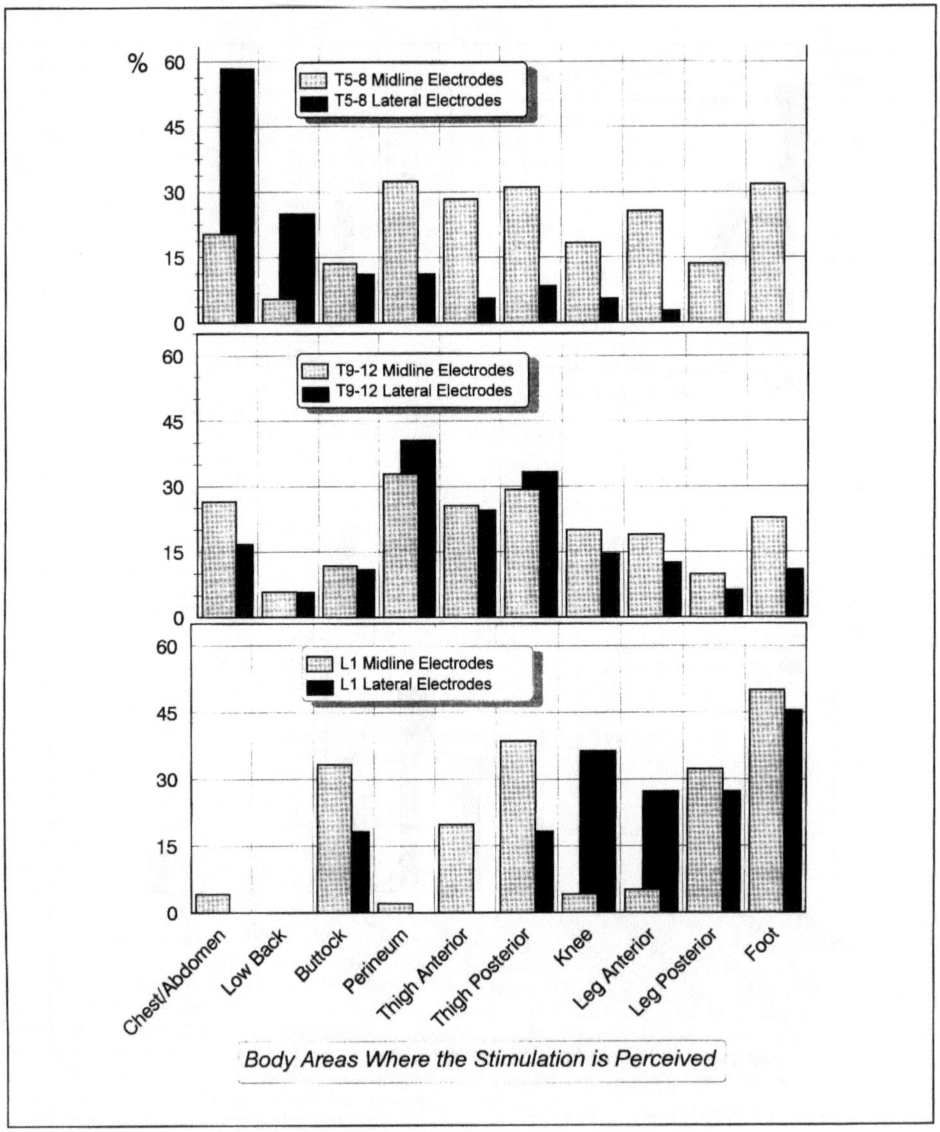

Fig. 7. Distribution of paresthesiae from spinal cord stimulation of perception threshold

the arm/forearm and the hand. When the area to be covered includes the ulnar distribution of the upper extremity and the upper chest/axilla area, the site of implant is at C7–T1. Pain in the chest wall distribution commands a placement slightly caudal to the pain area with electrodes located on the side of the pain. A low thoracic placement at T9–10 is optimal to obtain stimulation in the lower lumbar area and both lower extremities. A slightly lateral placement at T11–12 will give rise to stimulation in the anterior thigh area, whereas a midline placement at the same level will generate paresthesiae exactly in the S1 distribution. At the L1 level most of the stimulation goes to the foot.

It is possible that with different electrodes arrangements, inter-contact distance and different electrical parameters, the paresthesiae distribution can be modified in a more discrete fashion. This might allow us in the future to more precisely direct the current flow and more consistently stimulate the desired body areas.

References

1. Barolat G, Zeme S, Ketcik B (1991) Multifactorial Analysis of Epidural Spinal Cord Stimulation. Stereotactic and Functional Neurosurg 56: 77–103
2. Barolat G et al. (1993) Mapping of sensory responses to epidural stimulation of the intraspinal neural structures in man. J Neurosurg 78: 233–239
3. He J, Barolat G, Strujk J, Holsheimer J (1994) Perception threshold and electrode position for spinal cord stimulation. Pain, In press
4. Law JD, Miller LV (1982) Importance of documentation of an epidural stimulating position. Appl Neurophisiol 45: 461–464
5. Strujk J,Holsheimer J, Barolat G, He J (1993) Paresthesia threshold in spinal cord stimulation: a comparison of theoretical results with clinical data. IEEE Transactions on Rehabilitation Engineering 1: 101–108
6. Tulgar M, Barolat G, Ketcik B (1994) Analysis of parameters for epidural spinal cord stimulation. 1. Perception and tolerance thresholds resulting from 1,100 combinations. Stereotactic and Functional Neurosurg 61: 129–139
7. Tulgar M, Barolat G, Ketcik B (1994) Analysis of parameters for epidural spinal cord stimulation. 2. Usange ranges resulting from 3,000 combinations Stereotactic and Functional Neurosurg 61: 140–145
8. Tulgar M, He J, Barolat G, Ketcik B, Strujk H, Holsheimer J (1994) Analysis of parameters for epidural spinal cord stimulation. 3. Topographical distribution of paresthesiae Stereotactic and Functional Neurosurg 61: 146–155

Author's address:
Prof. Giancarlo Barolat, MD
Division of Functional Neurosurgery
Thomas Jefferson University
1015 Chestnut Street, Suite 1400
Philadelphia, Pa 19107
USA

Epidural spinal cord electrical stimulation (ESES) effect on penile flow: an experimental study

V. Sciacca[1], G. Mattioli[2], P. Oppido[2], G. Di Giugno[2]

[1] Dept. of Surgery, University "La Sapienza", Rome, Italy
[2] Dept. of Neurological Sciences, University "La Sapienza", Rome, Italy

Introduction

Epidural spinal cord electrical stimulation (ESES), introduced for the control of chronic pain of different ethiologies (10, 14) represents an alternative method of treating patients with critical limb ischaemia (CLI) neither amenable to vascular reconstructions nor responsive to medical treatment (2, 3, 6, 8, 13). The good results achieved in limb salvage (1, 7) are related mainly to combined effect of ESES on pain (control) and microcirculation (improvement) through several mechanisms of action centrally and peripherically (segmentary) mediated (4, 9).

The anectodal reports of full erection in elderly patients treated with ESES for lower limb arterial insufficiency and the old experimental experience of penile erection in dogs, caused by electrical stimulation of visceral (parasympathetic) nervous branches from the sacral spinal cord (5), stimulated us to investigate penile blood flow during epidural electrical stimulation in rabbits.

Material and methods

Seven New Zealand rabbits (mean body weight 2.5 Kgs), under general anesthesia after endotracheal intubation in mechanical ventilation, were submitted to L6–7 laminectomy. A monopolar Itrel (Medtronic, Minneapolis, Min., USA) electrode was inserted and advanced proximally to L1–2 level. Electrical activity of the periacqueduct central gray matter (CGM) was recorded through stereotaxic electrode implantation. A laser-Doppler implantable probe (TSI, St. Paul, Min., USA) was infixed in the penis (cavernous body) to evaluate flow modifications (PLDF) during ESES.

Electroencephalogram (EEG), electrocardiogram (EKG), intracranial pressure (ICP), and arterial blood pressure (BP) were monitored. The ESES and CGM electrodes were connected to an external stimulator with the following impulse parameters: frequency 85 pps, width 85 μs, voltage 4–6.5 V.

Results

The ESES caused a significant PLDF increase (Figs. 1, 2) evident only during stimulation with low voltage (4 and 5 volts), but longlasting (ca. 15 s) with higher voltage

Research partially supported by MURST CAP. 05150111 "Stimolazione midollare ed arteriopatie periferiche"

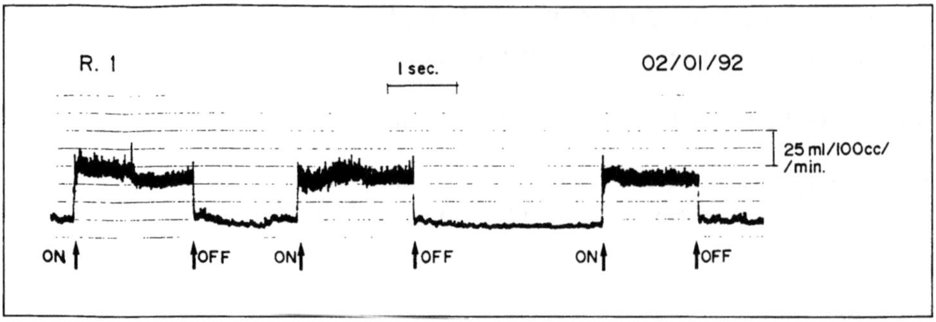

Fig. 1. Penile laser-Doppler flow modification during ESES with 4.5 V impulse.

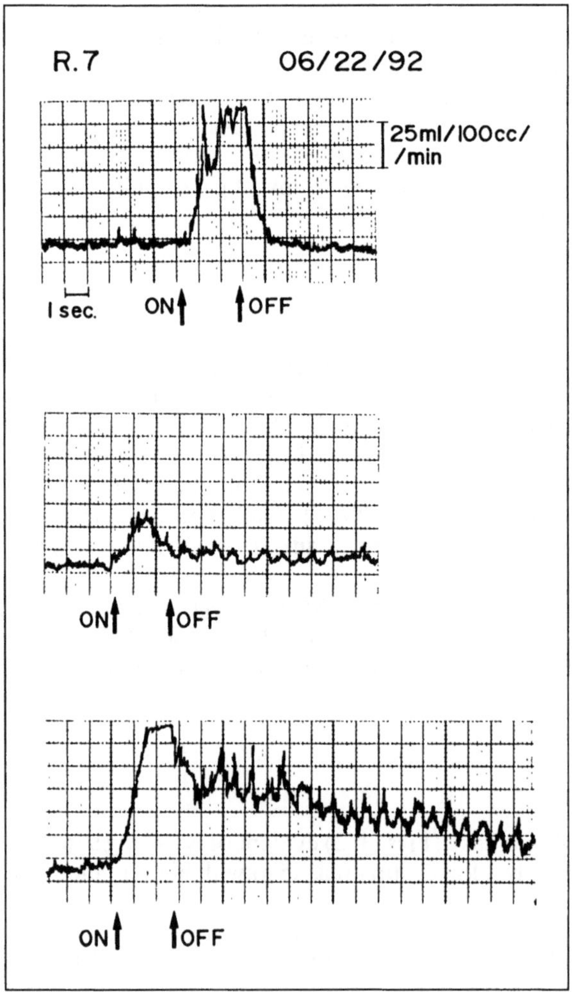

Fig. 2. Penile laser-Doppler flow modifications with different voltages: at top 4 V, middle 5 V, bottom 6.5 V. Notice the long-lasting effect on PLDF with higher voltage.

stimulation (6.5 volts). The CGM electrical activity amplitude increased while EEG was partially desynchronized during ESES (Fig. 3), with simultaneous rapid increase of ICP (Fig. 4). Likewise, direct CGM electrical stimulation caused an increase of PLDF (Fig. 5). Neither bradycardia nor moderate arterial hypertension, caused by ESES, influenced PLDF.

Discussion

This experimental model, previously utilized for the study of heart-brain relationship to ascertain the role of the central nervous system in sudden cardiac death (12), had been applied here to evaluate the ESES effect on penile microcirculation and realize the causes of spontaneous erection reported by some elderly patients submitted to ESES for critical limb ischemia.

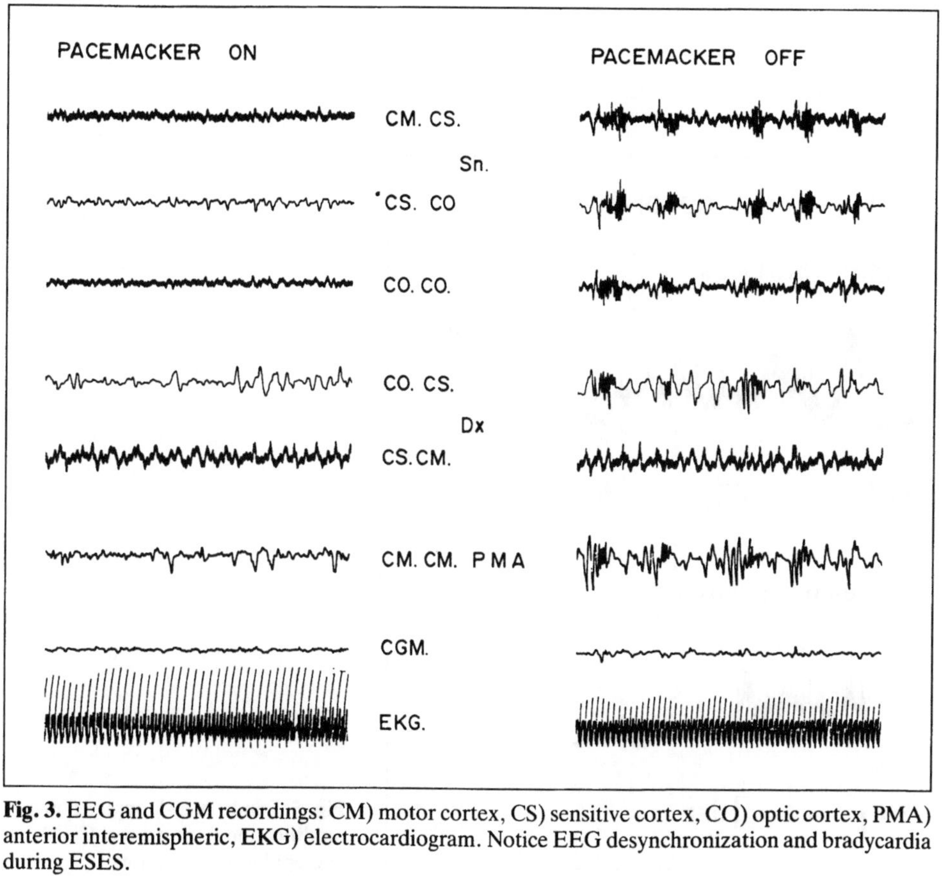

Fig. 3. EEG and CGM recordings: CM) motor cortex, CS) sensitive cortex, CO) optic cortex, PMA) anterior interemispheric, EKG) electrocardiogram. Notice EEG desynchronization and bradycardia during ESES.

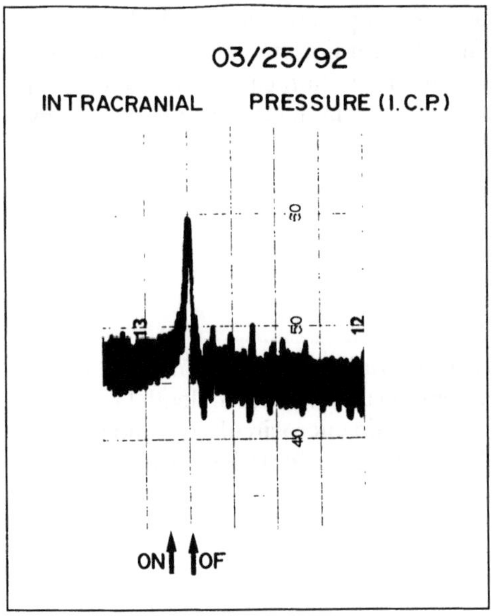

Fig. 4. Modification of intracranial pressure during ESES.

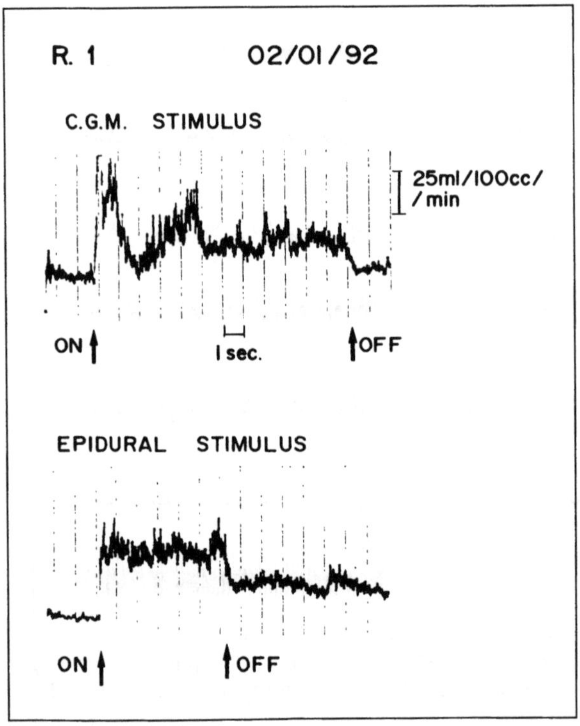

Fig. 5. Penile laser-Doppler flow modification during direct CGM and epidural stimulation.

Although the ESES demonstrated the ability to increase PLDF, the penile erection is a complex physiologic response that is dependent upon the integration of vascular, endocrine, and neurologic mechanisms. Many aspects of neurohumoral control of erection are still uncertain, but it is clear that psychogenic and reflexogenic stimuli are produced by a neurally mediated vasodilation of the penile blood vessels leading to the increase in blood flow and distension of the cavernous tissue (11, 15).

Various levels of the central nervous system and three sets of peripheral nerves (thoracolumbar sympathetic, sacral parasympathetic, and sacral somatic) have a role in erectile function. The neuromodulation effect of ESES may influence both central and peripheral nervous centers involved in erection. In this experimental model, the ESES mechanism of action seems to be related to the electrical activity of CGM, so-called neurovegetative brain, control area of sympathetic and parasympathetic autonomic system: direct CGM stimulation achieved the same effect of ESES on PLDF.

This experimental study is still in progress aiming to localize the appropriate level of ESES and to adjust ESES parameters for maximal PLDF increase.

The clinical application of ESES in arteriogenic male impotence may represent in the future a further application of this neuromodulation procedure.

References

1. Augustinsson LE, Holm J, Carlsson CA et al. (1985) Epidural electrical stimulation in severe limb ischemia. Evidence of pain relief, increased blood flow and a possible limb saving effect. Ann Surg 202: 104–110
2. Cook AW, Oygar A, Baggenstos O et al. (1976) Vascular disease of the extremities. Electrical stimulation of spinal cord and posterior roots. NY State J Med 76: 366–368
3. Dooley DM, Kaspark M (1976) Modification of blood flow to the extremities by electrical stimulation of the nervous system. South Med J 69: 1309–1311
4. Duggan AW (1992) Controls of nociceptive transmission in the spinal cord in Galley D, Illis LS, Krainick JU et al., ed. Monduzzi, Bologna, Italy, I Int. Congr. INS, Rome, pgg. 185–192
5. Eckhard C (1863) Untersuchungen uber die erection des penis beim hunde. Beit Anat Physiol 3: 123–150
6. Graber NJ, Lifson A (1987) The use of spinal cord stimulation for severe limb threatening ischemia. A preliminary report. Ann Vasc Surg 1: 345–349
7. Jacobs MJ, Jorning PJ, Beckers RC et al. (1990) Foot salvage and improvement of microvascular blood flow as a result of epidural spinal cord electrical stimulation. J Vasc Surg 12: 354–360
8. Jevegard L, Augustinsson LE, Carlsson CA et al. (1987) Long-term results by epidural spinal electrical stimulation (ESES) in patients with inoperable severe lower limb ischemia. Eur J Vasc Surg 1: 345–349
9. Linderoth B (1992) Neurophysiological mechanisms involved in vasodilation and ischemic pain relief by spinal cord stimulation in Galley D, Illis LS, Krainick JU et al., ed. Monduzzi, Bologna, Italy, I Int. Congr. INS, Rome, pgg 27–40
10. Long DH (1977) Electrical stimulation for control of pain. Arch Surg 112: 884–888
11. Lue TF, Takamura T, Schmidt RA et al. (1983) Hemodynamics of erection in the monkey. J Urol 130: 1237–1241
12. Mattioli GL, Rosa G, Ferrante L et al. (1990) Relazione cuore cervello: un modello sperimentale con implicazioni nelle epilessie generalizzate. Boll Lega Ital Epil 79/71: 405–411
13. Mingoli A, Sciacca V, Tamorri M et al. (1993) Clinical results of epidural spinal cord electrical stimulation in patients affected with limb-threatening chronic arterial obstructive disease. Angiology 44: 21–25

14. Shealy CN. Mortimer JT. Reswick JB (1967) Electrical inhibition of pain by stimulation of the dorsal columns: Preliminary clinical report. Anesth Analg (Cleve) 46: 489–491
15. Weiss HD (1980) The physiology of human penile erection. Ann Intern Med 76: 793–799

Author's address:
Prof. Vincenzo Sciacca. MD
Associate Professor of Surgery
Istituto I Clinical Chirurgica
Policlinico Umberto I
Università di Roma "La Sapienza"
Viale del Policlinico
00161 Rome
Italy

MIX
Papier aus verantwortungsvollen Quellen
Paper from responsible sources
FSC® C105338

If you have any concerns about our products,
you can contact us on
ProductSafety@springernature.com

In case Publisher is established outside the EU,
the EU authorized representative is:
Springer Nature Customer Service Center GmbH
Europaplatz 3, 69115 Heidelberg, Germany

Printed by Libri Plureos GmbH
in Hamburg, Germany